Bootstrap Methods

Gerhard Dikta · Marsel Scheer

Bootstrap Methods

With Applications in R

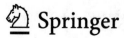 Springer

Gerhard Dikta
Department of Medical Engineering
and Technomathemathics
FH Aachen – University of Applied Sciences
Jülich, Nordrhein-Westfalen, Germany

Marsel Scheer
Bayer AG
Cologne, Nordrhein-Westfalen, Germany

ISBN 978-3-030-73482-4   ISBN 978-3-030-73480-0   (eBook)
https://doi.org/10.1007/978-3-030-73480-0

RStudio is a trademarks of RStudio, PBC

This Springer imprint is published by the registered company Springer Nature Switzerland AG
The registered company address is: Gewerbestrasse 11, 6330 Cham, Switzerland

To our families:

Renate and Jan
Natalie, Nikolas and Alexander
for their support and patience

Preface

Efron's introduction of the classical bootstrap in 1979 was the starting point of an immense and lasting research activity. Accompanied and supported by the improvement of PCs' computing power, these methods are now an established approach in applied statistics. The appealing simplicity makes it easy to use this approach in different fields of science where statistics is applied.

The intention of this manuscript is to discuss the bootstrap concept in the context of statistical testing, with a focus on its use or support in statistical modeling. Furthermore, we would like to address different reader preferences with the content.

Specifically, we have thought of two types of readers. On the one hand, users of statistics who have a solid basic knowledge of probability theory and who would like to have a goal-oriented and short-term problem solution provided. On the other hand, however, this book is also intended for readers who are more interested in the theoretical background of a problem solution and who have advanced knowledge of probability theory and mathematical statistics.

In most cases, we start a topic with some introductory examples, basic mathematical considerations, and simple implementations of the corresponding algorithm. A reader who is mainly interested in applying a particular approach may stop after such a section and apply the discussed procedures and implementations to the problem in mind. This introductory part to a topic is mainly addressed to the first type of reader. It can also be used just to motivate bootstrap approximations and to apply them in simulation studies on a computer. The second part of a topic covers the mathematical framework and further background material. This part is mainly written for those readers who have a strong background in probability theory and mathematical statistics.

Throughout all chapters, computational procedures are provided in R. R is a powerful statistical computing environment, which is freely available and can be downloaded from the R-Project website at www.r-project.org. We focus only on a few but very popular packages from the so-called tidyverse, mainly ggplot2 and dplyr. This hopefully helps readers, who are not familiar with R, understand the implementations more easily, first because the packages make the source code quite intuitive to read and second because of their popularity a lot of helpful information can be found on the Internet. However, the repository of additional R-packages that have been created by the R-community is immense, also with respect to non-statistical aspects, that makes it worth to learn and work with R. The R-programs considered in the text are made available on the website https://www.springer.com/gp/book/9783030734794.

The first three chapters provide introductory material and are mainly intended for readers who have never come into contact with bootstrapping. Chapter 1 gives a short introduction to the bootstrap idea and some notes on R. In the Chap. 2, we summarize some results about the generation of random numbers. The Chap. 3 lists some well-known results of the classical bootstrap method.

In Chap. 4, we discuss the first basic statistical tests using the bootstrap method. Chapters 5 and 6 cover bootstrap applications in the context of linear and generalized linear regression. The focus is on goodness-of-fit tests, which can be used to detect contradictions between the data and the fitted model. We discuss the work of Stute on marked empirical processes and transfer parts of his results into the bootstrap context in order to approximate p-values for the individual goodness-of-fit tests. Some of the results here are new, at least to the best of our knowledge. Although the mathematics behind these applications is quite complex, we consider these tests as useful tools in the context of statistical modeling and learning. Some of the subsections focus exactly on this modeling topic.

In the appendix, some additional aspects of R with respect to bootstrap applications are illustrated. In the first part of this appendix, some applications of the "boot" R-package of Brian Ripley, which can be obtained from the R-project's website, are demonstrated. The second part describes the "simTool" R-package of Marsel Scheer, which was written to simplify the implementation of simulation studies like bootstrap replications in R. This package also covers applications of parallel programming issues. Finally, the usage of our "bootGOF" R-package is illustrated, which provides a tool to perform goodness-of-fit tests for (linear) models as discussed in Chap. 6.

Jülich, Germany   Gerhard Dikta
January 2021   Marsel Scheer

Acknowledgements

The first three chapters of this manuscript were written during the time when the first author was employed as a Research Assistant at the Chair for Mathematical Stochastics of the Justus Liebig University in Gießen. They were prepared for a summer course at the Department of Mathematical Sciences at the University of Wisconsin-Milwaukee, which the first author taught in 1988 (and several times later on) after completing his doctorate.

Special thanks must be given to Prof. Dr. Winfried Stute, who supervised the first author in Giessen. Professor Stute realized the importance of the bootstrap method at a very early stage and inspired and promoted interest in it among the first author. In addition, Prof. Stute together with Prof. Gilbert Walter from the Department of Mathematical Science of the University of Wisconsin-Milwaukee initiated a cooperation between the two departments, which ultimately formed the basis for the long-lasting collaboration between the first author and his colleagues from the statistics group in Milwaukee.

Financially, this long-term cooperation was later on supported by the Department of Medical Engineering and Technomathematics of the Fachhochschule Aachen and by the Department of Mathematical Sciences of the University of Wisconsin-Milwaukee, and we would like to thank Profs. Karen Brucks, Allen Bell, Thomas O'Bryan, and Richard Stockbridge for their kind assistance.

Finally, the first author would like to thank his colleagues from the statistics group in Milwaukee, Jay Beder, Vytaras Brazauskas, and especially Jugal Ghorai, and, from Fachhochschule Aachen, Martin Reißel for their helpful discussions and support.

Also, the second author gives special thanks to Prof. Dr. Josef G. Steinebach from the Department of Mathematics of the University of Cologne for his excellent lectures in Statistics and Probability Theory.

We are both grateful to Dr. Andreas Kleefeld, who kindly provided us with many comments and corrections to a preliminary version of the book.

Contents

1 Introduction 1
  1.1 Basic Idea of the Bootstrap 1
  1.2 The R-Project for Statistical Computing 5
  1.3 Usage of R in This Book 5
      1.3.1 Further Non-Statistical R-Packages 6
  References 7

2 Generating Random Numbers 9
  2.1 Distributions in the R-Package Stats 9
  2.2 Uniform df. on the Unit Interval 10
  2.3 The Quantile Transformation 11
  2.4 The Normal Distribution 15
  2.5 Method of Rejection 16
  2.6 Generation of Random Vectors 19
  2.7 Exercises 20
  References 20

3 The Classical Bootstrap 21
  3.1 An Introductory Example 21
  3.2 Basic Mathematical Background of the Classical Bootstrap 27
  3.3 Discussion of the Asymptotic Accuracy of the Classical
      Bootstrap 32
  3.4 Empirical Process and the Classical Bootstrap 34
  3.5 Mathematical Framework of Mallow's Metric 36
  3.6 Exercises 44
  References 45

4 Bootstrap-Based Tests 47
  4.1 Introduction 47
  4.2 The One-Sample Test 49
  4.3 Two-Sample Tests 53

4.4   Goodness-of-Fit (GOF) Test   60
4.5   Mathematical Framework of the GOF Test   65
4.6   Exercises   70
References   72

5   Regression Analysis   73
5.1   Homoscedastic Linear Regression under Fixed Design   74
      5.1.1   Model-Based Bootstrap   77
      5.1.2   LSE Asymptotic   84
      5.1.3   LSE Bootstrap Asymptotic.......................   88
5.2   Linear Correlation Model and the Bootstrap................   90
      5.2.1   Classical Bootstrap   93
      5.2.2   Wild Bootstrap   96
      5.2.3   Mathematical Framework of LSE   99
      5.2.4   Mathematical Framework of Classical
              Bootstrapped LSE 101
      5.2.5   Mathematical Framework of Wild Bootstrapped LSE..... 104
5.3   Generalized Linear Model (Parametric) 106
      5.3.1   Mathematical Framework of MLE 121
      5.3.2   Mathematical Framework of Bootstrap MLE 133
5.4   Semi-parametric Model.............................. 142
      5.4.1   Mathematical Framework of LSE 147
      5.4.2   Mathematical Framework of Wild Bootstrap LSE 153
5.5   Exercises 162
References 164

6   Goodness-of-Fit Test for Generalized Linear Models 165
6.1   MEP in the Parametric Modeling Context 167
      6.1.1   Implementation 168
      6.1.2   Bike Sharing Data 171
      6.1.3   Artificial Data 177
6.2   MEP in the Semi-parametric Modeling Context 187
      6.2.1   Implementation 190
      6.2.2   Artificial Data 192
6.3   Comparison of the GOF Tests under the Parametric
      and Semi-parametric Setup 194
6.4   Mathematical Framework: Marked Empirical Processes 197
      6.4.1   The Basic MEP................................ 198
      6.4.2   The MEP with Estimated Model Parameters
              Propagating in a Fixed Direction 203
      6.4.3   The MEP with Estimated Model Parameters
              Propagating in an Estimated Direction 207

6.5   Mathematical Framework: Bootstrap of Marked Empirical
      Processes 214
      6.5.1   Bootstrap of the BMEP 218
      6.5.2   Bootstrap of the EMEP 221
6.6   Exercises 229
References 230

Appendix A: boot Package 231

Appendix B: simTool Package 237

Appendix C: bootGOF Package 249

Appendix D: Session Info 253

Index 255

Abbreviations

a.e.	Almost everywhere
a.s.	Almost sure
BMEP	Basic marked empirical process
CLT	Central limit theorem
CvM	Cramér-von Mises
df.	Distribution function
edf.	Empirical distribution function of an i.i.d. sample
EMEP	Estimated marked empirical process
EMEPE	Estimated marked empirical process in estimated direction
GA	General assumptions
GC	Glivenko-Cantelli theorem
GLM	Generalized linear model
GOF	Goodness-of-fit
i.i.d.	Independent and identically distributed
KS	Kolmogorov-Smirnov
MEP	Marked empirical process
MLE	Maximum likelihood estimate
pdf.	Probability density function
PRNG	Pseudo-random number generators
qf.	Quantile function
rv.	Random variable
RSS	Resampling scheme
SLLN	Strong law of large numbers
W.l.o.g.	Without loss of generality
WLLN	Weak law of large numbers
w.p.1	With probability one

Notations

$A := B$	A is defined by B
$A \equiv B$	A and B are equivalent
$\mathcal{B}_n^*$	Borel σ-algebra on $\mathbb{R}^n$
$C[0,1]$	Space of continuous, real-valued function on the unit interval
$D[0,1]$	Skorokhod space on the unit interval
$\mathbb{E}(X)$	Expectation of the random variable X
$\mathbb{E}_n^*(X^*)$	Expectation of the bootstrap random variable X
$\mathrm{EXP}(\alpha)$	Exponential distribution with parameter $\alpha > 0$
F_n	Empirical distribution function
$I_{\{x \in A\}}$	Indicator function
$I_{\{A\}}(x)$	Indicator function
I_p	Identity matrix of size $p \times p$
$\langle \cdot, \cdot \rangle$	Inner product of a Hilbert space
$a \wedge b$	Minimum of a and b
$\mathcal{N}(\mu, \sigma^2)$	Normal distribution with expectation μ and variance σ^2
$\mathbb{P}_n^*$	Probability measure corresponding to bootstrap rvs. based on n original observations
$\mathbb{P}^*$	Probability measure corresponding to the wild bootstrap
R_n	Basic marked empirical process (BMEP)
R_n^1	Marked empirical process with estimated parameters propagating in fixed direction (EMEP)
$\bar{R}_n^1$	Marked empirical process with estimated parameters propagating in an estimated direction (EMEPE)
$\mathrm{UNI}(a,b)$	Uniform distribution on the interval $[a,b]$
UNI	Standard uniform distribution on the interval, i.e., $UNI(0,1)$
$\mathrm{VAR}(X)$	Variance of the random variable X
$\mathrm{VAR}_n^*(X^*)$	Variance of the bootstrap random variable X
$\mathrm{WEIB}(\alpha, \beta)$	Weibull distribution with parameter α and β
$X \sim F$	Random variable X is distributed according to F

Chapter 1
Introduction

In this introduction, we discuss the basic idea of the bootstrap procedure using a simple example. Furthermore, the Statistical Software R and its use in the context of this manuscript is briefly covered. Readers who are familiar with this material can skip this chapter.

A short summary of the contents of this manuscript can be found in the Preface and is not listed here again.

1.1   Basic Idea of the Bootstrap

Typical statistical methods, such as constructing a confidence interval for the expected value of a random variable or determining critical values for a hypothesis test, require knowledge of the underlying distribution. However, this distribution is usually only partially known at most. The statistical method we use to perform the task depends on our knowledge of the underlying distribution.

Let us be more precise and assume that

$$X_1, \ldots, X_n \sim F$$

is a sequence of independent and identically distributed (i.i.d.) random variables with common distribution function (df.) F. Consider the statistic

---

Electronic supplementary material   The online version of this chapter (https://doi.org/10.1007/978-3-030-73480-0_1) contains supplementary material, which is available to authorized users.

$$\bar{X}_n := \frac{1}{n} \sum_{i=1}^{n} X_i$$

to estimate the parameter $\mu_F = \mathbb{E}(X)$, that is, the expectation of X.

To construct a confidence interval for μ_F or to perform a hypothesis test on μ_F, we consider the df. of the studentized version of $\bar{X}_n$, that is,

$$\mathbb{P}_F\left(\sqrt{n}(\bar{X}_n - \mu_F)/s_n \leq x\right), \qquad x \in \mathbb{R}, \tag{1.1}$$

where

$$s_n^2 := \frac{1}{n-1} \sum_{i=1}^{n} (X_i - \bar{X}_n)^2$$

is the unbiased estimator of $\sigma^2 = \mathrm{VAR}(X)$, that is, the variance of X. Note that we write $\mathbb{P}_F$ here to indicate that F is the data generating df.

If we know that F comes from the class of normal distributions, then the df. under (1.1) belongs to a t_{n-1}–distribution, i.e., a Student's t distribution with $n-1$ degrees of freedom. Using the known quantiles of the $t_{n-1}-$ distribution exact confidence interval can be determined. For example, an exact 90% confidence interval for μ_F is given by

$$\left[\bar{X}_n - \frac{s_n \, q_{0.95}}{\sqrt{n}}, \; \bar{X}_n + \frac{s_n \, q_{0.95}}{\sqrt{n}}\right], \tag{1.2}$$

where $q_{0.95}$ is the 95% quantile of the t_{n-1} distribution.

But in most situations we are not able to specify a parametric distribution class for F. In such a case, we have to look for a suitable approximation for (1.1). If it is ensured that $\mathbb{E}(X^2) < \infty$, the central limit theorem (CLT) guarantees that

$$\sup_{x \in \mathbb{R}} \left| \mathbb{P}_F\left(\sqrt{n}(\bar{X}_n - \mu_F)/s_n \leq x\right) - \Phi(x) \right| \longrightarrow 0, \quad \text{for } n \to \infty, \tag{1.3}$$

where Φ denotes the standard normal df. Based on the CLT, we can now construct an asymptotic confidence interval. For example, the 90% confidence interval under (1.2) has the same structure when we construct it using the CLT. However, $q_{0.95}$ now is the 95% quantile of the standard normal distribution. The interval constructed in this way is no longer an exact confidence interval. It can only be guaranteed that the confidence level of 90% is reached with $n \to \infty$. It should also be noted that for $q_{0.95}$ the 95% quantile of the $t_{n-1}-$ distribution can also be chosen, because for $n \to \infty$, the $t_{n-1}-$ df. converges to the standard normal df.

So far we have concentrated exclusively on the studentized mean. Let us generalize this to a statistic of the type

$$T_n(F) = T_n(X_1, \ldots, X_n; F),$$

where $X_1, \ldots, X_n \sim F$ are i.i.d. Then the question arises how to approximate the df.

$$\mathbb{P}_F\big(T_n(F) \leq x\big), \qquad x \in \mathbb{R} \tag{1.4}$$

if F is unknown. This is where Efron's bootstrap enters the game. The basic idea of the bootstrap method is the assumption that the df. of T_n is about the same when the data generating distribution F is replaced by another data generating distribution $\hat{F}$ which is close to F and which is known to us. If we can find such a df. $\hat{F}$,

$$\mathbb{P}_{\hat{F}}(T_n(\hat{F}) \leq x), \qquad x \in \mathbb{R} \tag{1.5}$$

may also be an approximation of Eq. (1.4). We call this df. for the moment a *bootstrap approximation* of the df. given under Eq. (1.4). However, this approach only makes sense if we can guarantee that

$$\sup_{x \in \mathbb{R}} \Big| \mathbb{P}_F\big(T_n(F) \leq x\big) - \mathbb{P}_{\hat{F}}\big(T_n(\hat{F}) \leq x\big) \Big| \longrightarrow 0, \quad \text{for } n \to \infty. \tag{1.6}$$

Now let us go back to construct a 90% confidence interval for μ_F based on the bootstrap approximation. For this, we take the studentized mean for T_n and assume that we have a data generating df. $\hat{F}$ that satisfies (1.6). Since $\hat{F}$ is known, we can now, at least theoretically, calculate the 5% and 95% quantiles of the df.

$$\mathbb{P}_{\hat{F}}\big(\sqrt{n}(\bar{X}_n - \mu_{\hat{F}})/s_n \leq x\big),$$

which we denote by $q_{n,0.05}$ and $q_{n,0.95}$, respectively, to derive

$$\Big[\bar{X}_n - \frac{s_n\, q_{n,0.95}}{\sqrt{n}}\, , \ \bar{X}_n - \frac{s_n\, q_{n,0.05}}{\sqrt{n}}\Big], \tag{1.7}$$

an asymptotic 90% confidence interval for μ_F.

If we want to use such a bootstrap approach, we have

(A) to choose the data generating df. $\hat{F}$ such that the bootstrap approximation (1.6) holds,
(B) to calculate the df. of T_n, where the sample is generated under $\hat{F}$.

Certainly (A) is the more demanding part, in particular, the proof of the approximation (1.6). Fortunately, a lot of work has been done on this in the last decades. Also, the calculation of the df. under (B) may turn out to be very complex. However, this is of minor importance, because the bootstrap df. in Eq. (1.6) can be approximated very well by a Monte Carlo approach. It is precisely this opportunity to perform a Monte Carlo approximation, together with the rapid development of powerful PCs that has led to the great success of the bootstrap approach.

To demonstrate such a Monte Carlo approximation for the df. of Eq. (1.5), we proceed as follows:

(a) Construct m i.i.d. (bootstrap) samples independent of one another of the type

$$X^*_{1;1} \cdots X^*_{1;n}$$

$$\vdots \quad \vdots \quad \vdots$$

$$X^*_{m;1} \cdots X^*_{m;n}$$

with common df. $\hat{F}$.

(b) Calculate for each sample $k \in \{1, 2, \ldots, m\}$

$$T^*_{k;n} := T_n(X^*_{k;1}, \ldots, X^*_{k;n}; \hat{F})$$

to obtain $T^*_{1;n}, \ldots, T^*_{m;n}$.

(c) Since the $T^*_{1;n}, \ldots, T^*_{m;n}$ are i.i.d. , the Glivenko-Cantelli theorem (GC) guarantees

$$\sup_{x \in \mathbb{R}} \left| \mathbb{P}_{\hat{F}}\left(T_n(\hat{F}) \leq x\right) - \frac{1}{m} \sum_{k=1}^{m} I_{\{T^*_{k;n} \leq x\}} \right| \longrightarrow 0, \quad \text{for } m \to \infty, \qquad (1.8)$$

where $I_{\{x \in A\}} \equiv I_{\{A\}}(x)$ denotes the indicator function of the set A, that is,

$$I_{\{x \in A\}} = \begin{cases} 1 & : x \in A \\ 0 & : x \notin A \end{cases}.$$

The choice of an appropriate $\hat{F}$ depends on the underlying problem, as we will see in the following chapters. In the context of this introduction, F_n, the *empirical df.* (edf.) of the sample $X_1, \ldots, X_n$, defined by

$$F_n(x) := \frac{1}{n} \sum_{i=1}^{n} I_{\{X_i \leq x\}}, \qquad x \in \mathbb{R}, \qquad (1.9)$$

is a good choice for $\hat{F}$ since, by the Glivenko-Cantelli theorem, we get with probability one (w.p.1)

$$\sup_{n \in \mathbb{R}} \left| F_n(x) - F(x) \right| \xrightarrow[n \to \infty]{} 0.$$

If we choose F_n for $\hat{F}$ then we are talking about the *classical bootstrap* which was historically the first to be studied.

1.2   The R-Project for Statistical Computing

The programming language R, see R Core Team (2019), is a widely used open-source software tool for data analysis and graphics which runs on the commonly used operating systems. It can be downloaded from the R-project's website at www.r-project.org. The R Development Core Team also offers some documentation on this website:

- R installation and administration,
- An introduction to R,
- The R language definition,
- R data import/export, and
- The R reference index.

Additionally to this material, there is a large and strongly growing number of textbooks available covering the R programming language and the applications of R in different fields of data analysis, for instance, Beginning R or Advanced R.

Besides the R software, one also should install an editor or an integrated development environment (IDE) to work with R conveniently. Several open-source products are available on the web, like

- RStudio, see RStudio Team (2020), at www.rstudio.org;
- RKWard, at http://rkward.sourceforge.net;
- Tinn-R, at http://www.sciviews.org/Tinn-R; and
- Eclipse based StatET, at http://www.walware.de/goto/statet.

1.3   Usage of R in This Book

Throughout the book we implement, for instance, different resampling schemes and simulation studies in R. Our implementations are free from any checking of function arguments. We provide R-code that focuses solely on an understandable implementation of a certain algorithm. Therefore, there is plenty of room to improve the implementations. Some of these improvements will be discussed within the exercises.

R is organized in packages. A new installation of R comes with some pre-installed packages. And the packages provided by the R-community makes this programming language really powerful. More than 15000 packages (as of 2020/Feb) are available (still growing). But especially for people starting with R this is also a problem. The CRAN Task View https://cran.r-project.org/web/views summarizes certain packages within categories like "Graphics", "MachineLearning", or "Survival". We decided to use only a handful of packages that are directly related to the main objective of this book, like the `boot`-package for bootstrapping, or (in the opinion of the authors) are too important and helpful to be ignored, like `ggplot2`, `dplyr`, and `tidyr`. In addition, we have often used the `simTool` package from Marsel Scheer to carry out simulations. This package is explained in the appendix. Furthermore, we decided to use the pipe operator, i.e., %>%. There are a few critical voices about this operator, but the authors as the most R users find it very comfortable to work with the pipe operator. People familiar with Unix systems will recognize the concept and probably appreciate it. A small example will demonstrate how the pipe operator works. Suppose we want to apply a function A to the object x and the result of this operation should be processed further by the function B. Without the pipe operator one could use

```
B(A(x))
# or
tmp = A(x)
B(tmp)
```

With the pipe operator this becomes

```
A(x) %>%
    B
# or
x %>%
  A %>%
  B
```

Especially with longer chains of functions using pipes may help to obtain R-code that is easier to understand.

1.3.1 Further Non-Statistical R-Packages

There are a lot of packages that are worth to look at. Again the CRAN Task View may be a good starting point. The following list is focused on writing reports, developing R-packages, and increasing the speed of R-code itself. By far this list is not exhaustive:

- knitr for writing reports (this book was written with knitr);
- readxl for the import of excel files;
- testthat for creating automated unit tests. It is also helpful for checking function arguments;
- covR for assessing test coverage of the unit tests;
- devtools for creating/writing packages;
- data.table amazingly fast aggregation, joins, and various manipulations of large datasets;
- roxygen2 for creating help pages within packages;
- Rcpp for a simple integration of C++ into R;
- profvis a profiling tool that assess at which line of code R spends its time;
- checkpoint, renv for package dependency.

Of course, further packages for importing datasets, connecting to databases, creating interactive graphs and user interfaces, and so on exist. Again, the packages provided by the R-community make this programming language really powerful.

Finally, we want to strongly recommend the R-package `drake`. According to the package-manual: *It analyzes your workflow, skips steps with up-to-date results, and orchestrates the rest with optional distributed computing.* We want to briefly describe how this works in principle. One defines a plan with steps one wants to perform:

```
plan <- drake::drake_plan(
  raw = import_data("/foo/bar/data.csv"),
  wrangled = preprocess(raw),
  model1 = fit1(wrangled),
  model2 = fit2(wrangled)
)
```

This plan can then be executed/processed by `drake`.

```
drake::make(plan)
```

This creates the four objects raw, wrangled, model1, and model2. Assume now that we change the underlying source code for one of the model-fitting functions, then there is, of course, no need to rerun the preprocess step. Since `drake` analyzed our defined plan it automatically skips the import and preprocessing for us. This can be extremely helpful if the preprocess step is computationally intensive. Or imagine the situation that we refactor the data-import function. If these changes do not modify the raw object created in the first step, then again there is no need to rerun the preprocess step or to refit the models. Again `drake` automatically detects that and skips the preprocessing. Furthermore, looking at the definition of model1 and model2, we see that there is no logical need to process them sequentially and with `drake` one can easily do the computation in parallel. The package does also a lot of other helpful things in the background, for instance, it measures the time used to perform a single step of the plan. Although we do not use `drake` in this book we encourage the reader to try out the package. A good starting point is the excellent user manual accessible under https://books.ropensci.org/drake.

References

R Core Team (2019) R: A language and environment for statistical computing. R Foundation for Statistical Computing, Vienna, Austria, https://www.R-project.org/
RStudio Team (2020) RStudio: integrated development environment for R. RStudio, PBC, Boston, MA, http://www.rstudio.com/

Chapter 2
Generating Random Numbers

To perform a Monte Carlo approximation, we have to generate random variables (rv.) on a computer according to a given df. F. In this chapter, we will discuss some commonly used procedures and their application under R.

Since most of the widely used distributions are implemented in R, random variables according to these distributions can easily be generated directly in R through the corresponding built-in R functions. In the first section of this chapter, we will give a brief overview on those distributions which are implemented in the R `stats` package.

However, if a specific distribution is needed which is neither supported by R itself nor by any additional package, one can try the "quantile transformation method" or the "method of rejection". Both approaches are considered in this chapter. For a detailed discussion of random number generation, we refer to Devroye (1986) and Ripley (1987). In Eubank and Kupresanin (2011, Chapter 4), this is also considered in the R-context.

2.1 Distributions in the R-Package Stats

The standard R-package `stats` contains several standard probability distributions. We can list them from a R-workspace by typing the command

```
help(distributions)
```

For all these distributions, the corresponding cumulative distribution function, density function, quantile function, and random generation function are implemented and can be called by

- dxxx(...)—density function;
- pxxx(...)—distribution function;

© Springer Nature Switzerland AG 2021
G. Dikta and M. Scheer, *Bootstrap Methods*,
https://doi.org/10.1007/978-3-030-73480-0_2

- qxxx(...)—quantile function; and
- rxxx(...)—random number generator function.

In the notation above, "xxx" is the name in R of the corresponding distribution and (...) a placeholder for the required parameters of the function call. The following example lists some calls regarding a normal distribution with expected value $\mu = 2$ and variance $\sigma^2 = 4$, here abbreviated as $\mathcal{N}(2, 4)$.

R-Example 2.1 Note that in the corresponding function calls under R, the standard deviation (sd=2) is used while in the notation $\mathcal{N}(2, 4)$ the variance $\sigma^2 = 4$ is given. The R name "xxx" of the normal distribution is "norm".

```
#call the help for rnorm
help(rnorm)
#density function at x = 2
dnorm(x = 2, mean = 2, sd = 2)
```

```
## [1] 0.1994711
```

```
#distribution function at q = 2
pnorm(q = 2, mean = 2, sd = 2)
```

```
## [1] 0.5
```

```
#0.5-quantile
qnorm(p = 0.5, mean = 2, sd = 2)
```

```
## [1] 2
```

```
#3 normal random variables
rnorm(n = 3, mean = 2, sd = 2)
```

```
## [1] 1.008104 3.768502 2.064348
```

2.2 Uniform df. on the Unit Interval

A rv. U is *uniformly* distributed on the interval $[a, b]$, where $-\infty < a < b < \infty$, if

$$\mathbb{P}(U \leq u) = \begin{cases} 0 & : u < a \\ (u - a)/(b - a) & : a \leq u \leq b \\ 1 & : u > b. \end{cases}$$

We denote this distribution here by $UNI(a, b)$ and use UNI to abbreviate UNI $(0, 1)$, the *standard uniform distribution*, which is also referred to as the *uniform distribution*.

The uniform distribution is the most important one in generating rv. As we will see in the next section, we can generate a rv. $X \sim F$ for every df. F if we can generate a rv. $U \sim UNI$.

There is a large literature on generating sequences of independent and uniformly distributed rvs. which we will not discuss here. Eubank and Kupresanin (2011, Chapter 4) is a good reference for pseudo-random number generators (PRNG), which specifically addresses R.

Remark 2.2 In this manuscript, we usually take "Mersenne twister" as PRNG. If a normally distributed rv. is to be created, this is done using the "inversion" method. For reasons of reproducibility, a starting value ("set.seed") is set before each simulation. This seed also contains the name of the PRNG used and the name of the method for generating normal distributed rvs. A typical call looks like

```
set.seed(123,kind ="Mersenne-Twister",normal.kind ="Inversion")
```

With the `simTool` package, simulations can also be run in parallel. In this case, "L'Ecuyer-CMRG" is set globally as PRNG!

2.3 The Quantile Transformation

The following theorem says that we can generate a rv. X according to an arbitrary df. F if we apply a certain transformation to a generated rv. $U \sim UNI$.

Theorem 2.3 *Let F be the df. of a rv. X and define for $0 < u < 1$*

$$F^{-1}(u) = \inf\{x \in \mathbb{R} \mid F(x) \geq u\} \tag{2.1}$$

the quantile function (qf.). If $U \sim UNI$ then:

$$X := F^{-1}(U) \sim F.$$

Proof At first note that the qf. equals the inverse function of F if F is strictly increasing. If this is not the case, F^{-1} is still well defined and therefore qf. is a generalized inverse of an increasing function.

We have to show that

$$\mathbb{P}(F^{-1}(U) \leq x) = F(x), \quad \forall x \in \mathbb{R}.$$

For this choose $x \in \mathbb{R}$ and $0 < u < 1$ arbitrarily. Then the following equivalence holds:

$$F^{-1}(u) \leq x \iff u \leq F(x) \tag{2.2}$$

"$\Leftarrow$:" If $u \leq F(x)$, apply the definition of F^{-1} to get $F^{-1}(u) \leq x$.
"$\Rightarrow$:" Assume now $F^{-1}(u) \leq x$ and continue indirectly. For this assume further that $u > F(x)$. Since F is continuous from above there exists $\varepsilon > 0$ such that $u > F(x + \varepsilon)$. Apply the definition of F^{-1} to get $F^{-1}(u) \geq x + \varepsilon$. This contradiction leads to $F^{-1}(u) \leq x$.
Now, apply (2.2) to get for arbitrary $x \in \mathbb{R}$:

$$\mathbb{P}(F^{-1}(U) \leq x) = \mathbb{P}(U \leq F(x)) = F(x) = \mathbb{P}(X \leq x),$$

where the second equality follows from $U \sim UNI$. This finally proves the theorem. $\square$

Example 2.4 Let $U \sim UNI$ and

$$F(x) := \begin{cases} 0 & : x \leq 0 \\ 1 - \exp(-\alpha x) & : x > 0 \end{cases}$$

the df. of the exponential distribution with parameter $\alpha > 0$, abbreviated by $EXP(\alpha)$. Calculate the inverse of F to get

$$F^{-1}(u) = -\frac{\ln(1 - u)}{\alpha}.$$

The last theorem guarantees that $F^{-1}(U) \sim EXP(\alpha)$.

R-Example 2.5 This example shows the generation of 1000 $EXP(2)$ variables with R based on the quantile transformation derived in Example 2.4.

```
gen.exp <- function(n, alpha){
  #n - number of observations
  #alpha - distribution parameter

  return(-log(1 - runif(n)) / alpha)
}

# set the seed for the pseudo random number generator
# for reproducible results
set.seed(123,kind ="Mersenne-Twister",normal.kind ="Inversion")

# generate 1000 EXP(2) random variables
obs <- gen.exp(n = 1000, alpha = 2)

# draw a histogram with 50 cells
hist(obs, breaks = 50, freq = FALSE,
     main = "Histogram of 1000 EXP(2)",
     xlab = "", ylab = "density",
```

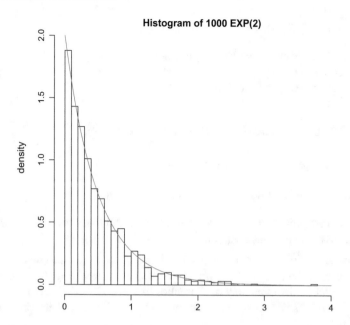

Fig. 2.1 Histogram of 1000 *EXP*(2) distributed random variables and the *EXP*(2)-density

```
    xlim=c(0,4),
    ylim=c(0,2))

# add the density function of a EXP(2) distributed random
# variable to the plot
curve(dexp(x, rate = 2), add = TRUE, col = "red")
```

In the first statement, the R-function "gen.exp" is defined with two parameters; n and $alpha$, which implements the result derived in Example 2.4. It returns a vector of n independent realizations of the $EXP(alpha)$ distribution. In the second statement, the seed is set for the pseudo-random number generator which is here "Mersenne-Twister" to obtain reproducible results. "gen.exp" is applied with $n = 1000$ and $alpha = 2$. The resulting vector is stored in the variable "obs" in statement three. With the fourth statement a histogram of the generated variables is produced and with the last statement this histogram is overlaid with the true density function of the $EXP(2)$ distribution, see Fig. 2.1.

In the following lemma, some further properties of the quantile function are listed:

Lemma 2.6 *Let F be an arbitrary df. and denote by* F^{-1} *the corresponding quantile function. We have for* $x, x_1, x_2 \in \mathbb{R}$ *and* $0 < u < 1$:

1. $F(x) \geq u \iff F^{-1}(u) \leq x$.
2. $F(x) < u \iff F^{-1}(u) > x$.

3. $F(x_1) < u \le F(x_2) \iff x_1 < F^{-1}(u) \le x_2$.

Proof (i) Already shown under (2.2) of Theorem 2.3.
(ii) Consequence of part (i).
(iii) Consequence of part (i) and (ii).

$\square$

Lemma 2.7 *Let F be an arbitrary df. and $0 < u < 1$. Then*

$$F \circ F^{-1}(u) \ge u.$$

If $u \in F(\mathbb{R})$ the inequality above changes to an equality.

Proof The inequality can be obtained from Lemma 2.6 (ii), since $F \circ F^{-1}(u) < u$ would result in the obvious contradiction $F^{-1}(u) > F^{-1}(u)$.

Now assume in addition that $u \in F(\mathbb{R})$, i.e., there exists $x \in \mathbb{R}$ such that $u = F(x)$. Therefore, by definition of F^{-1}, we get $F^{-1}(u) \le x$. Applying F to both sides of this inequality, the monotony of F implies that $F \circ F^{-1}(u) \le F(x) = u$. Thus, $F \circ F^{-1}(u) > u$ is not possible and according to the first part of the proof we get $F \circ F^{-1}(u) = u$. $\square$

Corollary 2.8 *Let X be a rv. with continuous df. F. Then*

$$F(X) \sim UNI.$$

Proof According to Theorem 2.3, we can assume that

$$X = F^{-1}(U),$$

where $U \sim UNI$. Thus, it remains to show that $F \circ F^{-1}(U) \sim UNI$. For this choose $0 < u < 1$ arbitrarily. Then continuity of F and the last lemma leads to

$$\mathbb{P}(F \circ F^{-1}(U) \le u) = \mathbb{P}(U \le u) = u$$

which proves the corollary. $\square$

We finalize the section by another inequality of the quantile function.

Lemma 2.9 *For each df. F and $x \in \mathbb{R}$, we have*

$$F^{-1} \circ F(x) \le x.$$

If in addition x fulfills the extra condition that for all $y < x$, $F(y) < F(x)$ holds, then the inequality above changes to an equality.

Proof If $F^{-1} \circ F(x) > x$ for $x \in \mathbb{R}$, then Lemma 2.6 (ii) immediately yields the contradiction $F(x) < F(x)$. Thus, the inequality stated above is correct.

Now, assume the extra condition of the lemma for the point $x \in \mathbb{R}$. According to the part just shown, we have to prove that $F^{-1}(F(x)) < x$ cannot be correct. Assuming that this inequality is correct, Lemma 2.7 implies

$$F(x) \leq F \circ F^{-1}(F(x)) < F(x)$$

which is obviously a contradiction.   □

2.4   The Normal Distribution

Theorem 2.3 of the last section shows how the quantile function can be used to generate a rv. according to a given df. F. However, the quantile function might be difficult to calculate. Therefore, the procedure suggested under Theorem 2.3 is only used in standard situations where F is invertible and the inverse can easily be obtained. In those cases where it is not possible to calculate F^{-1} directly, other procedures should be applied.

In the case of the standard normal distribution, i.e., the rv. $X \sim \mathcal{N}(0, 1)$, the df. Φ has the density ϕ with

$$\Phi(x) = \mathbb{P}(X \leq x) = \int_{-\infty}^{x} \phi(t)\, dt = \frac{1}{\sqrt{2\pi}} \int_{-\infty}^{x} \exp\left(-\frac{t^2}{2}\right) dt$$

which can be obtained only numerically. Thus, quantile transformation is not applicable to generate such a rv.

As the next lemma will show, we can generate a rv. $Z \sim \mathcal{N}(\mu, \sigma^2)$, i.e., Z has df. F with

$$F(x) = \frac{1}{\sqrt{2\pi\sigma^2}} \int_{-\infty}^{x} \exp\left(-\frac{(t - \mu)^2}{2\sigma^2}\right) dt, \tag{2.3}$$

through a linear transformed rv. $X \sim \mathcal{N}(0, 1)$.

Lemma 2.10 *Let $X \sim \mathcal{N}(0, 1)$. Then $Z := \sigma \cdot X + \mu$ is distributed according to $\mathcal{N}(\mu, \sigma^2)$.*

Proof Let $\mu \in \mathbb{R}$, $\sigma > 0$, and $z \in \mathbb{R}$ be given. Then

$$\mathbb{P}(Z \leq z) = \mathbb{P}(\sigma X + \mu \leq z) = \mathbb{P}(X \leq (z - \mu)/\sigma)$$
$$= \frac{1}{\sqrt{2\pi}} \int_{-\infty}^{(z-\mu)/\sigma} \exp\left(-\frac{t^2}{2}\right) dt.$$

Now, differentiate both sides w.r.t. z to obtain by the chain rule and the Fundamental Theorem of Calculus the density function

$$f(z) = \frac{1}{\sqrt{2\pi\sigma^2}} \exp\left(-\frac{(z-\mu)^2}{2\sigma^2}\right).$$

But f is precisely the density function of a rv. which is $\mathcal{N}(\mu, \sigma^2)$ distributed. □

In the next theorem, the *Box-Muller* algorithm to generate $\mathcal{N}(0, 1)$ distributed rv. is given.

Theorem 2.11 Box-Muller algorithm. *Let $U, V \sim UNI$ be two independent rv. uniformly distributed on the unit interval. Then the rv.*

$$X = \sqrt{-2\log(U)}\cos(2\pi V), \quad Y = \sqrt{-2\log(U)}\sin(2\pi V)$$

are independent from one another and both are $\mathcal{N}(0, 1)$ distributed.

Proof The proof is omitted here but can be found in Box and Muller (1958). □

2.5 Method of Rejection

As already discussed in the last section, quantile transformation is not always applicable in practise. In this section, we discuss a method which is applicable in a situation where the df. F has a density function f.

Theorem 2.12 Method of Rejection. *Let F, G be df. with probability density functions f, g. Furthermore, let $M > 0$ be such that*

$$f(x) \le Mg(x), \quad \forall x \in \mathbb{R}.$$

To generate a rv. $X \sim F$ perform the following steps:

(i) Generate $Y \sim G$.
(ii) Generate $U \sim UNI$ independent of Y.
(iii) If $U \le f(Y)/(M \cdot g(Y))$, return Y. Else reject Y and start again with step (i).

Proof We have to prove that $X \sim F$. Note first that

$$\mathbb{P}(X \le x) = \mathbb{P}\left(Y \le x \,\Big|\, U \le \frac{f(Y)}{M \cdot g(Y)}\right) = \frac{\mathbb{P}\left(Y \le x,\, U \le \frac{f(Y)}{M \cdot g(Y)}\right)}{\mathbb{P}\left(U \le \frac{f(Y)}{M \cdot g(Y)}\right)}.$$

For the numerator on the right-hand side, we obtain by conditioning w.r.t. Y

$$\mathbb{P}\left(Y \le x,\, U \le \frac{f(Y)}{M \cdot g(Y)}\right) = \int_{-\infty}^{x} \mathbb{P}\left(U \le \frac{f(Y)}{M \cdot g(Y)} \,\Big|\, Y = y\right) G(dy)$$

$$= \int_{-\infty}^{x} \mathbb{P}\left(U \le \frac{f(y)}{M \cdot g(y)}\right) G(dy),$$

where the last equality follows from the independence of U and Y. Since $U \sim UNI$, the last integral is equal to

$$\int_{-\infty}^{x} \frac{f(y)}{M \cdot g(y)} g(y) dy = \frac{1}{M} \int_{-\infty}^{x} f(y) \, dy = \frac{F(x)}{M}.$$

Since the denominator is the limit of the numerator for $x \to \infty$ and $F(x) \to 1$ for $x \to \infty$, the denominator must be identical to $1/M$. This finally proves the theorem. $\qquad\square$

Generally, one chooses the rv. $Y \sim G$ in such a way that Y can be easily generated by quantile transformation. The constant $M > 0$ should then be chosen as small as possible to minimize the cases of rejection.

In the following example, we apply the rejection method to generate a rv. $X \sim \mathcal{N}(0, 1)$. For the df. G, we choose the Cauchy distribution given under Exercise 2.16.

Example 2.13 At first, we have to find a proper constant M

$$\frac{f(x)}{g(x)} = \frac{1}{\sqrt{2\pi}} \exp\left(-\frac{x^2}{2}\right) \bigg/ \left(\frac{1}{\pi(1+x^2)}\right) = \sqrt{\pi/2} \exp\left(-\frac{x^2}{2}\right) (1+x^2).$$

The function $\exp\left(-\frac{x^2}{2}\right)(1+x^2)$ is symmetric around 0 and has a global maximum at $x = 1$. Thus, the constant

$$M := \frac{2\sqrt{\pi/2}}{\sqrt{e}} = \sqrt{\frac{2\pi}{e}}$$

can be used.

R-Example 2.14 The results of the last example can be implemented in R like

```
set.seed(123,kind ="Mersenne-Twister",normal.kind ="Inversion")
gen.norm.rm <- function(n){
  # n - number of observations

  # constant used during the method of rejection
  M = sqrt(2 * pi * exp(-1))

  # actual method of rejection, returning one observation
  MethodOfRejection <- function() {
    repeat{
      Y = rcauchy(1)
      if(runif(1) <= dnorm(Y) / (M * dcauchy(Y)))
        return(Y)
    }
  }
}
```

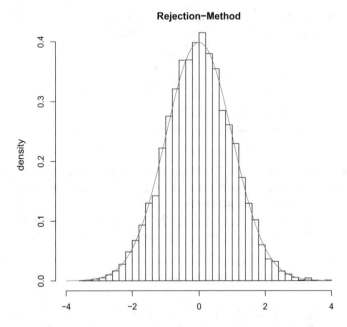

Fig. 2.2 Histogram of 10000 $\mathcal{N}(0, 1)$ rvs. generated with the rejection method and the $\mathcal{N}(0, 1)$-density

```
    # calling MethodOfRejection n times
    replicate(n, MethodOfRejection())
}
obs <- gen.norm.rm(n = 10000)
hist(obs, breaks = 50, freq = FALSE, xlab = "", xlim=c(-4,4),
                ylab = "density",
        main = "Rejection-Method")
curve(dnorm(x), col = "red", add = TRUE)
```

In the source code above, we define the function "gen.norm.rm" which returns a vector of n independent standard normal rvs. by applying the rejection method as described in Example 2.13. The function is called with $n = 10000$ and the result is stored in the variable "obs". The last two lines produce the histogram in Fig. 2.2. Within "gen.norm.rm" the functions "rcauchy", "runif", "dnorm", and "dcauchy" from the stats library are called. For the meaning of these functions, compare Sect. 2.1.

2.6 Generation of Random Vectors

In this section, we discuss the generation of two-dimensional random vectors (X, Y). If the variables are independent of one another, the methods stated above can be used. Thus, the remaining difficulty is the generation of dependent rv.

In the case of a known regression function, e.g.,

$$Y = f(X) + \varepsilon,$$

where X is independent of ε and $\mathbb{E}(\varepsilon) = 0$, we can also use the methods described above. To be precise, we generate the rv. X and ε independent of one another and substitute the results into the right-hand side of the regression equation above to obtain the rv. Y. Finally, (X, Y) is returned.

If no regression function is given but the regular conditional df. of Y given $X = x$ is known for each $x \in \mathbb{R}$, i.e.,

$$\mathscr{B}^* \ni B \longrightarrow \mathbb{P}(Y \in B \mid X = x),$$

where $\mathscr{B}^*$ denotes the Borel sets, then the *Rosenblatt Transformation* can be applied. For this transformation, let $G(y \mid x) := \mathbb{P}(Y \leq y \mid X = x)$ denote the conditional df. of Y given $X = x$ and F the df. of X. Then

$$(X, Y) \sim (F^{-1}(U), G^{-1}(V \mid F^{-1}(U))), \tag{2.4}$$

where U, V are independent rv. which are uniformly distributed on the unit interval.

Proof The proof is based on some standard operations of conditional distributions.

$$
\begin{aligned}
\mathbb{P}\left(F^{-1}(U) \leq t, G^{-1}(V \mid F^{-1}(U)) \leq y\right) &= \int_{-\infty}^{t} \mathbb{P}(G^{-1}(V \mid x) \leq y) \, F(dx) \\
&= \int_{-\infty}^{t} \mathbb{P}(V \leq G(y \mid x)) \, F(dx) \\
&= \int_{-\infty}^{t} G(y \mid x) \, F(dx) \\
&= \int_{-\infty}^{t} \mathbb{P}(Y \leq y \mid X = x) \, F(dx) \\
&= \mathbb{P}(X \leq t, Y \leq y).
\end{aligned}
$$

$\square$

2.7 Exercises

Exercise 2.15 Assume that $X_1, \ldots, X_n$ is an i.i.d. sequence of rvs. with common continuous df. F and let F_n denote the associated empirical distribution function; compare with (1.9).

(i) Determine $n\,F_n(X_i)$ and $F_n^{-1}(i/n)$, for $1 \le i \le n$.
(ii) Find the distribution of $F_n^{-1}(U)$ given the observations $X_1, \ldots, X_n$, if $U \sim UNI$ is independent of the sequence.
(iii) Implement a R-function to generate rvs. according to F_n.

Exercise 2.16 The density function of the Cauchy distribution is defined by

$$\mathbb{R} \ni x \longrightarrow f(x) := \frac{1}{\pi(1 + x^2)}.$$

Determine the corresponding df. F and F^{-1}.

Exercise 2.17 The Weibull distribution to the parameter (α, β), where $\alpha > 0$ and $\beta > 0$, abbreviated by $WEIB(\alpha, \beta)$, possess the df.

$$F(x) := \begin{cases} 1 - \exp(-(x/\alpha)^\beta) & : x \ge 0 \\ 0 & : \text{otherwise} \end{cases}$$

(i) Use the quantile transformation to define a procedure for generating Weibull distributed rvs.
(ii) Implement your Weibull generator in R.
(iii) Generate 10000 independent $WEIB(2, 2)$ variables in R with your generator and visualize the result in a histogram together with the corresponding density function.

Exercise 2.18 Let f, g be the pdfs. in the rejection method and $M > 0$ the corresponding constant. Determine the probability that the rejection method succeeds in the first step, i.e., no rejection.

References

Box GEP, Muller ME (1958) A note on the generation of random normal deviates. Ann Math Stat 29(2):610–611

Devroye L (1986) Non-uniform random variate generation. Springer, New York

Eubank R, Kupresanin A (2011) Statistical computing in C++ and R. Chapman and Hall/CRC Press, New York

Ripley BD (1987) Stochastic simulation. Wiley series in probability and mathematical statistics. Wiley, New York

Chapter 3
The Classical Bootstrap

In Chap. 1, we briefly introduced the idea of bootstrapping. Now, together with the first applications, we will also give some theoretical results of the classical bootstrap approximation as first published simultaneously by Bickel and Freedman (1981) and Singh (1981). The methods of proof in these two papers are different and we follow mainly the work of Singh (1981) here. However, in Sect. 3.5, we will go into more detail about a proof concept applied in Bickel and Freedman (1981).

The first two sections of this chapter contain programming examples and the essential theorems for the classical bootstrap procedure. The last four sections give a deeper insight into the mathematical background. They are rather intended for readers who have a deeper knowledge of probability theory and mathematical statistics.

3.1 An Introductory Example

Recall from Chap. 1 the basic idea of the bootstrap. Starting with an i.i.d. sample

$$X_1, \ldots, X_n \sim F$$

with common unknown df. F we consider a statistic $T_n(F) = T_n(X_1, \ldots, X_n; F)$ whose df. we want to approximate. For the approximation, we use the df. of $T_n(\hat{F})$, where $\hat{F}$ is a known df. which is close to F.

In the situation of the *classical bootstrap* (cb.), the edf. F_n is used for $\hat{F}$. Hence

$$T_n(\hat{F}) = T_n(F_n) = T_n(X_1^*, \ldots, X_n^*; F_n),$$

where

© Springer Nature Switzerland AG 2021
G. Dikta and M. Scheer, *Bootstrap Methods*,
https://doi.org/10.1007/978-3-030-73480-0_3

$$X_1^*, \ldots, X_n^* \sim F_n \tag{3.1}$$

is an i.i.d. sample with common df. F_n. We call $X_1^*, \ldots, X_n^*$ the *bootstrap sample*. The underlying probability measure will be denoted here by $\mathbb{P}_n^* \equiv \mathbb{P}_{F_n}$. Note that the probability measure of the bootstrap distribution, $\mathbb{P}_n^*$, depends on the original observations $X_1, \ldots, X_n$, thus it is random! Furthermore, it changes from n to $n+1$. Notice, in (3.1), we notationally suppress the fact that the bootstrap sample changes its distribution with n. Hence, in an asymptotics setting, i.e., $n \to \infty$, it would be more precise to write

$$X_{1,n}^*, \ldots, X_{n,n}^* \sim F_n. \tag{3.2}$$

Nevertheless, for notational convenience we simply write $X_1^*, \ldots, X_n^*$ for the triangular scheme (3.2).

In the following set of examples, we will describe how the classical bootstrap can be used to construct a confidence interval for the expectation of an rv. Note that this is just an introductory example.

Example 3.1 Confidence interval for the expectation μ, part 1. Recall the situation of Sect. 1.1 and assume that we want to construct a confidence interval for the expectation $\mu = \mathbb{E}(X)$ of an rv. $X \sim F$ whose variance $\mathrm{VAR}(X) = \sigma^2 < \infty$ is unknown to us but expected to be finite. We observe an i.i.d. sample $X_1, \ldots, X_n$ and use the CLT to construct a 90% asymptotic confidence interval for μ. Based on Eq. (1.3), we get

$$\mathbb{P}\big(\Phi^{-1}(0.05) \le \sqrt{n}(\bar{X}_n - \mu)/s_n \le \Phi^{-1}(0.95)\big) \approx 0.9.$$

Here Φ^{-1} denotes the quantile function of the $\mathcal{N}(0, 1)$ distribution. Since $\Phi^{-1}(0.05)$ is equal to $-\Phi^{-1}(0.95)$, the confidence interval can be obtained from the result above. After some algebraic rearrangements, we get

$$\mathbb{P}\big(\mu \in \big[\bar{X}_n - s_n \times \Phi^{-1}(0.95)/\sqrt{n}, \ \bar{X}_n + s_n \times \Phi^{-1}(0.95)/\sqrt{n}\big]\big) \approx 0.9.$$

In this classical construction, the quantiles of the approximating normal distribution Φ are taken to approximate the corresponding quantiles of $\mathbb{P}_F\big(\sqrt{n}(\bar{X}_n - \mu)/s_n \le x\big)$. It is Eq. (1.3) which allows this construction.

Now assume that the following approximation is a.s. correct:

$$\sup_{x \in \mathbb{R}} \left| \mathbb{P}\big(\sqrt{n}(\bar{X}_n - \mu)/s_n \le x\big) - \mathbb{P}_n^*\big(\sqrt{n}(\bar{X}_n^* - \bar{X}_n)/s_n^* \le x\big) \right| \longrightarrow 0, \quad \text{as } n \to \infty, \tag{3.3}$$

where

$$\bar{X}_n^* := \frac{1}{n} \sum_{i=1}^{n} X_i^*, \qquad s_n^{*2} := \frac{1}{n-1} \sum_{i=1}^{n} \big(X_i^* - \bar{X}_n^*\big)^2.$$

As in the construction above, we can use $q_{0.05}$ and $q_{0.95}$ the 0.05 and 0.95 quantile of the approximating df. of $\sqrt{n}(\bar{X}_n^* - \bar{X}_n)/s_n^*$ (with respect to the probability measure $\mathbb{P}_n^*$), respectively, to get

$$\mathbb{P}\left(q_{0.05} \leq n^{1/2}(\bar{X}_n - \mu)/s_n \leq q_{0.95}\right) \approx 0.9. \tag{3.4}$$

With some minor algebraic rearrangements, we finally derive

$$\left[\bar{X}_n - s_n \times q_{0.95}/\sqrt{n}, \ \bar{X}_n - s_n \times q_{0.05}/\sqrt{n}\right], \tag{3.5}$$

the bootstrap confidence interval for μ.

But we still have to determine the two quantiles $q_{0.05}$ and $q_{0.95}$. In principle, it is possible to calculate these quantiles since we know the underlying distribution. With respect to the computing time involved, this will be impossible in most cases. However, since we know the underlying df. we can now use a *Monte Carlo* approach (mc.) to get at least an acceptable approximation for these quantiles. To see how this works in practice, we continue with Example 3.1.

Example 3.2 Confidence interval for the expectation μ, part 2. We start with a resampling scheme for the bootstrap data:

Resampling scheme 3.3 Classical bootstrap.

(A) $X_1, \ldots, X_n$ *observed data.*
(B) *Calculate $q_{0.05}$ and $q_{0.95}$ the 0.05 and 0.95 quantile of $\mathbb{P}_n^*(\sqrt{n}(\bar{X}_n^* - \bar{X}_n)/s_n^* \leq x)$, where $X_1^*, \ldots, X_n^*$ are i.i.d. according to F_n, the edf. of the observed data.*
(C) *Take $[\bar{X}_n - s_n \times q_{0.95}/\sqrt{n}, \bar{X}_n - s_n \times q_{0.05}/\sqrt{n}]$ as a confidence interval.*

To apply a Monte Carlo approximation for step (B), one can use the following basic approach:

(B1) Generate m bootstrap datasets $X_{\ell;1}^*, \ldots, X_{\ell;n}^* \sim F_n$, $1 \leq \ell \leq m$ and calculate
$T_{\ell;n} := \sqrt{n}(\bar{X}_{\ell;n}^* - \bar{X}_n)/s_{\ell;n}^*$.
(B2) Take $T_{[0.05 \times m]:m;n}$ and $T_{[0.95 \times m]:m;n}$ as an approximation for $q_{0.05}$ and $q_{0.95}$ in the interval under (C), where $(T_{\ell:m;n})_{1 \leq \ell \leq m}$ are the ordered $(T_{\ell;n})_{1 \leq \ell \leq m}$, that is, $T_{1;n} \leq T_{2;n} \leq \ldots \leq T_{m;n}$.

R-Example 3.4 Confidence interval for the expectation μ, part 3. The following R-code shows how this Monte Carlo approximation is applied under R to find the quantiles. Note that the unbiased estimates

$$s_n^2 := \frac{1}{n-1} \sum_{i=1}^{n} (X_i - \bar{X}_n)^2, \quad s_n^{*2} := \frac{1}{n-1} \sum_{i=1}^{n} (X_i^* - \bar{X}_n^*)^2$$

are used in the R-code. Further, the sample quantiles obtained from the R-function "quantile" differ slightly from the sample quantiles defined in step (B2).

```r
step.B1 <- function(x, m = 1000){
  # x - observed data
  # m - number of MC replications

  # Realize step (B1).
  # generates m classical bootstrap data sets
  # calculates the standardized statistic and returns
  # them as a vector

  n <- length(x)
  mean.observed.x <- mean(x)

  # studentize x.boot according to step (B1)
  studentize <- function(x.boot){
    sqrt(n) * (mean(x.boot) - mean.observed.x) / sd(x.boot)
  }

  # step (B1)
  replicate(m, {
    x.boot <- sample(x, n, replace=TRUE)
    studentize(x.boot)
  })
}

ci <- function(x, conf.level){
  # x - observed data
  # conf.level - confidence level
  # returns left and right bound of the confidence interval
  # as a vector

  alpha   <- 1 - conf.level
  t.boot <- step.B1(x, m=999)

  # quantiles based on the MC simulation, see step (B) and (B2)
  ql.boot <- quantile(t.boot, alpha / 2)
  qr.boot <- quantile(t.boot, 1 - alpha / 2)

  n <- length(x)
  mean.observed.x <- mean(x)
  sd.observed.x   <- sd(x)

  # calculations according to step (C)
  left  <- mean.observed.x - qr.boot * sd.observed.x / sqrt(n)
  right <- mean.observed.x - ql.boot * sd.observed.x / sqrt(n)

  ret <- c(left, right)
  names(ret) <- c("lower", "upper")
  ret
}

set.seed(123,kind ="Mersenne-Twister",normal.kind ="Inversion")
#x is a vector with the observed data
x <- rnorm(20, mean = 5, sd = 2)
```

```
ci(x = x, conf.level = 0.90)
```

```
##      lower    upper
## 4.583343 6.052707
```

A more convenient way to obtain the confidence interval is to apply the function "boot.ci" from the boot package.

```
bootstrap.ci <- function(x, conf.level, R){
  # x - observed data
  # conf.level - confidence level
  # R number of MC simulations

  # calculate mean and variance for the bootstrapped sample
  mean_and_var <- function(d, i){
    # d - observed data
    # i - boot::boot tells us which indices to be used to
    #     obtain the resampling version of the observed data

    d_boot <- d[i]
    c(mean_boot <- mean(d_boot), variance_boot = var(d_boot))
  }

  # resampled mean and variance
  b <- boot::boot(x, mean_and_var, R = R)

  # type = "stud" stands for studentized statistics
  ret <- boot::boot.ci(b, conf = conf.level, type = "stud",
                     # var.t0 - variance of the observed data
                     var.t0 = var(x),
                     # var.t - variances for every
                     #         resampled data sets
                     var.t = b$t[,2])$student[4:5]

  names(ret) <- c("lower", "upper")
  ret
}
```

```
set.seed(123,kind ="Mersenne-Twister",normal.kind ="Inversion")
bootstrap.ci(rnorm(20, mean=5, sd=2), conf.level=0.9, R=999)
```

```
##      lower    upper
## 4.510934 6.097640
```

The slight differences between the two calculated confidence intervals originate from two facts. First, the resampled data are generated differently; cf. the parameter "simple" in the help page of the function "boot". Second, the quantiles are calculated differently, cf. Davison and Hinkley (1997, p. 195).

Table 3.1 Observed coverage and mean interval length of 80% and 90% confidence intervals, based on resampling scheme 3.3 and normal approximation. The underlying distribution functions of the random samples ($n=10$) are $Exp(0.1)$ and $UNI(0,6)$

fun	conf.level	proc	obsCoverage	meanIntervalWidth
rexp	0.8	bootstrap.ci	0.80	10.51
rexp	0.8	normal.ci	0.71	7.35
rexp	0.9	bootstrap.ci	0.90	14.36
rexp	0.9	normal.ci	0.84	9.76
runif	0.8	bootstrap.ci	0.85	1.51
runif	0.8	normal.ci	0.75	1.38
runif	0.9	bootstrap.ci	0.94	2.08
runif	0.9	normal.ci	0.86	1.77

Example 3.5 Confidence interval for the expectation μ, part 4. According to this classical bootstrap approach, we constructed confidence intervals and compared them with the corresponding ones constructed by approximation with the normal distribution. The result of this simulation study is given below in Table 3.1. For the distribution function, we choose the uniform df. on the interval [0, 6] and the exponential df. with parameter 0.1.

```
normal.ci <- function(x, conf.level){
  # x - observed data
  # conf.level - confidence level

  # calculate confidence interval based on the
  # central limit theorem

  mean_observed_x <- mean(x)
  sd_observed_x   <- sd(x)
  n <- length(x)
  q <- qnorm((1-conf.level)/2)

  c(lower = mean_observed_x + q * sd_observed_x / sqrt(n),
    upper = mean_observed_x - q * sd_observed_x / sqrt(n))
}

# data will be generated using the uniform distribution
# and the exponential distribution
dg <- bind_rows(
  simTool::expand_tibble(fun = "runif", n = 10, max = 6),
  simTool::expand_tibble(fun = "rexp",  n = 10, rate = 0.1)) %>%
  as.data.frame

# 80% and 90% confidence intervals will be calculated by using
# the function boostrap.ci() and normal.ci()
pg <- bind_rows(
  simTool::expand_tibble(proc = "bootstrap.ci",
                         conf.level = c(0.8, 0.9), R = 999),
  simTool::expand_tibble(proc = "normal.ci",
```

```
                        conf.level = c(0.8, 0.9))) %>%
  as.data.frame

# create data sets according to data.frame dg
# calculate confidence intervals according to data.frame pg
# do this 1000 times on 4 cpus on the local machine
eg <- simTool::eval_tibbles(dg, pg, replications = 1000,
                            ncpus = 4,
                            cluster_seed = rep(123456, 6),
                            discard_generated_data = TRUE,
                            simplify = FALSE,
                            # convert the resulting vectors
                            # to a tibble
                            post_analyze = tibble::enframe)

results <- eg$simulation %>%
  # put the lower and upper limit
  # into two columns
  tidyr::unnest(results) %>%
  tidyr::spread(key = name, value = value) %>%
  # calculate the width of every constructed
  # confidence interval and determine if it
  # covers the true mean
  dplyr::mutate(width = upper - lower,
        mu = ifelse(fun == "rexp", 10, 3),
        muCovered = lower <= mu & mu <= upper) %>%
  dplyr::group_by(fun, conf.level, proc) %>%
  # calculate the covarage and mean length of the
  # confidence intervals conditioned on the different
  # distribution function, the confidence level of
  # the interval and the function used to calculate
  # the confidence interval
  dplyr::summarize(obsCoverage = mean(muCovered),
                meanIntervalWidth = mean(width))
```

3.2 Basic Mathematical Background of the Classical Bootstrap

In this section, we give some mathematical justifications for the validity of the classical bootstrap approximations. We start with an example to show that the bootstrap approximation is not always correct!

Example 3.6 Let $X_1, \ldots, X_n \sim UNI$ be an i.i.d. sample with $UNI \equiv F$ as common df. The right-hand point of the support of F is obviously $1(= T(F))$. To "estimate" $T(F)$, we take the largest observation $T_n(F) \equiv T_n(X_1, \ldots, X_n; F) = X_{n:n}$, where

$$X_{1:n} \leq X_{2:n} \leq \ldots \leq X_{n:n}$$

denotes the order statistic corresponding to the observations. As we will see in Exercise 3.26,

$$
\begin{aligned}
\mathbb{P}_F(n(T(F) - T_n(F)) \leq x) &= \mathbb{P}_F(n(1 - X_{n:n}) \leq x) \\
&\longrightarrow 1 - \exp(-x), \quad \text{as } n \to \infty,
\end{aligned}
$$

for all $x \geq 0$. In particular, we get for $x = 0$ that

$$
\mathbb{P}_F(n(T(F) - T_n(F)) \leq 0) = \mathbb{P}_F(n(1 - X_{n:n}) \leq 0) \longrightarrow 0.
$$

Now we mimic this situation for the bootstrap approximation. Having observed the sample $X_1, \ldots, X_n$, the right-hand point of the support of F_n is obviously the largest observation, thus $T(F_n) \equiv X_{n:n}$. To "estimate" $T(F_n)$ from the bootstrap sample $X_1^*, \ldots, X_n^*$ we have to take the largest bootstrap observation, thus $T_n(F_n) = X_{n:n}^*$. But now we get (see Exercise 3.26)

$$
\begin{aligned}
\mathbb{P}_n^*(n(T(F_n) - T_n(F_n)) \leq 0) &= \mathbb{P}_n^*(n(X_{n:n} - X_{n:n}^*) \leq 0) \\
&\longrightarrow 1 - \exp(-1), \quad \text{as } n \to \infty.
\end{aligned}
$$

This shows that the bootstrap approximation is not correct here.   □

This disillusioning example points out clearly that we cannot expect a bootstrap approximation to be always possible. Furthermore, it tells us that we have to prove its correctness before we are allowed to use it.

In the following considerations, the sample size and the resampling size will be n, and the bootstrap sample will be taken from F_n the edf. corresponding to the i.i.d. sample $X_1, \ldots, X_n \sim F$. The bootstrap sample will be denoted as usual by $X_1^*, \ldots, X_n^* \sim F_n$ and we skip the second index n here. Furthermore, we use $\mathbb{E}(X) = \mu$, $\text{VAR}(X) = \sigma^2$,

$$
\mathbb{E}_n^*(X^*) = \int x \, F_n(\mathrm{d}x) = \frac{1}{n} \sum_{i=1}^{n} = \bar{X}_n, \quad \text{VAR}_n^*(X^*) = \frac{1}{n} \sum_{i=1}^{n} (X_i - \bar{X}_n)^2 = s_n^2,
$$

and finally

$$
\bar{X}_n^* = \frac{1}{n} \sum_{i=1}^{n} X_i^*, \quad s_n^{*2} = \frac{1}{n} \sum_{i=1}^{n} (X_i^* - \bar{X}_n^*)^2.
$$

Note that now $1/n$ is used for s_n^2 and s_n^{*2} instead of $1/(n-1)$. In asymptotic considerations, this is irrelevant. With this definition s_n^2 becomes the variance of the bootstrap variable. This has, as will be seen later, advantages in theoretical considerations.

The Weak Law of Large Number (WLLN) guarantees that

$$\mathbb{P}\left(\left|\frac{1}{n}\sum_{i=1}^{n}h(X_i)-\int h(x)\,F(dx)\right|>\varepsilon\right)\longrightarrow 0,\quad\text{for every }\varepsilon>0,$$

whenever the integral is defined. As to the bootstrap sample, we show

Theorem 3.7 Weak Law of Large Numbers for the classical bootstrap. *Assume that $\int|h(x)|\,F(dx)<\infty$. Then with probability one (w.p.1):*

$$\mathbb{P}_n^*\left(\left|n^{-1}\sum_{i=1}^{n}h(X_i^*)-\int h(x)\,F(dx)\right|>\varepsilon\right)\longrightarrow 0,\quad\text{as }n\to\infty,$$

for every $\varepsilon>0$.

Proof Assume w.l.o.g. that the F−integral of h vanishes, otherwise we consider $h-\int h\,dF$. The bootstrap variables form a triangular array of independent rvs. within each row with common df. F_n. Define for $n\in\mathbb{N}$

$$h_n(x)=h(x)\,\mathrm{I}_{\{|h(x)|<n\}}$$

to get

$$\mathbb{P}_n^*\left(\left|\frac{1}{n}\sum_{i=1}^{n}h(X_i^*)\right|>\varepsilon\right)\le\mathbb{P}_n^*\left(\left|\frac{1}{n}\sum_{i=1}^{n}h_n(X_i^*)\right|>\varepsilon\right)+\mathbb{P}_n^*\left(\bigcup_{i=1}^{n}\{|h(X_i^*)|\ge n\}\right).$$

The second probability on the right-hand side is bounded by

$$n\,\mathbb{P}_n^*\left(|h(X_1^*)|\ge n\right)$$

and the first by

$$\mathbb{P}_n^*\left(\left|\frac{1}{n}\sum_{i=1}^{n}h_n(X_i^*)-\mathbb{E}_n^*(h_n(X_1^*))\right|>\varepsilon/2\right)+\mathrm{I}_{\{|\mathbb{E}_n^*(h_n(X_1^*))|>\varepsilon/2\}}.$$

Apply Chebyshev's inequality to get

$$\mathbb{P}_n^*\left(\left|\frac{1}{n}\sum_{i=1}^{n}h_n(X_i^*)-\mathbb{E}_n^*(h_n(X_1^*))\right|>\varepsilon/2\right)\le\frac{4}{n\varepsilon^2}\mathrm{VAR}_n^*(h_n(X_1^*)).$$

Thus, the proof is complete if we can show that

$$\lim_{n\to\infty} n\mathbb{P}_n^*\big(|h(X_1^*)| \geq n\big) = 0 \quad \mathbb{P} - a.s. \tag{3.6}$$

$$\lim_{n\to\infty} \mathbb{E}_n^*(h_n(X_1^*)) = 0 \quad \mathbb{P} - a.s. \tag{3.7}$$

$$\lim_{n\to\infty} \frac{1}{n} \text{VAR}_n^*(h_n(X_1^*)) = 0 \quad \mathbb{P} - a.s. \tag{3.8}$$

hold. Now, apply Markov's inequality to get

$$n\mathbb{P}_n^*\big(|h(X_1^*)| \geq n\big) = n\mathbb{P}_{F_n}\{x : |h(x)| \geq n\} \leq \int_{\{x:\,|h(x)|\geq n\}} |h(x)|\, F_n(dx).$$

Fix for a moment $K \geq 0$ as a constant integer and apply the SLLN and the last inequality to get w.p.1

$$\limsup_{n\to\infty} n\mathbb{P}_n^*\big(|h(X_1^*)| \geq n\big) \leq \limsup_{n\to\infty} \int_{\{x:\,|h(x)|\geq K\}} |h(x)|\, F_n(dx) = \int_{\{x:\,|h(x)|\geq K\}} |h(x)|\, F(dx).$$

But the right-hand side can be made arbitrarily small by letting $K \uparrow \infty$ since $\int |h(x)|\, F(dx) < \infty$ by assumption. Thus (3.6) holds.

To verify (3.7), we first observe that w.p.1

$$\lim_{n\to\infty} \int h(x)\, F_n(dx) = \int h(x)\, F(dx) = 0$$

according to SLLN. Combine this result with

$$\limsup_{n\to\infty} \int_{\{x:\,|h(x)|\geq n\}} |h(x)|\, F_n(dx) \leq \int_{\{x:\,|h(x)|\geq K\}} |h(x)|\, F(dx)$$

and use the same argument as in the proof of (3.6) to show that (3.7) holds. According to (3.7) it remains to show that w.p.1.

$$\frac{1}{n} \mathbb{E}_n^*\big(h_n^2(X_1^*)\big) \longrightarrow 0.$$

Note that

$$\frac{1}{n} \mathbb{E}_n^*\big(h_n^2(X_1^*)\big) \leq \frac{1}{n} \sum_{k=1}^{n} k^2\, \mathbb{P}_n^*\big(k - 1 \leq |h(X_1^*)| < k\big)$$

$$\leq \frac{2}{n} \sum_{k=1}^{n} \sum_{j=1}^{k} j\, \mathbb{P}_n^*\big(k - 1 \leq |h(X_1^*)| < k\big)$$

$$\leq \frac{2}{n} \sum_{j=1}^{n} j\, \mathbb{P}_n^* \big(j - 1 \leq \big|h(X_1^*)\big| < n\big)$$

$$\leq 2 \sup_{j \in \mathbb{N}} \big|x_{nj} - x_j\big| + \frac{2}{n} \sum_{j=1}^{n} j\, \mathbb{P}\big(j - 1 \leq \big|h(X_1)\big|\big),$$

where $x_{nj} = j\, \mathbb{P}_n^*\big(j - 1 \leq \big|h(X_1^*)\big|\big)$ and $x_j = j\, \mathbb{P}\big(j - 1 \leq \big|h(X_1)\big|\big)$ for $n, j \in \mathbb{N}$. But the last sum is a Cesaro average, cf. Billingsley (1995, A30), of a sequence which tends to 0 w.p.1 by virtue of $\int |h(x)|\, F(dx) < \infty$. Hence, it remains to show that $\sup_{j \in \mathbb{N}} \big|x_{nj} - x_j\big| = o(1)$ almost surely, as $n \to \infty$. Note that for every fixed $j_0 \in \mathbb{N}$, $\big|x_{nj_0} - x_{j_0}\big| = o(1)$ almost surely, as $n \to \infty$, according to the SLLN. If the uniform convergence would not hold, a subsequence $(j_n)_{n \in \mathbb{N}}$ must exist such that $\big|x_{nj_n} - x_{j_n}\big| \geq c$ for all $n \in \mathbb{N}$ and some $c > 0$. But this is impossible due to $\int |h(x)|\, F(dx) < \infty$ and (3.6). This finally completes the proof. $\qquad\square$

The next theorem shows that the approximation given under (3.3) is correct. Our proof here is based on Singh (1981).

Theorem 3.8 Central limit theorem for the classical bootstrap. *Let* $\mathbb{E}(X^2) < \infty$ *and set* $\mu = \mathbb{E}(X)$. *Then w.p.1*

$$\sup_{x \in \mathbb{R}} \Big| \mathbb{P}\big(n^{1/2}(\bar{X}_n - \mu) \leq x\big) - \mathbb{P}_n^*\big(n^{1/2}(\bar{X}_n^* - \bar{X}_n) \leq x\big) \Big| \longrightarrow 0, \quad \text{as } n \to \infty.$$

Proof By the CLT, the continuity of Φ, the standard normal df., we get from a classical argument, cf. Loève (1977, p. 21), that it suffices to prove

$$\mathbb{P}_n^*\big(n^{1/2}(\bar{X}_n^* - \bar{X}_n)/s_n \leq x\big) \longrightarrow \Phi(x), \quad \text{as } n \to \infty, \text{ for each } x \in \mathbb{R},$$

w.p.1. For this, we have to check the validity of Lindeberg's condition, cf. Serfling (1980, 1.9.3):

$$s_n^{-2} \int_{\{|X_1^* - \bar{X}_n| \geq \varepsilon n^{1/2} s_n\}} (X_1^* - \bar{X}_n)^2 \, d\mathbb{P}_n^* \longrightarrow 0, \quad \text{as } n \to \infty, \text{ for each } \varepsilon > 0,$$

where the left-hand term equals

$$s_n^{-2} n^{-1} \sum_{i=1}^{n} (X_i - \bar{X}_n)^2 \mathbf{I}_{\{|X_i - \bar{X}_n| \geq \varepsilon n^{1/2} s_n\}}. \tag{3.9}$$

Note that for all $\tilde{\varepsilon} > 0$

$$\sum_{i \geq 1} \mathbb{P}\left(\frac{|X_i|}{\sqrt{i}} > \tilde{\varepsilon}\right) = \sum_{i \geq 1} \int_{[i-1, i[} \mathbb{P}\left(\frac{X^2}{\tilde{\varepsilon}} > i\right) dx \leq \int_0^\infty \mathbb{P}\left(\frac{X^2}{\tilde{\varepsilon}} > x\right) dx = \frac{\mathbb{E}(X^2)}{\tilde{\varepsilon}} < \infty.$$

Therefore, according to the Borel-Cantelli Lemma:

$$\limsup_{i \to \infty} \frac{|X_i|}{\sqrt{i}} = 0, \qquad \text{w.p.1.}$$

Since $s_n \to \sigma$ and $\bar{X}_n \to \mu$ w.p.1 according to SLLN, the last result ensures w.p.1 that, for $n \equiv n(\omega)$ sufficiently large,

$$\left| X_i - \bar{X}_n \right| \geq \varepsilon n^{1/2} s_n$$

can only hold for finitely many i. Hence, the indicator function under (3.9) can only be 1 in finitely many cases. This completes the proof. $\square$

This result, however, is not exactly what we stated under (3.3).

Corollary 3.9 *Under the assumptions of Theorem 3.8, we get w.p.1*

$$\sup_{x \in \mathbb{R}} \left| \mathbb{P}\left(n^{1/2}(\bar{X}_n - \mu)/s_n \leq x \right) - \mathbb{P}_n^*\left(n^{1/2}(\bar{X}_n^* - \bar{X}_n)/s_n^* \leq x \right) \right| \longrightarrow 0, \quad \text{as } n \to \infty.$$

Proof As we have discussed in the proof of Theorem 3.8, we have to show

$$\mathbb{P}_n^*\left(n^{1/2}(\bar{X}_n^* - \bar{X}_n)/s_n^* \leq x \right) \longrightarrow \Phi(x), \quad \text{as } n \to \infty, \tag{3.10}$$

w.p.1, for each $x \in \mathbb{R}$, while we already know that

$$\mathbb{P}_n^*\left(n^{1/2}(\bar{X}_n^* - \bar{X}_n)/s_n \leq x \right) \longrightarrow \Phi(x), \quad \text{as } n \to \infty,$$

w.p.1, for each $x \in \mathbb{R}$. Since

$$\mathbb{P}_n^*\left(\left| s_n/s_n^* - 1 \right| > \varepsilon \right) \longrightarrow 0, \quad \text{as } n \to \infty,$$

w.p.1, for every $\varepsilon > 0$, according to an application of Theorem 3.7, (3.10) follows from Slutsky's theorem, cf. Serfling (1980, Theorem 1.5.4). $\square$

3.3   Discussion of the Asymptotic Accuracy of the Classical Bootstrap

In this section, we review some of Singh (1981) the results on the classical bootstrap without any proof. We have already seen in Theorem 3.8 that the CLT holds for the standardized mean when the classical bootstrap is used. But this result does not tell us anything about the quality of the approximation.

Again, going through the proof of Theorem 3.8, we find it to be in line with the classical argumentation. The same is true for the next theorem which gives us the rate of convergence. Note that in the classical situation an appropriate bound is given by the Berry-Esséen theorem, cf. Loève (1977, p. 300):

$$\sup_{x \in \mathbb{R}} \left| \mathbb{P}\left(n^{1/2}(\bar{X}_n - \mu) \leq x\right) - \Phi(x/\sigma) \right| \leq K\rho\,\sigma^{-3}n^{-1/2},$$

where K is a universal constant and $\rho = \mathbb{E}(|X - \mu|^3)$. Based on the Berry-Esséen theorem and the Law of Iterated Logarithm (LIL), i.e.,

$$\limsup_{n \to \infty} \frac{\sum_{i=1}^{n}(X_i - \mu)}{(2\sigma^2 n \log(\log(n)))^{1/2}} = 1, \qquad \text{w.p.1},$$

cf. Serfling (1980, 1.10 Theorem A), Singh proved the following result:

Theorem 3.10 *Let* $\mathbb{E}(X^4) < \infty$. *Then w.p.1*

$$\limsup_{n \to \infty} n^{1/2}(\log(\log(n)))^{-1/2} \sup_{x \in \mathbb{R}} \left| \mathbb{P}\left(n^{1/2}(\bar{X}_n - \mu) \leq x\right) - \mathbb{P}_n^*\left(n^{1/2}(\bar{X}_n^* - \bar{X}_n) \leq x\right) \right|$$
$$= (2\sigma^2\sqrt{2\pi e})^{-1}\left(2\mathrm{VAR}((X - \mu)^2)\right)^{1/2}.$$

As we already mentioned in the introduction, the bootstrap is a vehicle to approximate the df. of a given statistic. Theorem 3.8 shows that the classical bootstrap approximation holds in the case of arithmetic mean. But the normal approximation also holds due to CLT. In a particular situation, we have to decide which approximation is preferable. Therefore, we have to compare the order of convergence of these two approximations. Theorem 3.10 says that w.p.1

$$\sup_{x \in \mathbb{R}} \left| \mathbb{P}\left(n^{1/2}(\bar{X}_n - \mu) \leq x\right) - \mathbb{P}_n^*\left(n^{1/2}(\bar{X}_n^* - \bar{X}_n) \leq x\right) \right| = O\left(\left(\frac{\ln(\ln(n))}{n}\right)^{1/2}\right). \tag{3.11}$$

The Berry-Esséen theorem shows that

$$\sup_{x \in \mathbb{R}} \left| \mathbb{P}\left(n^{1/2}(\bar{X}_n - \mu)/\sigma \leq x\right) - \Phi(x) \right| = O(n^{-1/2}). \tag{3.12}$$

But (3.11) and (3.12) are not comparable since for (3.12) we have to know the variance σ^2 which is unknown in most situations and which is not used in (3.11). If $\mathbb{E}(|X|^3) < \infty$, Singh (1981) showed by applying an Edgeworth expansion that w.p.1

$$\sup_{x \in \mathbb{R}} \left| \mathbb{P}\left(n^{1/2}(\bar{X}_n - \mu)/\sigma \leq x\right) - \mathbb{P}_n^*\left(n^{1/2}(\bar{X}_n^* - \bar{X}_n)/s_n \leq x\right) \right| = o(n^{-1/2}), \tag{3.13}$$

which is better than the approximation under (3.12). Furthermore, Abramovitch and Singh (1985) proved under the assumption $\mathbb{E}(X^6) < \infty$ that w.p.1

$$\sup_{x \in \mathbb{R}} \left| \mathbb{P}\big(n^{1/2}(\bar{X}_n - \mu)/s_n \le x\big) - \mathbb{P}_n^*\big(n^{1/2}(\bar{X}_n^* - \bar{X}_n)/s_n^* \le x\big) \right| = o(n^{-1/2}), \quad (3.14)$$

where $s_n^{*2} = n^{-1} \sum_{i=1}^{n} (X_i^* - \bar{X}_n^*)^2$.

In summary, one might think that the classical bootstrap approximation is always better than the normal approximation since it incorporates the Edgeworth terms automatically. However, if, for instance, F, the underlying df. is symmetric around μ, we get

$$\sup_{x \in \mathbb{R}} \left| \mathbb{P}\big(n^{1/2}(\bar{X}_n - \mu)/\sigma \le x\big) - \Phi(x) \right| = o(n^{-1/2}), \quad (3.15)$$

which shows the same order of convergence that we find under (3.14). Furthermore, (3.15) still holds if we replace σ by s_n, cf. Abramovitch and Singh (1985).

Remark 3.11 A detailed discussion of the bootstrap and its relation to Edgeworth expansions can be found in Hall (1992).

3.4 Empirical Process and the Classical Bootstrap

Assume throughout this section that $X_1, \ldots, X_n \sim F$ is an i.i.d. sample with common continuous df. F, and let

$$\alpha_n(x) := n^{1/2}(F_n(x) - F(x)) \qquad (3.16)$$

be the *empirical process*. The classical invariance principle of this process says, cf. Billingsley (1968, Theorem 16.4), that

$$\alpha_n \xrightarrow[n \to \infty]{} B^o(F), \qquad \text{in distribution}$$

in the Skorokhod topology, where $B^o(F)$ is a transformed Brownian bridge, i.e., a centered Gaussian process with covariance structure given by

$$\mathbb{E}\big(B^o(F)(s) \cdot B^o(F)(t)\big) = F(s)(1 - F(t)), \quad s \le t.$$

To analyze the distribution of this process, one often takes a special version of α_n given by

$$\bar{\alpha}_n(F(x)), \qquad x \in \mathbb{R},$$

where $\bar{\alpha}_n(u) = n^{1/2}(\bar{F}_n(u) - u)$ is the *uniform empirical process* based on an uniform sample $U_1, \ldots, U_n \sim UNI$. Note that

$$\alpha_n(x) = n^{1/2}\left(n^{-1}\sum_{i=1}^{n} I_{\{]-\infty,x]\}}(X_i) - F(x)\right)$$

$$= n^{1/2}\left(n^{-1}\sum_{i=1}^{n} I_{\{]-\infty,x]\}}(F^{-1}(U_i)) - F(x)\right)$$

$$= n^{1/2}\left(n^{-1}\sum_{i=1}^{n} I_{\{]0,F(x)]\}}(U_i) - F(x)\right)$$

$$= \bar{\alpha}_n(F(x)).$$

In the following, we will consider the empirical process built according to the classical bootstrap resampling scheme. Denote this process by

$$\alpha_n^*(x) := n^{1/2}(F_n^*(x) - F_n(x)).$$

Theorem 3.12 *Assume F to be continuous. Then w.p.1*

$$\alpha_n^* \xrightarrow[n\to\infty]{} B^o(F), \qquad \text{in distribution}$$

in the Skorokhod topology.

Proof Since we know from the classical invariance principle that $\bar{\alpha}_n(F)$ converges to this limit process, it is enough to find a version of the empirical bootstrap process which is close to $\bar{\alpha}_n(F)$. To be precise, take for α_n^* the version given by

$$\alpha_n^* = \bar{\alpha}_n(F_n),$$

where now the same sample $U_1, \ldots, U_n$ is used as for the process $\bar{\alpha}_n(F)$. For notational reason, we use $\bar{\mathbb{P}}$ for the probability measure corresponding to this uniform sample. Let $\varepsilon > 0$ be arbitrarily chosen. Then

$$\bar{\mathbb{P}}\left(\sup_{x\in\mathbb{R}} |\bar{\alpha}_n(F_n(x)) - \bar{\alpha}_n(F(x))| \geq \varepsilon\right) \leq \bar{\mathbb{P}}(\bar{w}_n(\|F_n - F\|) > \varepsilon),$$

where

$$\bar{w}_n(\delta) := \sup_{|t-s|\leq\delta} |\bar{\alpha}_n(t) - \bar{\alpha}_n(s)|$$

denotes the modulus of continuity. Since $\|F_n - F\| \to 0$ $\mathbb{P}$−a.s. we can apply a general result on the oscillation of the uniform empirical process given by Stute (1982, (0.3)), to obtain w.p.1

$$\bar{\mathbb{P}}(\bar{w}_n(\|F_n - F\|) > \varepsilon) \xrightarrow[n\to\infty]{} 0,$$

which finally proves the theorem.   □

Remark 3.13 The proof of this theorem can be found in Swanepoel (1986) and in Dikta (1987, Appendix). Further bootstrap versions of important processes are also discussed there.

3.5   Mathematical Framework of Mallow's Metric

To analyze the classical bootstrap of the mean, Bickel and Freedman (1981) used a different concept than Singh (1981). Parts of their analysis are based on the relation of the classical bootstrap approximation to Mallow's metric. In this section, we will outline their approach and start with an important minimization result given in Major (1978, Theorem 8.1).

Theorem 3.14 *Let F and G be distribution functions such that $\int |x|\, F(\mathrm{d}x)$ and $\int |x|\, G(\mathrm{d}x)$ are finite. Assume that H is a two-dimensional df. on $(\mathbb{R}^2, \mathscr{B}_2^*)$, the product space equipped with the Borel $\sigma-$algebra, with marginal df. F and G, respectively, and define $\mathscr{M}$ to be the collection of all those H's. Then for every convex function $f : \mathbb{R} \longrightarrow \mathbb{R}$*

$$\inf_{H \in \mathscr{M}} \int f(x - y)\, H(\mathrm{d}x, \mathrm{d}y) = \int_0^1 f(F^{-1}(u) - G^{-1}(u))\, \mathrm{d}u. \qquad (3.17)$$

Proof By an application of the separation theorem for convex functions, compare Rockafellar (1997, Corollary 11.5.1), we can find appropriate constants c and d such that $f(x - y) \geq c(x - y) + d$. This shows that $\int f(x - y)\, H(\mathrm{d}x, \mathrm{d}y)$ might be infinite but is always defined for every $H \in \mathscr{M}$.

In the first step of the proof, we assume that F and G define discrete distributions with common support on $x_1 < x_2 < \ldots < x_n$. Since $\{\int f(x - y)\, H(\mathrm{d}x, \mathrm{d}y) : H \in \mathscr{M}\}$ is closed and bounded in $\mathbb{R}$, the infimum under (3.17) is attained for some H. Fix such a minimizer, denote it by $H \in \mathscr{M}$, and let $X \sim F$ and $Y \sim G$ be defined over some probability space $(\Omega, \mathscr{A}, \mathbb{P})$ with joint df. H. Denote $\mathbb{P}(X = x_i, Y = x_k)$ by $p_{i,k}$, for $1 \leq i, k \leq n$. Then we can assume that the following property (3.18) holds:

$$\min(p_{i,j}, p_{k,\ell}) = 0, \quad \text{for all } k < i \text{ and } j < \ell. \qquad (3.18)$$

To prove this property assume that it is not correct for this H. Then we can find some $k < i$ and $j < \ell$ such that

$$p = \min(p_{i,j}, p_{k,\ell}) > 0.$$

We now define a new distribution $\tilde{H}$ by

$$\tilde{p}_{i,\ell} = p_{i,\ell} + p, \quad \tilde{p}_{k,j} = p_{k,j} + p, \quad \tilde{p}_{i,j} = p_{i,j} - p, \quad \tilde{p}_{k,\ell} = p_{k,\ell} - p,$$
$$\tilde{p}_{s,t} = p_{s,t} \quad \text{otherwise.}$$

Note that the marginal distributions of $\tilde{H}$ are identical to those of H and that

$$x_k - x_\ell < x_k - x_j < x_i - x_j \quad \text{and} \quad x_k - x_\ell < x_i - x_\ell < x_i - x_j.$$

With $0 < \alpha < 1$ defined by

$$\alpha = \frac{(x_k - x_j) - (x_i - x_j)}{(x_k - x_\ell) - (x_i - x_j)}$$

we get

$$x_k - x_j = \alpha(x_k - x_\ell) + (1 - \alpha)(x_i - x_j),$$

and also, since

$$(1 - \alpha) = \frac{(x_i - x_\ell) - (x_i - x_j)}{(x_k - x_\ell) - (x_i - x_j)},$$

$$x_i - x_\ell = (1 - \alpha)(x_k - x_\ell) + \alpha(x_i - x_j).$$

Convexity of f now yields

$$f(x_k - x_j) + f(x_i - x_\ell) \le \alpha f(x_k - x_\ell) + (1 - \alpha)f(x_i - x_j)$$
$$+ (1 - \alpha)f(x_k - x_\ell) + \alpha f(x_i - x_j)$$
$$= f(x_k - x_\ell) + f(x_i - x_j),$$

and, therefore,

$$\int f(x - y)\, \tilde{H}(dx, dy) - \int f(x - y)\, H(dx, dy)$$
$$= p\left(f(x_k - x_j) + f(x_i - x_\ell) - f(x_k - x_\ell) - f(x_i - x_j)\right) \le 0.$$

Overall, this shows that switching from H to $\tilde{H}$ does not increase the integral but fulfills (3.18) for this particular choice of i, j, k, ℓ. Furthermore, if $\tilde{H}$ should not have the property (3.18), we can apply the same procedure as above and, after finitely many steps, we end up with a df. such that fulfills the required property (3.18), and that minimizes $\int f(x - y) H(dx, dy)$ over $\mathcal{M}$.

Define the matrix $P_n = (p_{i,j})_{1 \le i, j \le n}$. Then property (3.18) says that for every coefficient $p_{i,j} > 0$ of P_n all the other northeast and southwest coefficients have to be zero. One can easily check (by induction on n) that this property together with the given marginal distributions uniquely determines the matrix P_n and, therefore, the joint distribution of (X, Y). Now check that the joint distribution of

$(F^{-1}(U), G^{-1}(U))$ has the property (3.18) when U is uniformly distributed on the unit interval. Therefore, (3.17) is correct in the discrete case.

In the next step, we assume that F and G are concentrated on the interval $[-T, T]$. Since f as a convex function on $\mathbb{R}$ is continuous and F and G are concentrated on a bounded interval, we can assume without loss of generality that f is bounded and that the infimum on the left-hand side of (3.17) is finite. Thus, we can find for an arbitrary $\varepsilon > 0$ a df. $H_0 \in \mathcal{M}$ such that

$$\inf_{H \in \mathcal{M}} \int f(x - y) H(dx, dy) > \int f(x - y) H_0(dx, dy) - \varepsilon.$$

The Rosenblatt transformation 2.4 guarantees that two rvs. (X, Y) on some probability space $(\Omega, \mathcal{A}, \mathbb{P})$ exist with joint df. H_0. Define, for every $n \in \mathbb{N}$,

$$\left(X_n, Y_n \right) = \left(\frac{[nX]}{n}, \frac{[nY]}{n} \right),$$

where $[t]$ denotes the integer part of t, and use F_n and G_n to denote the df. of X_n and Y_n, respectively. Obviously, $\left(X_n, Y_n \right) \longrightarrow (X, Y)$ w.p.1 and F_n and G_n define discrete distributions. Since the w.p.1 convergence also implies the convergence in distribution, the proof of the elementary Skorokhod theorem, compare Billingsley (1995, Theorem 25.6), shows that $F_n^{-1}(u) \longrightarrow F^{-1}(u)$ and $G_n^{-1}(u) \longrightarrow G^{-1}(u)$. This convergence holds for all $0 < u < 1$ out of a set with Lebesgue measure 1. Now, apply Lebesgue's dominated convergence theorem to get with the first part of our proof

$$\int f(x - y) H_0(dx, dy) = \lim_{n \to \infty} \int f(X_n - Y_n) \, d\mathbb{P}$$

$$\geq \liminf_{n \to \infty} \int_0^1 f\left(F_n^{-1}(u) - G_n^{-1}(u) \right) du$$

$$= \int_0^1 f\left(F^{-1}(u) - G^{-1}(u) \right) du.$$

Overall, this shows that

$$\inf_{H \in \mathcal{M}} \int f(x - y) H(dx, dy) > \int_0^1 f\left(F^{-1}(u) - G^{-1}(u) \right) du - \varepsilon,$$

which proves (3.17) for F and G concentrated on intervals of the type $[-T, T]$.

In the third step of the proof, we now can take arbitrary F and G. Without loss of generality, we assume that the infimum in (3.17) is finite. As in the second step, we can find, for an arbitrary $\varepsilon > 0$, a df. $H_0 \in \mathcal{M}$ and random variables (X, Y) on some probability space $(\Omega, \mathcal{A}, \mathbb{P})$ with joint df. H_0 such that

$$\inf_{H \in \mathcal{M}} \int f(x-y) \, H(dx, dy) > \int f(x-y) \, H_0(dx, dy) - \varepsilon.$$

Now set $A_n = \{|X| \le n\} \cap \{|Y| \le n\}$ and define $X_n = X \cdot I_{\{A_n\}}$ and $Y_n = Y \cdot I_{\{A_n\}}$, for $n \in \mathbb{N}$, and note that w.p.1 $X_n \longrightarrow X$ and $Y_n \longrightarrow Y$, respectively. Furthermore,

$$\left| f(X_n - Y_n) \right| \le \left| f(X - Y) \right| + \left| f(0) \right|$$

for every $n \in \mathbb{N}$, and the bound on the right-hand side is integrable with respect to the chosen probability. Thus, Lebesgue's dominated convergence theorem is applicable. With the same argumentation used in the second step, we finally can complete the proof of (3.17) for these arbitrary F and G.   □

If the convex function f is defined by $f(x) = |x|^p$, for $p \ge 1$, we get an important application of the last theorem which leads to the following definition.

Definition 3.15 For $p \ge 1$, denote with $\mathscr{F}_p$ the class of all df. F with $\int |x|^p \, F(dx) < \infty$. Let $F, G \in \mathscr{F}_p$. Then

$$d_p(F, G) := \left(\int_0^1 |F^{-1}(u) - G^{-1}(u)|^p \, du \right)^{1/p} \tag{3.19}$$

defines *Mallow's p-metric*. For notational convenience, we will also use $d_p(X, Y)$, where $X \sim F$ and $Y \sim G$ and the joint distribution of (X, Y) minimizes the L^p distance over $\mathscr{M}$.

Corollary 3.16 *If we put $X = F^{-1}(U)$ and $Y = G^{-1}(U)$, where $U \sim UNI$, then*

$$d_p(F, G) = \|X - Y\|_p,$$

where the basic probability space is the unit interval with the Lebesgue measure and $\| \cdot \|_p$ denotes the L^p-norm.

Remark 3.17 For any scalars a, b let $F_{a,b}$ be the df. of $aX + b$, where $X \sim F$. For $F, G \in \mathscr{F}_p$, we then get

$$d_p(F_{a,b}, G_{a,b}) = |a| d_p(F, G).$$

Proof Apply Theorem 3.14 to get

$$\begin{aligned} d_p(F_{a,b}, G_{a,b}) &= \inf_{X \sim F, Y \sim G} \|(aX + b) - (aY + b)\|_p \\ &= |a| \inf_{X \sim F, Y \sim G} \|X - Y\|_p \\ &= |a| d_p(F, G). \end{aligned}$$

□

As the next lemma shows, Mallow's metric is closely related to weak convergence, where we now use the term "weak convergence" instead of "convergence in distribution", since we are dealing here with dfs. and not with rvs.

Lemma 3.18 *Assume that $F_n, F \in \mathscr{F}_p$, where F_n denotes not necessarily an edf. Then the following criteria are equivalent:*

(i) $d_p(F_n, F) \longrightarrow 0$, as $n \to \infty$.

(ii) *As $n \to \infty$, $F_n \longrightarrow F$ weakly and $\int |x|^p F_n(dx) \longrightarrow \int |x|^p F(dx)$.*

(iii) $F_n \longrightarrow F$ *weakly, as $n \to \infty$ and $\{|X_n|^p : n \geq 1\}$ is uniformly integrable, where $X_n \sim F_n$.*

(iv) $\int \varphi \, dF_n \longrightarrow \int \varphi \, dF$, *as $n \to \infty$ for all continuous φ such that $\varphi(x) = O(|x|^p)$ as $x \to \pm\infty$.*

Proof (i)$\Rightarrow$(ii): According to the last corollary we can use the rv.

$$X_n = F_n^{-1}(U), \quad X = F^{-1}(U).$$

Then,

$$\left| \left(\int |x|^p F_n(dx) \right)^{1/p} - \left(\int |x|^p F(dx) \right)^{1/p} \right| = \left| \|X_n\|_p - \|X\|_p \right| \leq \|X_n - X\|_p$$
$$= d_p(F_n, F) \longrightarrow 0$$

which shows the convergence of the integrals under (ii). It also guarantees the L^p−convergence of X_n to X which implies the weak convergence. This completes the proof of (ii).

(ii)$\Rightarrow$(iii): We only have to show uniform integrability. For this, we fix a point $a > 0$ such that a and $-a$ are continuity points of F. Then, we get

$$\int\limits_{\{|x|>a\}} |x|^p F_n(dx) = \int |x|^p F_n(dx) - \int\limits_{\{|x|\leq a\}} |x|^p F_n(dx) \equiv I_n.$$

Since $\pm a$ are continuity points of F, the assumed weak convergence of $F_n \to F$ together with a slight modification of Billingsley (1995, Theorem 29.1) guarantees that

$$\int\limits_{\{|x|\leq a\}} |x|^p F_n(dx) \longrightarrow \int\limits_{\{|x|\leq a\}} |x|^p F(dx).$$

This combined with the assumed convergence of the p-th moments yields

$$I_n \longrightarrow \int |x|^p F(dx) - \int\limits_{\{|x|\leq a\}} |x|^p F(dx) = \int\limits_{\{|x|>a\}} |x|^p F(dx).$$

The integral on the right-hand side can be made arbitrarily small by increasing a, which proves the uniform integrability.

(iii)$\Rightarrow$(iv): Let φ be as under (iv). Again, we take a fixed such that $\pm a$ are continuity points of F to get from the weak convergence of $F_n \to F$ that

$$\int_{\{|x| \leq a\}} \varphi(x) \, F_n(dx) \longrightarrow \int_{\{|x| \leq a\}} \varphi(x) \, F(dx).$$

Since $\varphi = O(|x|^p)$ there exists a constant c such that

$$|\varphi(x)| \leq c|x|^p,$$

for all x such that $|x| \geq a$. Thus,

$$\int_{\{|x| > a\}} |\varphi(x)| \, F_n(dx) \leq c \int_{\{|x| > a\}} |x|^p \, F_n(dx).$$

Furthermore, the assumed uniform integrability implies that we can choose for every given $\varepsilon > 0$ a continuity point $a = a(\varepsilon)$ of F such that

$$\sup_{n \geq 1} c \int_{\{|x| > a\}} |x|^p \, F_n(dx) \leq \varepsilon$$

which completes the proof of (iv).

(iv)$\Rightarrow$(i): Obviously, (iv) implies (ii). Therefore, it suffices to show (ii)$\Rightarrow$(i). But the weak convergence of F_n to F implies the almost sure convergence of $X_n = F_n^{-1}(U)$ to $X = F^{-1}(U)$ w.r.t. the Lebesgue measure on the unit interval ($U \sim UNI$), cf. the proof of Billingsley (1995, Theorem 25.6). Since $\mathbb{E}(|X_n|^p) \longrightarrow \mathbb{E}(|X|^p) < \infty$, as $n \to \infty$, according to (iv), we finally get from Loève (1977, L^p–Convergence Theorem) that $\|X_n - X\|_p \to 0$, as $n \to \infty$. This completes the proof of (i). $\square$

In the special case that F_n is the edf. of an i.i.d. sample, we get the following corollary.

Corollary 3.19 *Assume $F \in \mathscr{F}_p$ and let F_n be the edf. Then, $d_p(F_n, F) \longrightarrow 0$ w.p.1.*

Proof The Glivenko-Cantelli theorem says that w.p.1

$$\sup_{x \in \mathbb{R}} |F_n(x) - F(x)| \longrightarrow 0.$$

Thus, w.p.1, $F_n \to F$ weakly. Furthermore, from the SLLN, we conclude

$$\int |x|^p \, F_n(dx) \longrightarrow \int |x|^p \, F(dx)$$

w.p.1. Now, apply the last lemma to complete the proof.   □

In the following lemma, we bound Mallow's distance of two sums of independent rv. by Mallow's distance of the summands.

Lemma 3.20 *Assume that $X_1, \ldots, X_n$ and $Y_1, \ldots, Y_n$ are two sequences of independent rv. in $\mathscr{F}_p$. Then,*

$$d_p\left(\sum_{i=1}^{n} X_i, \sum_{i=1}^{n} Y_i\right) \leq \sum_{i=1}^{n} d_p(X_i, Y_i).$$

Proof Take $U_1, \ldots, U_n \sim UNI$ as an i.i.d. sample and set

$$\tilde{X}_i := F_i^{-1}(U_i), \quad \tilde{Y}_i := G_i^{-1}(U_i)$$

for $i = 1, \ldots, n$, where $X_i \sim F_i$ and $Y_i \sim G_i$, for $1 \leq i \leq n$. According to the definition of $d_p(X, Y)$, we get for each $i = 1, \ldots, n$

$$d_p(X_i, Y_i) = d_p(\tilde{X}_i, \tilde{Y}_i) = \|\tilde{X}_i - \tilde{Y}_i\|_p.$$

Now, apply Corollary 3.16 and Minkowski's inequality to obtain

$$d_p\left(\sum_{i=1}^{n} X_i, \sum_{i=1}^{n} Y_i\right) \leq \left\|\sum_{i=1}^{n} \tilde{X}_i - \sum_{i=1}^{n} \tilde{Y}_i\right\|_p \leq \sum_{i=1}^{n} \|\tilde{X}_i - \tilde{Y}_i\|_p$$

$$= \sum_{i=1}^{n} d_p(\tilde{X}_i, \tilde{Y}_i) = \sum_{i=1}^{n} d_p(X_i, Y_i),$$

which finally proves the lemma.   □

If $p = 2$, the last lemma improves in the presence of equal means.

Lemma 3.21 *Assume in addition to the assumptions of Lemma 3.20 that $\mathbb{E}(X_i) = \mathbb{E}(Y_i)$, for $1 \leq i \leq n$ and $p \geq 2$. Then,*

$$d_2^2\left(\sum_{i=1}^{n} X_i, \sum_{i=1}^{n} Y_i\right) \leq \sum_{i=1}^{n} d_2^2(X_i, Y_i).$$

Proof Take $(\tilde{X}_i, \tilde{Y}_i)$ as in the proof of Lemma 3.20. From Corollary 3.16 and Bienaymé's equality, we get

$$d_2^2\left(\sum_{i=1}^{n} X_i, \sum_{i=1}^{n} Y_i\right) \leq \left\|\sum_{i=1}^{n} \tilde{X}_i - \tilde{Y}_i\right\|_2^2 = \sum_{i=1}^{n} \|\tilde{X}_i - \tilde{Y}_i\|_2^2 = \sum_{i=1}^{n} d_2^2(X_i, Y_i).$$

                                                                                               □

Corollary 3.22 *Let $F, G \in \mathscr{F}_p$ with $p \geq 2$. Assume that $X_1, \ldots, X_n$ are i.i.d. with common df. F and $Y_1, \ldots, Y_n$ are i.i.d. with common df. G, respectively. Furthermore, we assume that $\mathbb{E}(X_1) = \mathbb{E}(Y_1)$. Then,*

$$d_2^2\left(n^{-1/2}\sum_{i=1}^n X_i, n^{-1/2}\sum_{i=1}^n Y_i\right) \leq n^{-1}\sum_{i=1}^n d_2^2(X_i, Y_i) = d_2^2(F, G).$$

Remark 3.23 According to the CLT and Lemma 3.18 (ii), for standardized F and $G = \Phi$, the left-hand side of the inequality under Corollary 3.22 tends to zero as $n \to \infty$. Since the right-hand side of this inequality is fixed for each $n \geq 1$ and positive for $G \neq F$, this inequality cannot be used to prove the CLT. However, if G depends on n in such a way that $d_2^2(F, G_n) \to 0$, as $n \to \infty$, we can use this inequality to prove weak convergence. In the particular case of the classical bootstrap, $G_n = F_n$ is the edf. of the i.i.d. sample $X_1, \ldots, X_n$, while $Y_1, \ldots, Y_n$ forms a bootstrap sample, then $d_2^2(F, F_n) \to 0$ w.p.1. Together with the CLT, this proves the CLT for the standardized bootstrap sample under the classical resampling scheme.

Sometimes, however, the bootstrap sample comes from $\tilde{F}_n$, the edf. of a not necessarily independent sample $X_1^*, \ldots, X_n^*$. For example, in linear regression, we have the situation that the residuals $X_i^* = \tilde{\varepsilon}_i$, $1 \leq i \leq n$, are not independent. In such a case, the approach outlined above for F_n cannot be applied for $\tilde{F}_n$ unless it is guaranteed that in some sense $\tilde{F}_n$ is close to F_n. A condition which will work in this setup is given in the next lemma; compare also Freedman (1981).

Lemma 3.24 *Assume that $X_1, \ldots, X_n$ are i.i.d. with df. F and edf. F_n. Let $X_1^*, \ldots, X_n^*$ be a second i.i.d. sample with edf. $\tilde{F}_n$ such that w.p.1*

$$\frac{1}{n}\sum_{i=1}^n |X_i^* - X_i|^p \longrightarrow 0, \quad as \ n \to \infty \tag{3.20}$$

holds. If $F \in \mathscr{F}_p$ for some $p \geq 1$, then, w.p.1, $d_p(\tilde{F}_n, F) \longrightarrow 0$, as $n \to \infty$.

Proof Let $U \sim UNI$ be the uniform distribution on the unit interval. Since

$$\begin{aligned}
d_p(\tilde{F}_n, F) &= \|\tilde{F}_n^{-1}(U) - F^{-1}(U)\|_p \\
&\leq \|\tilde{F}_n^{-1}(U) - F_n^{-1}(U)\|_p + \|F_n^{-1}(U) - F^{-1}(U)\|_p \\
&= d_p(\tilde{F}_n, F_n) + d_p(F_n, F)
\end{aligned}$$

and, w.p.1, $d_p(F_n, F) \longrightarrow 0$, as $n \to \infty$, according to Corollary 3.19, we get from assumption (3.20) and Theorem 3.14

$$d_p(\tilde{F}_n, F_n) \leq \left(\frac{1}{n}\sum_{i=1}^n |X_i^* - X_i|^p\right)^{1/p} \longrightarrow 0, \quad as \ n \to \infty,$$

w.p.1. This completes the proof of the lemma. □

3.6 Exercises

Exercise 3.25 Repeat the simulation study from Example 3.5 without using the `simTool` package. Note in that simulation the functions "bootstrap.ci" and "normal.ci" are applied to any dataset that is generated.

Exercise 3.26 Recall the assumptions of Example 3.6 and show that for $x \geq 0$

$$\mathbb{P}(n(1 - X_{n:n}) \leq x) \longrightarrow 1 - \exp(-x), \quad \text{as } n \to \infty.$$

Furthermore, show for the bootstrap sample

$$\mathbb{P}_n^*(n(X_{n:n} - X_{n:n}^*) \leq 0) \longrightarrow 1 - \exp(-1), \quad \text{as } n \to \infty.$$

Exercise 3.27 Conduct a simulation that indicates

$$\mathbb{P}_n^*(n(X_{n:n} - X_{n:n}^*) \leq 0) \longrightarrow 1 - \exp(-1), \quad \text{as } n \to \infty,$$

see Exercise 3.26.

Exercise 3.28 Recall the scenario of Theorem 3.7 and assume in addition that

$$\int h^2(x) \, F(\mathrm{d}x) < \infty.$$

Use Chebyshev's inequality to verify the assertion of Theorem 3.7.

Exercise 3.29 Implement in R the simulation study of Example 3.5, without using the `simTool` package.

Exercise 3.30 Use R to generate $U_1, \ldots, U_{100}$ i.i.d. rvs. according to the uniform distribution. Based on this data,

 (i) plot the path of the corresponding empirical process;
(ii) generate a classical bootstrap sample to the data and plot the path of the corresponding empirical process.

Exercise 3.31 In the R-library `boot`, many bootstrap applications are already implemented. Read the corresponding help to this library and try to redo the simulation under Exercise 3.29 by using the functions of this library.

Exercise 3.32 Verify that for fixed discrete marginal distributions on $x_1 < x_2 < \ldots < x_n$ the property (3.18) used in the proof of Theorem 3.14 defines exactly one joint distribution.

Exercise 3.33 Verify that for fixed discrete marginal distributions on $x_1 < x_2 < \ldots < x_n$ with df. F and G, respectively, the joint distribution of $(F^{-1}(U), G^{-1}(U))$ has the property (3.18) used in the proof of Theorem 3.14. Here U is uniformly distributed on the unit interval.

Exercise 3.34 Let $F \in \mathscr{F}_p$, that is, $\int |x|^p \, F(dx) < \infty$. Verify that

(i) for a location family, $F_\theta(x) = F(x - \theta)$

$$d_p(F_{\theta_1}, F_{\theta_2}) = |\theta_1 - \theta_2|;$$

(ii) for a scale family, $F_\sigma(x) = F(\sigma x)$ with $\sigma > 0$

$$d_p(F_{\sigma_1}, F_{\sigma_2}) = |\sigma_1 - \sigma_2| \left(\int |x|^p \, F(dx) \right)^{1/p}.$$

Exercise 3.35 Verify that for two (centered) binomial distributions F_1 and F_2 with parameters (n, p_1) and (n, p_2), respectively,

$$d_2^2(F_1, F_2) \le n|p_1 - p_2|(1 - |p_1 - p_2|).$$

Exercise 3.36 Verify that for two (centered) Poisson distributions F_1 and F_2 with parameters λ_1 and λ_2, respectively,

$$d_2^2(F_1, F_2) \le |\lambda_1 - \lambda_2|.$$

References

Abramovitch L, Singh K (1985) Edgeworth corrected pivotal statistics and the bootstrap. Ann Stat 13(1):116–132

Bickel PJ, Freedman DA (1981) Some asymptotic theory for the bootstrap. Ann Stat 9(6):1196–1217

Billingsley P (1968) Convergence of probability measures. Wiley, New York

Billingsley P (1995) Probability and measure, 3rd edn. Wiley Series in Probability and Mathematical Statistics. Wiley, New York

Davison AC, Hinkley DV (1997) Bootstrap methods and their application, vol 1. Cambridge Series in Statistical and Probabilistic Mathematics. Cambridge University Press, Cambridge, UK

Dikta G (1987) Beiträge zur nichtparametrischen Schätzung der Regressionsfunktion. PhD thesis, Justus-Liebig-Universität Gießen

Freedman DA (1981) Bootstrapping regression models. Ann Stat 9(6):1218–1228

Hall P (1992) The bootstrap and Edgeworth expansion. Springer Series in Statistics. Springer, New York

Loève M (1977) Probability theory. I, 4th edn. Springer, New York

Major P (1978) On the invariance principle for sums of independent identically distributed random variables. J Multivar Anal 8(4):487–517

Rockafellar RT (1997) Convex analysis. Princeton Landmarks in Mathematics. Princeton University Press, Princeton, NJ

Serfling RJ (1980) Approximation theorems of mathematical statistics. Wiley Series in Probability and Mathematical Statistics. Wiley, New York

Singh K (1981) On the asymptotic accuracy of Efron's bootstrap. Ann Stat 9(6):1187–1195

Stute W (1982) The oscillation behavior of empirical processes. Ann Probab 10(1):86–107

Swanepoel JWH (1986) A note on proving that the (modified) bootstrap works. Commun Stat Theory Methods 15(11):3193–3203

Chapter 4
Bootstrap-Based Tests

In Shao and Tu (1995, p. 117) we read the following statement:

..., the methodology and theory for bootstrap hypothesis testing are not well developed, partly because of technical difficulties ....

This statement is mainly based on the fact that the bootstrap resampling scheme has to be closely adapted to the hypothesis and therefore different resampling schemes have to be considered in different test scenarios. Naturally, the underlying distribution theory will not be available for each possible case in general. Thus a practitioner confronted with bootstrap hypothesis testing has to consider two things. Firstly, a proper resampling scheme has to be defined which closely mirrors the hypothesis. Secondly, he or she has to insure that the approximation under the chosen resampling scheme is valid.

4.1 Introduction

We start with a short summary of some of the key ideas in significance testing. For this let $X_1, \ldots, X_n$ be random vectors each of dimension k (not necessarily i.i.d.) having joint df. $F^{(n)}$, and let $\mathscr{F}^{(n)}$ be the collection of possible $F^{(n)}$. Suppose that

$$\mathscr{F}^{(n)} = \mathscr{F}_0^{(n)} \cup \mathscr{F}_1^{(n)},$$

where the collections on the right-hand side are disjoint. Now, we would like to determine, based on the observations $X_1, \ldots, X_n$, whether the hypothesis $F^{(n)} \in \mathscr{F}_0^{(n)}$ is true, i.e., to test

$$H_0 : \quad F^{(n)} \in \mathscr{F}_0^{(n)} \quad \text{versus} \quad H_1 : \quad F^{(n)} \in \mathscr{F}_1^{(n)}. \tag{4.1}$$

© Springer Nature Switzerland AG 2021
G. Dikta and M. Scheer, *Bootstrap Methods*,
https://doi.org/10.1007/978-3-030-73480-0_4

H_0 is called the *null* hypothesis and H_1 the *alternative* hypothesis.

In special but highly relevant situations, the observations are i.i.d. w.r.t. a certain df. F. Then $F^{(n)}$ is totaly determined by F and the general test problem given under (4.1) reduces to

$$H_0 : \quad F \in \mathscr{F}_0 \quad \text{versus} \quad H_1 : \quad F \in \mathscr{F}_1. \tag{4.2}$$

Example 4.1 Consider i.i.d. $X_1, \ldots, X_n \sim F$.

(i) Let F_0 be a known df. Set $\mathscr{F}_0 = \{F_0\}$ and $\mathscr{F}_1 = \{G : G \neq F_0\}$. In this case $\mathscr{F}_0$ contains only one element and the distribution of $X_1, \ldots, X_n$ is known under H_0. Here, H_0 is usually called a simple null hypothesis.

(ii) Assume that F has a finite expectation μ_F and we want to check whether $\mu_F \in \Theta_0 \subset \mathbb{R}^k$. In this case $\mathscr{F}_0 = \{G : \mu_G \in \Theta_0\}$ and $\mathscr{F}_1 = \{G : \mu_G \notin \Theta_0\}$. Now, $\mathscr{F}_0$ contains infinitely many elements even if Θ_0 is a single point. Thus, the distribution of $X_1, \ldots, X_n$ is unknown under H_0. This type of H_0 is called a complex hypothesis and the test problem can be written as

$$H_0 : \quad \mu_F \in \Theta_0 \quad \text{versus} \quad H_1 : \quad \mu_F \in \Theta_1. \tag{4.3}$$

Here μ_F is the parameter of interest while the overall df. is only a nuisance or adjustment parameter.

Constructing a test for these problems is equivalent to finding a *rejection region* $\mathscr{R}_n$ such that we reject the hypothesis H_0 if and only if $(X_1, \ldots, X_n) \in \mathscr{R}_n$. Before we can determine such a $\mathscr{R}_n$, we have to look for a proper test statistic $T_n = T_n(X_1, \ldots, X_n)$ and

$$\mathscr{R}_n := \{x : T_n(x) \geq c_n\}, \tag{4.4}$$

where c_n is called the *critical value*. The rejection region is determined by controlling the probability of rejecting H_0 when H_0 is correct, i.e.,

$$\sup_{F^{(n)} \in \mathscr{F}_0^{(n)}} \mathbb{P}_{F^{(n)}}\big(T_n(X_1, \ldots, X_n) \in \mathscr{R}_n\big) \leq \alpha,$$

where α is the given *type 1 error*.

Assume that the rejection region is of the type given by (4.4) and let the observations be $X_1 = x_1, \ldots, X_n = x_n$. Based on the observed values, we can calculate $T_n(x_1, \ldots, x_n)$. The level of evidence against H_0 is measured by the significance probability

$$p = \sup_{G \in \mathscr{F}_0^{(n)}} \mathbb{P}_G\big(T_n(X_1, \ldots, X_n) \geq T_n(x_1, \ldots, x_n)\big)$$

often called the *p-value*.

Remark 4.2 In the case of a simple hypothesis, i.e., $H_0 : \mathscr{F}_0 = \{F_0\}$, the p-value of a given statistic $T_n(X_1, \ldots, X_n)$ can easily be approximated. For this, assume that

$X_1 = x_1, \ldots, X_n = x_n$ was observed and $t = T_n(x_1, \ldots, x_n)$ calculated. By defini-tion, the p-value equals $\mathbb{P}_{F_0}(T_n(X_1, \ldots, X_n) \geq t)$. Since we know F_0, we can try to calculate this probability. If this should be too complicated, we can use Monte Carlo approximation and obtain m independent i.i.d. samples

$$X_{\ell;1}, \ldots, X_{\ell;n} \quad \text{for } 1 \leq \ell \leq m,$$

where $X \sim F_0$ and calculate, based on these samples, $T_{1;n}, \ldots, T_{m;n}$. The SLLN then yields

$$\mathbb{P}_{F_0}(T_n(X_1, \ldots, X_n) \geq t) \approx \frac{1}{m} \sum_{\ell=1}^{m} \mathbb{I}_{\{[t,\infty[\}}(T_{\ell;n}) = 1 - G_m(t-), \quad (4.5)$$

where G_m denotes the edf. of $T_{1;n}, \ldots, T_{m;n}$, and $G_m(t-)$ the left-hand limit.

This approximation is also valid, if

$$\sup_{x \in \mathbb{R}} |\mathbb{P}_{F_0}(T_n(X_1, \ldots, X_n) \geq x) - \mathbb{P}_{\hat{F}_n}(T_n(X_1, \ldots, X_n) \geq x)| \underset{n \to \infty}{\longrightarrow} 0$$

holds and if we take

$$X_{\ell;1}, \ldots, X_{\ell;n} \quad \text{for } 1 \leq \ell \leq m,$$

as independent i.i.d. samples according to this $\hat{F}_n$. However, one should use $X \sim F_0$ instead of $X \sim \hat{F}_n$, since this guarantees that the data are generated under the null hypothesis.

Remark 4.3 As we just mentioned, a resampling scheme has to guarantee that the bootstrap data are generated under the null hypothesis or at least close to it. It is the distribution of the test statistic under the null hypothesis which has to be used to find the critical region or the p-value. If we want to use the approximation of the p-value given in (4.5) and the $T_{1;n}, \ldots, T_{m;n}$ are generated according to some resampling scheme, the sequence $T_{1;n}, \ldots, T_{m;n}$ must be i.i.d. and each $T_{\ell;n}$, for $1 \leq \ell \leq m$, should have a distribution that is equal or at least very close to the distribution of $T_n(X_1, \ldots, X_n)$, where $X_1, \ldots, X_n$ are from the null hypothesis.

In the next sections, we give some special examples which are discussed partly in Efron and Tibshirani (1993) and in Davison and Hinkley (1997), respectively.

4.2 The One-Sample Test

Example 4.4 **One-sample test, part 1.** Assume a *one-sample problem*, where we observed an i.i.d. sample $X_1, \ldots, X_n \sim F$. Furthermore, we denote the true expec-tation by $\mu = \mu_F$ and we assume that the variance exists. Now, we want to test

$$H_0: \quad \mu = 17 \quad \text{versus} \quad H_1: \quad \mu \neq 17.$$

Obviously, we have a complex null hypothesis, since $\mathscr{F}_0 = \{G : \mu_G = 17\}$. In this case we use the standardized test statistic

$$T_n \equiv T_n(X_1, \ldots, X_n) := \sqrt{n} \left| \frac{\mu_n - 17}{s_n} \right|,$$

where $\mu_n = n^{-1} \sum_{i=1}^{n} X_i$ and $s_n^2 = n^{-1} \sum_{i=1}^{n} (X_i - \mu_n)^2$, and the following resampling scheme:

Resampling Scheme 4.5

(A) *Generate independent bootstrap i.i.d. samples* $X_{\ell;1}^*, \ldots, X_{\ell;n}^*$ *for* $1 \leq \ell \leq m$
    according to the edf. F_n *of the observations* $X_1, \ldots, X_n$.
(B) *Calculate for each* $1 \leq \ell \leq m$, $\mu_{\ell;n}^* = n^{-1} \sum_{i=1}^{n} X_{\ell;i}^*$, $s_{\ell;n}^* = n^{-1} \sum_{i=1}^{n} (X_{\ell;i}^* - \mu_{\ell;n}^*)^2$, *and*

$$T_{\ell;n}^* = \sqrt{n} \left| \frac{\mu_{\ell;n}^* - \mu_n}{s_{\ell;n}^*} \right|.$$

(C) *Determine the p-value of* T_n *within the simulated* $T_{\ell;n}^*$, $1 \leq k \leq m$ *according to Eq.* (4.5).

Due to the CLT for the bootstrap when resampling is done according to the edf. of the observations, see Corollary 3.9, the resampling scheme given above will work in this scenario.

Remark 4.6 **One-sample test.** We already pointed out in Remark 4.3 that the resampling has to be done in such a way that the null hypothesis is mimicked, that is in this example, the expectation of X^* must be 17. Since we resampled according to F_n, the edf. based on our observations, the expectation of X^* equals μ_n which is not necessarily equal to 17. Thus, the resampling scheme given under 4.5 does not fulfill this requirement. However, if we resample according to the edf. $\hat{F}_n$ which is based on

$$Z_1 := X_1 - \mu_n + 17, \ldots, Z_n := X_n - \mu_n + 17$$

we easily obtain that $\mathbb{E}_{\hat{F}_n}(Z^*) = 17$. Furthermore, $Z^* = X^* - \mu_n + 17$ and $-\mu_n + 17$ is just a constant with respect to the bootstrap distribution. Thus, the standard deviations of both bootstrap samples, i.e., $Z_1^*, \ldots, Z_n^*$ and $X_1^*, \ldots, X_n^*$, are identical. Now, based on $Z_1^*, \ldots, Z_n^* \sim \hat{F}_n$ we have to calculate the statistic

$$T_n^* = T_n^*(Z_1^*, \ldots, Z_n^*) := \sqrt{n} \left| \frac{\frac{1}{n} \sum_{i=1}^{n} Z_i^* - 17}{s_n^*} \right|.$$

But

$$\frac{1}{n} \sum_{i=1}^{n} Z_i^* - 17 = \frac{1}{n} \sum_{i=1}^{n} (X^* - \mu_n + 17) - 17 = \mu_n^* - \mu_n.$$

Therefore, the Resampling Scheme 4.5 indeed incorporates the null hypothesis properly.

R-Example 4.7 One-sample test, part 2. The following R-code shows an implementation of the bootstrap approximated p-value based on (4.5) in the one-sample problem. Note that the unbiased estimates

$$\frac{1}{n-1}\sum_{i=1}^{n}(X_i - \bar{X}_n)^2, \quad \frac{1}{n-1}\sum_{i=1}^{n}(X_i^* - \bar{X}_n^*)^2$$

are used in the R-code instead of s_n^2 and s_n^{*2}, respectively. This modification does not affect the asymptotic result from Corollary 3.9, but it fits the usual variance estimation in classical methods.

```
oneSampleBootpvalue <- function(x, mu0, R = 999){
  # x    - observed data
  # mu0  - Mean under null hypothesis
  # R    - number of MC simulations

  # test statistic
  tstat <- function(d, i, mu0) {
    sqrt(length(i)) * abs(mean(d[i]) - mu0) / sd(d[i])
  }

  # test statistic for the observed data x
  t0 <- tstat(x, 1:length(x), mu0)

  # R resampled test statistics, where
  # mu0 = mean(x) will be passed to the function tstat
  bt <- boot::boot(x, tstat, R = R, mu0 = mean(x))$t[,1]

  # return p-value
  c(pvalue = mean(bt > t0))
}
```

Now, we apply this function to a dataset such that the null hypothesis is true

```
set.seed(123,kind ="Mersenne-Twister",normal.kind ="Inversion")
#H0 is correct
x <- rexp(100, rate = 1/17)
oneSampleBootpvalue(x, 17)
```

```
##      pvalue
## 0.6756757
```

and to a dataset, where the null hypothesis is not correct

```
#H0 is not correct
x <- rexp(100,rate = 1/14)
oneSampleBootpvalue(x, 17)
```

```
##       pvalue
## 0.07107107
```

R-Example 4.8 One-sample test, part 3. We utilize the `simTool` Package to generate exponential distributed data with expectation $\mu = 14$ and $\mu = 17$ and then test the null hypothesis that $\mu = 17$ with the function `oneSampelBootpvalue` defined in the R-Example 4.7. Figure 4.1 visualizes the result from this simulation study. According to Corollary 2.8, the p-values under the null hypothesis should be similar to the edf. of a uniform distributed random variable. As expected, the edf. under the alternative hypothesis shows a high percentage of small p-values.

```
dg <- simTool::expand_tibble(fun = "rexp", n = 100,
                             rate = c(1/14, 1/17))
pg <- simTool::expand_tibble(proc = "oneSampleBootpvalue",
                             mu0 = 17,
                             R = 999)
```

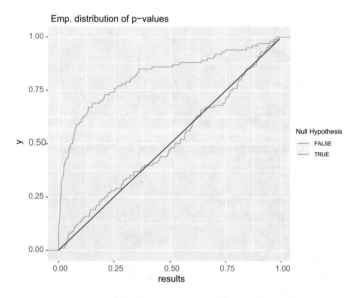

Fig. 4.1 Datasets are generated under the null hypothesis $\mu = 17$ and the alternative $\mu = 14$. p–values were obtained by *oneSampleBootpvalue* from R-Example 4.7. The figure shows the edf. of 100 p-values under the null hypothesis, edf. of 100 p-values under the alternativ, and the uniform distribution function (diagonal)

```
set.seed(123,kind ="Mersenne-Twister",normal.kind ="Inversion")
eg <- simTool::eval_tibbles(dg, pg, replications = 100)
eg$simulation %>%
  dplyr::mutate(null.hypothesis = (rate == 1/17)) %>%
  ggplot(aes(x = results, color = null.hypothesis)) +
  stat_ecdf() +
  stat_function(fun = identity, col = "black") +
  labs(color = "Null Hypothesis") +
  ggtitle("Emp. distribution of p-values")
```

4.3 Two-Sample Tests

In the two-sample test, the choice of an adequate test statistic depends on some general assumptions of the underlying two samples. In our first two-sample test, we assume an underlying location model.

Example 4.9 **Two-sample test under location model, part 1.**
In the *two-sample problem under the location model* we observe independent i.i.d. samples $X_1, \ldots, X_{n_1} \sim F$ and $Y_1, \ldots, Y_{n_2} \sim G$. Suppose now that

$$F(t) = H(t - \mu_x) \text{ and } G(t) = H(t - \mu_y) \quad \text{for every } t \in \mathbb{R}$$

for some unknown df. H, where $\mu_x = \mathbb{E}(X)$ and $\mu_y = \mathbb{E}(Y)$. Furthermore, we assume that the second moment w.r.t. H exists and we denote the corresponding variance by σ^2.

The assumptions guarantee that X and Y have the same variance and that $F = G$ is equivalent to $\mu_x = \mu_y$. Let our null hypothesis be $H_0 : \mu_x = \mu_y$ and suppose that we want to test H_0 versus $H_1 : \mu_x > \mu_y$.

A proper test statistic for this setup is given by

$$T_{n_1,n_2} := (1/n_1 + 1/n_2)^{-1/2} \frac{\bar{X}_{n_1} - \bar{Y}_{n_2}}{s_{n_1+n_2}},$$

where

$$\bar{X}_{n_1} := \frac{1}{n_1} \sum_{i=1}^{n_1} X_i, \quad \bar{Y}_{n_2} := \frac{1}{n_2} \sum_{i=1}^{n_2} Y_i,$$

and

$$s_{n_1+n_2}^2 := \frac{1}{n_1 + n_2} \left(\sum_{i=1}^{n_1} (X_i - \bar{X}_{n_1})^2 + \sum_{j=1}^{n_2} (Y_j - \bar{Y}_{n_2})^2 \right).$$

Since the df. of T_{n_1,n_2} is unknown to us even under H_0, we have to look for a proper approximation. For this we make the additional assumption that $n_2 \to \infty$ as $n_1 \to \infty$

and

$$\frac{n_1}{n_2} \longrightarrow \lambda, \quad \text{as } n_1 \to \infty,$$

where $0 < \lambda < \infty$. Note that SLLN guarantees that $s^2_{n_1+n_2} \to \sigma^2$, as $n_1 \to \infty$. Furthermore, under H_0 and the assumed independence of the samples the CLT implies that

$$
\begin{aligned}
T_{n_1,n_2} &= \sqrt{n_1} \frac{\bar{X}_{n_1} - \mu_x}{s_{n_1+n_2}} \frac{1}{\sqrt{1 + n_1/n_2}} - \sqrt{n_2} \frac{\bar{Y}_{n_2} - \mu_y}{s_{n_1+n_2}} \frac{1}{\sqrt{1 + n_2/n_1}} \\
&\longrightarrow \mathcal{N}\left(0, \frac{1}{1+\lambda} + \frac{1}{1+1/\lambda}\right) \\
&= \mathcal{N}(0, 1)
\end{aligned}
$$

in distribution, as $n_1 \to \infty$.

To apply the bootstrap, note that under H_0 both rvs. X and Y have the same df. Thus we can mimic the null hypothesis by resampling according to the edf. of the pooled sample. In particular:

Resampling Scheme 4.10

(A) *Generate independent bootstrap i.i.d. samples $Z^*_{\ell;1}, \ldots, Z^*_{\ell;n_1+n_2}$ for $1 \leq \ell \leq m$ according to the edf. of the observations $X_1, \ldots, X_{n_1}, Y_1, \ldots, Y_{n_2}$ and define for $1 \leq \ell \leq m$: $X^*_{\ell;i} := Z^*_{\ell;i}$, where $1 \leq i \leq n_1$, and $Y^*_{\ell;j} := Z^*_{\ell;n_1+j}$, where $1 \leq j \leq n_2$, respectively.*

(B) *Calculate for $1 \leq \ell \leq m$*

$$T^*_{\ell;n_1,n_2} := (1/n_1 + 1/n_2)^{-1/2} \frac{\bar{X}^*_{\ell;n_1} - \bar{Y}^*_{\ell;n_2}}{s^*_{\ell;n_1+n_2}},$$

where

$$\bar{X}^*_{\ell;n_1} = \frac{1}{n_1} \sum_{i=1}^{n_1} X^*_{\ell;i}, \quad \bar{Y}^*_{\ell;n_2} = \frac{1}{n_2} \sum_{j=1}^{n_2} Y^*_{\ell;j},$$

and

$$s^{*2}_{\ell;n_1+n_2} = \frac{1}{n_1+n_2}\left(\sum_{i=1}^{n_1}(X^*_{\ell;i} - \bar{X}^*_{\ell;n_1})^2 + \sum_{j=1}^{n_2}(Y^*_{\ell;j} - \bar{Y}^*_{\ell;n_2})^2\right)$$

(C) *Determine the p-value of T_n within the simulated $T^*_{\ell;n_1,n_2}$, $1 \leq \ell \leq m$ according to Eq. (4.5).*

The consistency of the aforementioned Resampling Scheme 4.10 can be seen as follows. Theorem 3.7 guarentees that, w.p.1, for every $\varepsilon > 0$,

$$\mathbb{P}^*_n\left(\left|s_{n_1+n_2}/s^*_{n_1+n_2} - 1\right| > \varepsilon\right) \longrightarrow 0, \quad \text{as } n_1 \to \infty,$$

holds true. Similar as in Corollary 3.9, this entails together with Theorem 3.8 and Slutsky's Theorem the consistency.

R-Example 4.11 Two-sample test under location model, part 2. The following R-code can be used for this two-sample test. Note that

$$\frac{1}{n_1 + n_2 - 2}\Big(\sum_{i=1}^{n_1}(X_i - \bar{X}_{n_1})^2 + \sum_{j=1}^{n_2}(Y_j - \bar{Y}_{n_2})^2\Big),$$

$$\frac{1}{n_1 + n_2 - 2}\Big(\sum_{i=1}^{n_1}(X_i^* - \bar{X}_{n_1}^*)^2 + \sum_{j=1}^{n_2}(Y_j^* - \bar{Y}_{n_2}^*)^2\Big)$$

are used here instead of $s_{n_1+n_2}^2$ and $s_{n_1+n_2}^{*2}$, respectively.

```
twoSampleLocModBootpValue <- function(x, y,
  alternative = c("two-sided", "less", "greater"), R = 999){

  # x - observed data (first sample)
  # y - observed data (second sample)
  # alternative - specifies the alternative hypothesis
  # R - number of MC simulations

  alternative <- match.arg(alternative)

  n1 <- length(x)
  n2 <- length(y)

  # test statistic
  tstat <- function(d, i){
    boot.xy <- d[i]

    # x and y are redfined in the scope of the
    # the function tstat. The orginial variables
    # passed to the function twoSampleLocModBootpValue
    # are not changed!
    x        <- boot.xy[1:n1]
    y        <- boot.xy[-(1:n1)]

    s        <- sqrt( ((n1-1) * var(x) + (n2 - 1) * var(y)) /
                      (n1 + n2 - 2) )
    mu.x     <- mean(x)
    mu.y     <- mean(y)
    (mu.x - mu.y) / s / sqrt(1 / n1 + 1 / n2)
  }

  xy <- c(x,y)

  # test statistics for the observed data
  t0 <- tstat(xy, 1:(n1 + n2))
```

```
# R resampled test statistics
bt <- boot::boot(xy, tstat, R = R)$t[,1]

# return p-value
if(alternative == "greater") return(c(pvalue = mean(bt > t0)))
if(alternative == "less") return(c(pvalue = mean(bt < t0)))
c(pvalue = mean(abs(bt) > abs(t0)))
}
```

Now, we apply this function to datasets such that the null hypothesis is true

```
# H0 correct, mu_x equals mu_y
set.seed(123,kind ="Mersenne-Twister",normal.kind ="Inversion")
twoSampleLocModBootpValue(rnorm(10, mean = 3, sd = 2),
                          rnorm(20, mean = 3, sd = 2),
                          alternative = "greater")
```

```
##      pvalue
## 0.3143143
```

and to datasets, where the null hypothesis is not correct

```
# H0 not correct
set.seed(123,kind ="Mersenne-Twister",normal.kind ="Inversion")
twoSampleLocModBootpValue(rnorm(10, mean = 3, sd = 2),
                          rnorm(20, mean = 2, sd = 2),
                          alternative = "greater")
```

```
##      pvalue
## 0.04504505
```

In the two-sample problem, we sometimes only want to compare the two expectations without making any additional assumptions about the corresponding df. F and G as we did in Example 4.9, where a location family was assumed. Even under the normality assumption, one might not want to accept that the variances of the two samples are equal. As a consequence, the simple t-test cannot be applied (Behrens-Fisher problem) and we have to look for a proper approximation.

Example 4.12 **Two-sample test under heterogeneity, part 1.** In this scenario, we observe independent i.i.d. samples $X_1, \ldots, X_{n_1} \sim F$ and $Y_1, \ldots, Y_{n_2} \sim G$ and we assume that $\mu_x = \mathbb{E}(X)$, $\mu_y = \mathbb{E}(Y)$, $\text{VAR}(X) = \sigma_x^2$, and $\text{VAR}(Y) = \sigma_y^2$ exist. To test the null hypothesis $H_0: \quad \mu_x = \mu_y$ versus $H_1: \quad \mu_x > \mu_y$, we now apply the test statistic:

$$T_{n_1,n_2} = \frac{\bar{X}_{n_1} - \bar{Y}_{n_2}}{\sqrt{s_x^2/n_1 + s_y^2/n_2}},$$

where

$$\bar{X}_{n_1} := \frac{1}{n_1} \sum_{i=1}^{n_1} X_i, \quad \bar{Y}_{n_2} := \frac{1}{n_2} \sum_{i=1}^{n_2} Y_i,$$

and

$$s_x^2 = \frac{1}{n_1} \sum_{i=1}^{n_1} (X_i - \bar{X}_{n_1})^2, \quad s_y^2 = \frac{1}{n_2} \sum_{j=1}^{n_2} (Y_j - \bar{Y}_{n_2})^2$$

are the corresponding sample variances.

As in the example above, the df. of T_{n_1,n_2} is unknown to us even under H_0 and again we have to look for a proper approximation. Assume, as in the example above, that $n_2 \to \infty$ as $n_1 \to \infty$ and that

$$\frac{n_1}{n_2} \longrightarrow \lambda, \quad \text{as } n_1 \to \infty,$$

where $0 < \lambda < \infty$. SLLN guarantees that the sample variances s_x^2 and s_y^2 tend to σ_x^2 and σ_y^2 $\mathbb{P}$−a.s. Finally, under H_0 and the assumed independence of the samples the CLT implies that

$$T_{n_1,n_2} = n_1^{1/2} \frac{\bar{X}_{n_1} - \mu_x}{s_x} \frac{1}{\sqrt{1 + (s_y^2 n_1)/(s_x^2 n_2)}} - n_2^{1/2} \frac{\bar{Y}_{n_2} - \mu_y}{s_y} \frac{1}{\sqrt{1 + (s_x^2 n_2)/(s_y^2 n_1)}}$$

$$\longrightarrow \mathcal{N}\left(0, \frac{1}{1 + \lambda \sigma_y^2/\sigma_x^2} + \frac{1}{1 + \sigma_x^2/(\sigma_y^2 \lambda)}\right)$$

$$= \mathcal{N}(0, 1)$$

in distribution, as $n_1 \to \infty$.

Now, we cannot use the edf. based on the pooled sample for the resampling procedure since this would not mimic the null hypothesis properly. In particular, we have to use

Resampling Scheme 4.13

(A) *Generate independent bootstrap i.i.d. samples* $X^*_{\ell;1}, \ldots, X^*_{\ell;n}$ *according to the edf. based on* $X_1 - \bar{X}_{n_1}, \ldots, X_{n_1} - \bar{X}_{n_1}$ *and* $Y^*_{\ell;1}, \ldots, Y^*_{\ell;n_2}$ *according to the edf. based on* $Y_1 - \bar{Y}_{n_2}, \ldots, Y_{n_2} - \bar{Y}_{n_2}$, *respectively, for* $1 \leq \ell \leq m$.

(B) *Calculate for* $1 \leq \ell \leq m$

$$T^*_{\ell;n_1,n_2} := \frac{\bar{X}^*_{\ell;n_1} - \bar{Y}^*_{\ell;n_2}}{\sqrt{s^{*2}_{\ell;x}/n_1 + s^{*2}_{\ell;y}/n_2}},$$

where

$$\bar{X}^*_{\ell;n_1} = \frac{1}{n_1} \sum_{i=1}^{n_1} X^*_{\ell;i}, \quad \bar{Y}^*_{\ell;n_2} = \frac{1}{n_2} \sum_{j=1}^{n_2} Y^*_{\ell;j},$$

and

$$s^{*2}_{\ell;x} = \frac{1}{n_1} \sum_{i=1}^{n_1} (X^*_{\ell;i} - \bar{X}^*_{\ell;n_1})^2, \quad s^{*2}_{\ell;y} = \frac{1}{n_2} \sum_{i=1}^{n_2} (Y^*_{\ell;i} - \bar{Y}^*_{\ell;n_2})^2.$$

(C) *Determine the p-value of T_n within the simulated $T^*_{\ell;n_1,n_2}$, $1 \le \ell \le m$ according to Eq. (4.5).*

Again, Theorem 3.7, the CLT for the bootstrap given in Theorem 3.8, and Slutsky's Theorem guarantee that the above resampling scheme will work.

R-Example 4.14 Two-sample test under heterogeneity, part 2. We use the following R-code for this two-sample test, where we modified the variance estimators s_x^2, s_y^2, s_x^{*2}, and s_y^{*2} by their corresponding unbiased estimators

$$\frac{1}{n_1 - 1} \sum_{i=1}^{n_1} (X_i - \bar{X}_{n_1})^2, \quad \frac{1}{n_2 - 1} \sum_{j=1}^{n_2} (Y_j - \bar{Y}_{n_2})^2,$$

$$\frac{1}{n_1 - 1} \sum_{i=1}^{n_1} (X_i^* - \bar{X}_{n_1}^*)^2, \quad \frac{1}{n_2 - 1} \sum_{j=1}^{n_2} (Y_j^* - \bar{Y}_{n_2}^*)^2.$$

```
twoSampleBootpvalue = function(x, y,
        alternative = c("two-sided", "less", "greater"), R = 999){

  # x - observed data (first sample)
  # y - observed data (second sample)
  # alternative - specifies the alternative hypothesis
  # R - number of MC simulations

  alternative <- match.arg(alternative)

  n1 <- length(x)
  n2 <- length(y)

  # test statistic
  tstat <- function(d, i){
    boot.xy <- d[i]
    x        <- boot.xy[1:n1]
    y        <- boot.xy[-(1:n1)]
    s        <- sqrt( var(x) / n1 + var(y) / n2 )
    mu.x     <- mean(x)
    mu.y     <- mean(y)
    (mu.x - mu.y) / s
  }
```

```
# test statistic for the observed data
xy <- c(x,y)
t0 <- tstat(xy, 1:(n1+n2))

# in order to facilitate step (A)
# x and y are centered
x  <- x - mean(x)
y  <- y - mean(y)
xy <- c(x,y)

# R resampled test statistics
# Note, the strata parameter explains boot() to resample
# from the first n1 entries and from the last n2 entries
# separately
bt <- boot::boot(xy, tstat, R = R,
                 strata = c(rep(1, n1), rep(2,n2)))$t[,1]

# return pvalue
if(alternative == "greater") return(c(pvalue = mean(bt > t0)))
if(alternative == "less") return(c(pvalue = mean(bt < t0)))
 c(pvalue = mean(abs(bt) > abs(t0)))
}
```

The following code shows an application of this two-sample bootstrap test.

```
set.seed(123,kind ="Mersenne-Twister",normal.kind ="Inversion")
#H0: mu.x = mu.y vs. H1: mu.x > mu.y
#H0 correct
twoSampleBootpvalue(rnorm(10, 3, 2), rnorm(20, 3, 3),
                    alternative = "greater")
```

```
 ##    pvalue
 ## 0.2952953
```

```
#H0: mu.x = mu.y vs. H1: mu.x > mu.y
#H0 not correct
twoSampleBootpvalue(rnorm(10, 3, 2), rnorm(20, 1, 3),
                    alternative = "greater")
```

```
 ##     pvalue
 ## 0.05905906
```

4.4 Goodness-of-Fit (GOF) Test

Let

$$\mathscr{F} = \{F(\cdot;\theta) : \theta \in \Theta\}$$

be a parametric family of df., that is, $F(\cdot;\theta)$ is totally determined by the parameter θ, and assume we observe an i.i.d. sample $X_1, \ldots, X_n$ with common df. F. In some situations it is important to know whether $H_0 : F \in \mathscr{F}$ or not.

A general recipe to test H_0 is to

1. compute the edf. F_n based on $X_1, \ldots, X_n$,
2. estimate θ_0 by some $\hat{\theta}_n$,
3. compare F_n with $F(\cdot;\hat{\theta}_n)$.

The comparison, or goodness-of-fit procedure, indicated under item 3 is often based on the *estimated empirical process*

$$\hat{\alpha}_n(x) = n^{1/2}(F_n(x) - F(x;\hat{\theta}_n)), \qquad x \in \mathbb{R}. \tag{4.6}$$

In particular, one considers the *Kolmogorov-Smirnov distance*

$$D_n = \sup_{x \in \mathbb{R}} |\hat{\alpha}_n(x)| \equiv \|\hat{\alpha}_n\|_\infty \tag{4.7}$$

or the *Cramér-von Mises distance*

$$W_n^2 = n \int (F_n(x) - F(x;\hat{\theta}_n))^2 \, F(dx;\hat{\theta}_n) = \int \hat{\alpha}_n^2(x) \, F(dx;\hat{\theta}_n). \tag{4.8}$$

While both test statistics are invariant w.r.t. continuous F if the correct F is used instead of $F(\cdot;\hat{\theta}_n)$, i.e., they are distribution free, this is not the case, when we use $F(\cdot;\hat{\theta}_n)$. Thus, critical values have to be computed for each individual $\mathscr{F}$. Among others, D'Agostino and Stephens (1986) provide in their book a comprehensive amount of available results for some selected parametric families.

Due to Theorem 4.17 of Sect. 4.5, we can use the bootstrap method to approximate the df. of the corresponding Cramér-von Mises (CvM) and Kolmogorov-Smirnov (KS) test statistics obtained from the estimated empirical process. Based on an i.i.d. sample $X_1, \ldots, X_n$, estimate $\hat{\theta}_n$ and obtain $Z_i = F(X_i;\hat{\theta}_n)$, for $1 \leq i \leq n$. The KS distance is then computed according to the following well-known formula:

$$D_n = \|\hat{\alpha}_n\| = n^{1/2} \max_{1 \leq i \leq n} \left(\frac{i}{n} - Z_{i:n}, Z_{i:n} - \frac{i-1}{n}\right). \tag{4.9}$$

For the CvM distance, set $Z_{0:n} = 0$, $X_{0:n} = -\infty$, $Z_{n+1:n} = 1$, and $X_{n+1:n} = \infty$. Now, observe that

$$W_n^2 = \int \hat{\alpha}_n^2(x) \, F(dx; \hat{\theta}_n) = n \int \left(F_n(x) - F(x; \hat{\theta}_n) \right)^2 F(dx; \hat{\theta}_n)$$

$$= n \sum_{i=0}^{n} \int_{[X_{i:n}, X_{i+1:n}[} \left(\frac{i}{n} - F(x; \hat{\theta}_n) \right)^2 F(dx; \hat{\theta}_n)$$

$$= n \sum_{i=0}^{n} \int_{[Z_{i:n}, Z_{i+1:n}[} \left(\frac{i}{n} - u \right)^2 du$$

$$= \frac{n}{3} \sum_{i=0}^{n} \left(\left(\frac{i}{n} - Z_{i:n} \right)^3 - \left(\frac{i}{n} - Z_{i+1:n} \right)^3 \right)$$

$$= \frac{n}{3} \left(\sum_{i=1}^{n} \left(\frac{i}{n} - Z_{i:n} \right)^3 - \sum_{i=0}^{n-1} \left(\frac{i}{n} - Z_{i+1:n} \right)^3 \right)$$

$$= \frac{n}{3} \left(\sum_{i=1}^{n} \left(\frac{i}{n} - Z_{i:n} \right)^3 - \sum_{i=1}^{n} \left(\frac{i-1}{n} - Z_{i:n} \right)^3 \right).$$

By some algebraic rearrangements, we finally end up with:

$$W_n^2 = \frac{1}{12n} + \sum_{i=1}^{n} \left(Z_{i:n} - \frac{2i-1}{2n} \right)^2. \tag{4.10}$$

To apply the bootstrap approximation we use the following resampling scheme:

Resampling Scheme 4.15

(A) *Based on the observations $X_1, \ldots, X_n$ calculate the estimator $\hat{\theta}_n$.*
(B) *Calculate D_n and W_n^2 according to (4.9) and (4.10), respectively.*
(C) *Generate independent bootstrap i.i.d. samples $X_{\ell;1}^*, \ldots, X_{\ell;n}^*$ according to $F(\cdot; \hat{\theta}_n)$, and obtain the estimator $\hat{\theta}_{\ell;n}^*$, for $1 \leq \ell \leq m$.*
(D) *Calculate for $1 \leq \ell \leq m$*

$$D_{\ell;n}^* := \|\hat{\alpha}_{\ell;n}^*\| = n^{1/2} \max_{1 \leq i \leq n} \left(\frac{i}{n} - Z_{\ell;i:n}^*, Z_{\ell;i:n}^* - \frac{i-1}{n} \right)$$

and/or

$$W_{\ell;n}^{*2} = \frac{1}{12n} + \sum_{i=1}^{n} \left(Z_{\ell;i:n}^* - \frac{2i-1}{2n} \right)^2,$$

where $Z_{\ell;i:n}^* = F(X_{\ell;i:n}^*; \hat{\theta}_{\ell;n}^*)$.
(E) *Determine the p-value of D_n within the simulated $D_{\ell;n}^*$, $1 \leq \ell \leq m$ and/or the p-value of W_n^2 within the simulated $W_{\ell;n}^{*2}$, $1 \leq \ell \leq m$, respectively.*

R-Example 4.16 To check for normality, one can use the following implementation of the two bootstrap based goodness-of-fit tests.

```r
# generic functions to calculate Kolmogorov-Smirnov distance
# and Cramer-von Mises distance
KS <- function(z){
  # z - appropriately transformed and sorted data
  len <- length(z)
  sqrt(len) * max(c((1:len) / len - z, z - (0:(len-1)) / len))
}
CvM <- function(z){
  # z - appropriately transformed and sorted data
  len <- length(z)
  1 / (12 * len) + sum( (z - (2 * (1:len) - 1) / (2 * len))^2 )
}


boot.gof.normal.p <- function(x, R = 999){
  # x - observed data
  # R - number of MC simulations

  # calculate KS and CvM distance
  gofStat <- function(d) {
    d  <- sort(d)
    z <- pnorm(d, mean = mean(d), sd = sd(d))
    c(KS(z), CvM(z))
  }

  # test statistics for observed data
  t0 <- gofStat(x)

  # generates normal distributed random variables
  # for the use in boot()
  ran.gen <- function(d, p){
    rnorm(length(d), mean = p[1], sd = p[2])
  }

  # R resampled KS and CvM distances
  # NOTE, boot() will pass x to the first argument
  # and mle to the second argument of ran.gen
  bt <- boot::boot(x, gofStat, sim = "parametric",
            ran.gen = ran.gen, mle = c(mean(x), sd(x)), R = R)$t

  # return pvalues
  c(ks.pvalue = mean(bt[,1] > t0[1]),
    cvm.pvalue = mean(bt[,2] > t0[2]))
}
```

Now, we apply this test to check for normality.

```
set.seed(123,kind ="Mersenne-Twister",normal.kind ="Inversion")
#data are normally distributed, H0 is correct
x <- rnorm(100, mean = 2, sd = 4)
boot.gof.normal.p(x)
```

```
##   ks.pvalue cvm.pvalue
##   0.5705706  0.8898899
```

```
#data are exponentially distributed, H0 is not correct
x <- rexp(100, rate = 2)
boot.gof.normal.p(x)
```

```
##   ks.pvalue cvm.pvalue
##           0          0
```

To check for a Weibull distribution the following implementations can be used.

```
mle.weibull <- function(x){
  # x - observed data

  # negative log-likelihood-function assuming
  # a weibull distribution
  nLL <- function(shape, scale)
    if (shape > 0 && scale >=0) {
      -sum(stats::dweibull(x, shape, scale, log = TRUE))
    } else {
      NA
    }

  # minimize the negative log-likelihood
  ret <- coef(stats4::mle(nLL, start = list(shape = 1, scale = 1),
        nobs = length(x)))

  # rename to increase readability later
  names(ret) <- paste("est", names(ret), sep=".")
  ret
}
```

```r
boot.gof.weibull.p <- function(x, R = 999){
  # x - observed data

  # calculate KS and CvM distance
  gofStat <- function(d) {
    d     <- sort(d)
    est   <- mle.weibull(d)
    shape <- est["est.shape"]
    scale <- est["est.scale"]
    d     <- pweibull(d, shape, scale)

    c(KS(d), CvM(d))
  }

  # test statistics for observed data
  t0 <- gofStat(x)

  # generates weibull distributed random variables
  # for the use in boot()
  ran.gen <- function(d, p){
    rweibull(length(d), shape = p[1], scale = p[2])
  }

  # R resampled KS and CvM distances
  # NOTE, boot() will pass x to the first argument
  # and mle to the second argument of ran.gen
  est <- mle.weibull(x)
  bt <- boot::boot(x, gofStat, sim = "parametric",
               ran.gen = ran.gen, mle = est, R = R)$t

  # return pvalues
  c(ks.pvalue = mean(bt[,1] > t0[1]),
    cvm.pvalue = mean(bt[,2] > t0[2]))
}


set.seed(123,kind ="Mersenne-Twister",normal.kind ="Inversion")
#H0 is correct
x <- rweibull(200, shape = 4, scale = 0.5)
boot.gof.weibull.p(x)



  ##   ks.pvalue cvm.pvalue
  ##   0.8588589  0.7337337

#H0 is not correct
x <- rbeta(200, shape1 = 4, shape2 = 5)
boot.gof.weibull.p(x)



  ##   ks.pvalue cvm.pvalue
  ##   0.02502503 0.07107107
```

Note, Excerise 4.20 is dedicated to locate computational bottlenecks within the function "boot.gof.weibull.p" using package `profvis` and improving the computation time.

4.5 Mathematical Framework of the GOF Test

A universal approach to approximate the critical values is given by the bootstrap as outlined in Stute et al (1993, Theorem 1.1). For this, the following regularity assumptions have to be made.

(A1) Under H_0, i.e., $F = F(\cdot; \theta_0)$ the estimator $\hat{\theta}_n$ has the following expansion:

$$n^{1/2}(\hat{\theta}_n - \theta_0) = n^{-1/2} \sum_{i=1}^{n} l(X_i, \theta_0) + r_n,$$

where $\mathbb{E}_{\theta_0}(l(X, \theta_0)) = 0$ and $\mathbb{E}_{\theta_0}(l^\top(X, \theta_0) l(X, \theta_0))$ exists. Furthermore, there exists a neighborhood V of θ_0 such that

$$\sup_{\theta \in V} \mathbb{P}_\theta(\|r_n\| > \varepsilon) \longrightarrow 0, \quad \text{as } n \to \infty,$$

for all $\varepsilon > 0$.

(A2) Moreover, as $\hat{\theta}_n \to \theta_0$, for each $x \in \mathbb{R}$

$$\int_{]-\infty,x]} l(t, \hat{\theta}_n) \, F(dt, \hat{\theta}_n) \longrightarrow \int_{]-\infty,x]} l(t, \theta_0) \, F(dt, \theta_0).$$

(A3) Furthermore, as $\hat{\theta}_n \to \theta_0$,

$$\int l^\top(x, \hat{\theta}_n) l(x, \hat{\theta}_n) \, F(dx, \hat{\theta}_n) \longrightarrow \int l^\top(x, \theta_0) l(x, \theta_0) \, F(dx, \theta_0).$$

In addition to these regularity assumptions, one also has to assume that $F(\cdot; \cdot)$ is sufficiently smooth. In particular, this means:

(B1) There exists an open neighborhood U of θ_0 such that

$$F(\cdot; \theta), \ \theta \in U \quad \text{is equicontinous}$$

and

$$g(x, \theta) = \frac{\partial F(x; \theta)}{\partial \theta} \quad \text{is uniformly continuous and bounded on } \mathbb{R} \times U.$$

Note, that (A1) is a typical expansion used to prove convergence in distribution of maximum likelihood estimators (MLE).

Durbin (1973) used a suitable transformation of the process so that the paths become elements of the Skorokhod space $D[0, 1]$. Then he proved under these assumptions that if H_0 is correct

$$\hat{\alpha}_n \longrightarrow Z$$

in distribution, where Z is a centered Gaussian process with continuous sample paths and covariance function

$$
\begin{aligned}
\text{COV}(Z(x_1), Z(x_2)) = {} & F(x_1, \theta_0) - F(x_1, \theta_0)F(x_2, \theta_0) \qquad (4.11) \\
& - \int_{]-\infty, x_1]} l^\top(x, \theta_0)g(x_1, \theta_0)\, F(dx, \theta_0) \\
& - \int_{]-\infty, x_2]} l^\top(x, \theta_0)g(x_2, \theta_0)\, F(dx, \theta_0) \\
& + \int l^\top(x, \theta_0)g(x_1, \theta_0)\, l^\top(x, \theta_0)g(x_2, \theta_0)\, F(dx, \theta_0),
\end{aligned}
$$

where $x_1 \leq x_2$.

Obviously, the limit distribution depends heavily on $F(\cdot; \theta_0)$ and is therefore different for different classes of parametric families.

Coming back to the bootstrap, we have to mimic H_0. This can be done by resampling according to $F(\cdot; \hat{\theta}_n)$. Thus the bootstrap sample $X_1^*, \ldots, X_n^* \sim F(\cdot; \hat{\theta}_n)$ is an i.i.d. sample and the appropriate bootstrap version of the estimated empirical process $\hat{\alpha}_n$ is given by

$$\hat{\alpha}_n^*(x) = n^{1/2}(F_n^*(x) - F(x; \hat{\theta}_n^*)),$$

where F_n^* is the edf. of the bootstrap sample and $\hat{\theta}_n^*$ the corresponding estimator of the parameter. Note that the correct parameter $\hat{\theta}_n$ is known for the bootstrap sample. Nevertheless, we have to estimate this parameter in order to mimic the situation of the original sample.

Theorem 4.17 *Under H_0, assume that (A1)–(A3) and (B1) are satisfied. Then, if $\hat{\theta}_n \to \theta_0$ w.p.1*

$$\hat{\alpha}_n^* \longrightarrow Z$$

in distribution with probability one. Here Z is a centered Gaussian process with continuous sample paths and covariance function given under (4.11).

Corollary 4.18 *Since Z has continuous sample paths and $\|\cdot\|_\infty$ is a continuous function on $C[0, 1]$, the continuous mapping theorem, Billingsley (1968, Theorem 5.1), yields that w.p.1*

$$\mathbb{P}_n^*(\|\hat{\alpha}_n^*\|_\infty \leq t) - \mathbb{P}(\|\hat{\alpha}_n\|_\infty \leq t) \longrightarrow 0, \quad \text{as } n \to \infty,$$

for each t such that $\mathbb{P}(\|Z\| = t) = 0$. *Thus under the stated assumptions, the distribution of D_n can be approximated by bootstrapping. Similarly, the bootstrap can be used to approximate the df. of W_n^2.*

Proof of Theorem 4.17 Unlike in Durbin (1973), we analyze the process untransformed, i.e., in the space $D[-\infty, \infty]$ itself, cf. Definition 6.3. As Remark 6.4 shows, $D[-\infty, \infty]$ can be identified with $D[0, 1]$. Recall the proof of Durbin (1973) and use the decomposition:

$$\hat{\alpha}_n(x) = n^{1/2}(F_n(x) - F(x; \theta_0)) + n^{1/2}(F(x; \theta_0) - F(x; \hat{\theta}_n))$$
$$\equiv I_1(n, x) + I_2(n, x).$$

Note, that $I_1(n, x)$ is just the empirical process at the point x. For the $I_2(n, x)$ term we get according to Taylor's expansion for an appropriate $\tilde{\theta}$ between $\hat{\theta}_n$ and θ_0

$$I_2(n, x) = -g^\top(x, \theta_0) n^{1/2}(\hat{\theta}_n - \theta_0) + \left(g^\top(x, \theta_0) - g^\top(x, \tilde{\theta})\right) n^{1/2}(\hat{\theta}_n - \theta_0)$$
$$= -g^\top(x, \theta_0) n^{1/2}(\hat{\theta}_n - \theta_0) + o_\mathbb{P}(1)$$
$$= -n^{-1/2} \sum_{i=1}^{n} g^\top(x, \theta_0) l(X_i, \theta_0) + o_\mathbb{P}(1),$$

where the $o_\mathbb{P}(1)$ term does not depend on x.
Overall, we have the representation, uniformly in x:

$$\hat{\alpha}_n(x) = n^{1/2}(F_n(x) - F(x; \theta_0)) - n^{-1/2} \sum_{i=1}^{n} g^\top(x, \theta_0) l(X_i, \theta_0) + o_\mathbb{P}(1). \quad (4.12)$$

The first term on the right-hand side is the empirical process $\alpha_n(x)$. Since $F(\cdot; \theta_0)$ is continuous and $\alpha_n(x) = \bar{\alpha}_n(F(x, \theta_0))$, where $\bar{\alpha}_n$ is the uniform empirical process (cf. Sect. 3.4), C-tightness of the uniform empirical process implies C-tightness of α_n. Furthermore, the second term on the right-hand side is C-tight due to the special representation of this term, the CLT, and the uniform continuity if $g(\cdot, \theta_0)$. Thus, the right-hand side is C-tight. Finally, the convergence of the finite-dimensional distributions (fidis.) follows from the multivariate CLT.
For the bootstrap, we will mimic the proof given above. At first, we give some results which will be needed.
We have w.p.1

$$\mathbb{P}_n^*(\|\hat{\theta}_n^* - \hat{\theta}_n\| > \varepsilon) \longrightarrow 0, \quad \text{as } n \to \infty, \quad (4.13)$$

for each $\varepsilon > 0$. Note that the bootstrap data was created under $\hat{\theta}_n$ and that $\hat{\theta}_n \longrightarrow \theta_0$, w.p.1. So we can assume that, w.p.1, for n sufficiently large, that $\hat{\theta}_n \in V$. Thus, according to (A1), we can focus on

$$\mathbb{P}_n^*(\|1/n \sum_{i=1}^{n} l(X_i^*, \hat{\theta}_n)\| > \varepsilon) \longrightarrow 0, \quad \text{as } n \to \infty,$$

to prove (4.13). To do this, apply Markov's inequality and get

$$\mathbb{P}_n^*\left(\left\|\frac{1}{n} \sum_{i=1}^{n} l(X_i^*, \hat{\theta}_n)\right\| > \varepsilon\right) \le \frac{1}{\varepsilon^2} \mathbb{E}_n^*\left(\left\|\frac{1}{n} \sum_{i=1}^{n} l(X_i^*, \hat{\theta}_n)\right\|^2\right)$$

$$= \frac{1}{n^2 \varepsilon^2} \sum_{i=1}^{n} \sum_{j=1}^{n} \mathbb{E}_n^*\left(l^\top(X_i^*, \hat{\theta}_n) l(X_j^*, \hat{\theta}_n)\right)$$

$$= \frac{1}{n^2 \varepsilon^2} \sum_{i=1}^{n} \mathbb{E}_n^*\left(l^\top(X_i^*, \hat{\theta}_n) l(X_i^*, \hat{\theta}_n)\right)$$

$$= \frac{1}{n \varepsilon^2} \mathbb{E}_n^*\left(l^\top(X^*, \hat{\theta}_n) l(X^*, \hat{\theta}_n)\right).$$

According to (A3) and (A1) the expectation on the right-hand side tends to a finite value w.p.1. Thus, the total right-hand side tends to 0, which completes the proof of (4.13).

Since $\hat{\theta}_n$ tends to θ_0 w.p.1, (4.13) yields that w.p.1

$$\mathbb{P}_n^*(\|\hat{\theta}_n^* - \theta_0\| > \varepsilon) \longrightarrow 0, \quad \text{as } n \to \infty, \tag{4.14}$$

for each $\varepsilon > 0$.

Under the given assumption, we further have a Glivenko-Cantelli type result, i.e.,

$$\|F(\cdot; \hat{\theta}_n) - F(\cdot; \theta_0)\|_\infty \longrightarrow 0, \quad \text{as } n \to \infty, \tag{4.15}$$

w.p.1. In particular, the convergence at each $x \in \mathbb{R}$ follows from Assumption (B1) and $\hat{\theta}_n \to \theta_0$ w.p.1. The uniform convergence is then a consequence of a standard argument, compare Loève (1977, pp. 20–21).

As already indicated, we will mimic the classical proof and obtain in our first step:

$$\hat{\alpha}_n^*(x) = n^{1/2}(F_n^*(x) - F(x; \hat{\theta}_n)) + n^{1/2}(F(x; \hat{\theta}_n) - F(x; \hat{\theta}_n^*))$$
$$\equiv I_1^*(n, x) + I_2^*(n, x).$$

The first term on the right-hand side is the original empirical process of the bootstrap sample, i.e., the empirical process corresponding to an i.i.d. sample w.r.t. $F(\cdot; \hat{\theta}_n)$. For the second term on the right-hand side, we apply Taylor's expansion to get for a proper chosen $\tilde{\theta}_n^*$ between $\hat{\theta}_n^*$ and $\hat{\theta}_n$

$$I_2^*(n, x) = -g^\top(x, \theta_0)\, n^{1/2}(\hat{\theta}_n^* - \hat{\theta}_n) + \left(g^\top(x, \theta_0) - g^\top(x, \tilde{\theta}_n^*)\right) n^{1/2}(\hat{\theta}_n^* - \hat{\theta}_n)$$

$$\equiv I_{2,1}^*(n, x) + I_{2,2}^*(n, x).$$

The $I_{2,2}^*$ term on the right-hand side can be neglected if we show that $n^{1/2}(\hat{\theta}_n^* - \hat{\theta}_n)$ is asymptotically normal w.p.1, since due to (4.14) and Assumption (B1) we have w.p.1

$$\mathbb{P}_n^*\left(\|g^\top(\cdot; \theta_0) - g^\top(\cdot, \tilde{\theta}_n^*)\|_\infty > \varepsilon\right) \longrightarrow 0, \quad \text{as } n \to \infty,$$

for each $\varepsilon > 0$. But

$$n^{1/2}(\hat{\theta}_n^* - \hat{\theta}_n) = n^{-1/2} \sum_{i=1}^n l(X_i^*, \hat{\theta}_n) + r_n^*$$

and r_n^* can asymptotically be neglected w.p.1 according to (A1) and $\hat{\theta}_n \to \theta_0$ w.p.1. Now, our sum $n^{-1/2} \sum_{i=1}^n l(X_i^*, \hat{\theta}_n)$ is in a suitable form, i.e., it consists of an i.i.d. sum of centered variables, c.f. (A1), for each n. To prove asymptotic normality for this representation, we have to apply the Cramér-Wold device. The Lindeberg condition can be verified with the same approach as under Theorem 3.8.
So far we have seen that uniformly in x, w.p.1,

$$\hat{\alpha}_n^*(x) = n^{1/2}(F_n^*(x) - F(x; \hat{\theta}_n)) - n^{-1/2} \sum_{i=1}^n l^\top(X_i^*, \hat{\theta}_n) g(x, \theta_0) + o_{\mathbb{P}_n^*}(1)$$

$$= \alpha_n^*(x) - n^{-1/2} \sum_{i=1}^n l^\top(X_i^*, \hat{\theta}_n) g(x, \theta_0) + o_{\mathbb{P}_n^*}(1) \tag{4.16}$$

holds.
To finalize the proof, we first use again Cramér-Wold device to show that the fidis converge to the same limit in distribution as the corresponding fidis of the original process w.p.1. To prove tightness, first observe that the process $\alpha_n^*(x) \equiv \bar{\alpha}_n(F(x; \hat{\theta}_n))$, where $\bar{\alpha}_n$ is the uniform empirical process. According to the Glivenko-Cantelli result given under (4.15), we can apply the same technique as under Theorem 3.12 to get, w.p.1, that

$$\alpha_n^* \longrightarrow B^o(F(\cdot; \theta_0))$$

in distribution. Therefore, α_n^* is tight w.p.1. The tightness of the second process

$$n^{-1/2} \sum_{i=1}^n l^\top(X_i^*, \hat{\theta}_n) g(x, \theta_0)$$

follows directly from the asymptotic normality of $n^{-1/2} \sum_{i=1}^n l^\top(X_i^*, \hat{\theta}_n)$ and Assumption (B1). $\square$

4.6 Exercises

Exercise 4.19 Repeat the simulation study from Example 4.8 without using the `simTool`-package.

Exercise 4.20 Use the `profvis`-package to obtain a similar output to Fig. 4.2. If we focus on the computational intensive steps we see, that we spend 5450 ms in "boot::boot()", where 5250 ms were used for calculating the MLE, i.e., "mle.weibull()". Note, this is not the time for calculating one MLE, but the time for all MLE calculations done in the bootstrap. Looking at "mle.weibull()" we see that it took 3490 ms in sum to calculate all the negative log-likelihoods. Therefore about 1760 ms are due to our choice of start parameters, i.e., *shape = 1* and *scale = 1*, for the estimation. Try to improve the performance, for instance, by

- using other optimization methods,
- using the equation $\log(-\log(1 - F(x))) = shape \log(x) - shape \log(scale)$ for Weibull-distributed random variables,
- using the MLE estimation of the original sample as a start parameter for the bootstrap sample.

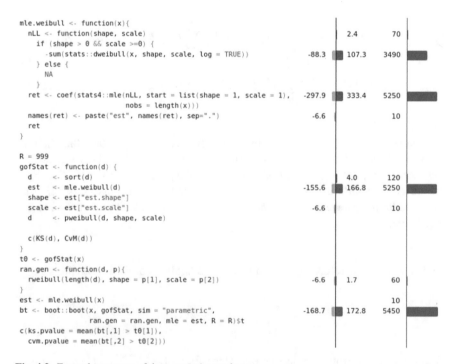

Fig. 4.2 Examplary output of the `profvis`-package

Exercise 4.21 In the two-sample problem of Example 4.12 we can also use the following modified resampling scheme:

(i) Generate independent bootstrap i.i.d. samples $X_{k,1}^*, \ldots, X_{k,n}^*$ according to the edf. based on $X_1, \ldots, X_n$ and $Y_{k,1}^*, \ldots, Y_{k,\ell}^*$ according to the edf. based on $Y_1, \ldots, Y_\ell$, respectively, for $1 \leq k \leq m$.

(ii) Calculate for $1 \leq k \leq m$

$$T_{n,k}^* := \frac{(\bar{X}_{n,k}^* - \bar{X}_n) - (\bar{Y}_{\ell,k}^* - \bar{Y}_\ell)}{\sqrt{s_{x,k}^{*2}/n + s_{y,k}^{*2}/\ell}},$$

where

$$\bar{X}_n = \frac{1}{n}\sum_{i=1}^{n} X_i, \quad \bar{Y}_\ell = \frac{1}{\ell}\sum_{j=1}^{\ell} Y_j$$

are the sample means of the observations.

(iii) Determine the p-value of T_n within the simulated $T_{n,k}^*$, $1 \leq k \leq m$ according to Eq. (4.5).

Give some arguments why this resampling scheme is equivalent to the resampling scheme given under 4.13.

Exercise 4.22 Use Resampling Scheme 4.10 with $m = 1000$ bootstrap replications to test $H_0 : \mu_x = \mu_y$ versus $H_1 : \mu_x \neq \mu_y$, where

X – sample	17.59	17.51	15.13	17.46	14.55	16.74	16.21	16.81	14.66	18.76
Y – sample	16.61	15.91	15.96	18.95	16.86	14.06	18.61	20.53	17.36	16.90

Exercise 4.23 Use Resampling Scheme 4.13 with $m = 1000$ bootstrap replications to test $H_0 : \mu_x = \mu_y$ versus $H_1 : \mu_x \neq \mu_y$, where

X – sample	2.11	2.30	6.41	8.95	0.13	4.06	4.86	2.37	2.68	10.83
Y – sample	0.16	1.12	2.08	0.49	0.22	1.55	1.85	3.07	-	-

Repeat the above test 100 times and determine the average p-value from these 100 simulations.

Exercise 4.24 To get an idea of the power of bootstrap based goodness-of-fit tests, generate an i.i.d. sample $X_1, \ldots, X_n \sim F$, where F is the χ^2 df. with one degree of freedom. Now, assume $H_0 : F \in \{EXP(\lambda) : \lambda > 0\}$.

(i) Write an R-function similar to "boot.gof.normal.p", see R-Example 4.16, to check the null hypothesis with the CvM and KS based bootstrap tests. Use ($m = 500$) for the bootstrap replications.

(ii) Apply your R-function to 1000 different original samples and store the corresponding 1000 p-values based on the KS-test and on the CvM-test in a vector. Use sample sizes $n = 20, 50, 100$.

(iii) Calculate the average p-value and the relative number of rejections for 0.1 as type 1 error for each sample size.
(iv) Visualize the vector of p-values obtained under 4.24 by a plot; compare R-Example 4.8 Fig. 4.1.

References

Billingsley P (1968) Convergence of probability measures. Wiley, New York
D'Agostino RB, Stephens MA (eds) (1986) Goodness-of-fit techniques, vol 68. Statistics: textbooks and monographs. Marcel Dekker Inc., New York
Davison AC, Hinkley DV (1997) Bootstrap methods and their application, vol 1. Cambridge series in statistical and probabilistic mathematics. Cambridge University Press, Cambridge, UK
Durbin J (1973) Distribution theory for tests based on the sample distribution function, vol 9. CBMS-NSF regional conference series in applied mathematics. Society for Industrial and Applied Mathematics, Philadelphia, PA
Efron B, Tibshirani RJ (1993) An introduction to the bootstrap, vol 57. Monographs on statistics and applied probability. Chapman and Hall, New York
Loève M (1977) Probability theory. I, 4th edn. Springer, New York
Shao J, Tu DS (1995) The jackknife and bootstrap. Springer series in statistics. Springer, New York
Stute W, Gonzáles Manteiga W, Presedo Quindimil M (1993) Bootstrap based goodness-of-fit tests. Metrika 40(3–4):243–256

Chapter 5
Regression Analysis

Assume we measure the insulin level $Y_1, \ldots, Y_n$ of n persons. Every person has a different weight $X_1, \ldots, X_n$. Can we somehow explain the insulin level using the weights? This is the general context of regression analysis. There are different reasons why such a question might be of interest. For instance, a scientist could be interested in understanding the mechanics behind insulin level, i.e., which factor influences the insulin level and how? Other scientists may only be interested in predicting the insulin level. One common way to achieve this is to find a way to express the conditional expectation of Y given X. Call the function $m(X) = \mathbb{E}(Y|X)$ the regression function. This chapter is dedicated to methods that estimate parametric forms $m(X, \vartheta)$ under various assumptions. We start with the classical linear models that assume that $m(X, \vartheta) = \vartheta^\top X$ is linear in X while Y follows a normal distribution first under independence assumptions and later under certain correlation assumptions. Afterward, we allow other distributions for Y like the negative-binomial distribution which lead to the classical generalized linear models. The chapter concludes with semi-parametric models, i.e., we do not explicitly assume a distribution for Y but the regression function $m(X, \vartheta)$ still depends on some (multi-dimensional) parameter ϑ.

Beside bootstrapping in the classical manner, that is sampling with replacement, other options are available. Therefore, after investigating the estimators (asymptotic) distribution we present resampling techniques that can be used to bootstrap the distribution. Of course, this allows again to estimate confidence intervals or to derive other statistics, but these results will also be used (in the next chapter) to construct goodness-of-fit statistics for the regression function itself. Usually, visual techniques are used to assess if the model fits the data well. The next chapter provides a more rigorous approach to that leveraging the results from this chapter.

© Springer Nature Switzerland AG 2021
G. Dikta and M. Scheer, *Bootstrap Methods*,
https://doi.org/10.1007/978-3-030-73480-0_5

5.1   Homoscedastic Linear Regression under Fixed Design

Linear models are important statistical tools and are very common in the scientific literature. In general, more sophisticated regression techniques originate from linear models. The purpose of linear models, or regression models in general, is to model or investigate the influence of some variables, usually called independent variables or covariates, onto another variable, usually called dependent variable. For instance, to model the price for a real estate (dependent variable) depending on the land area, year of construction, and so on (covariates). Here the focus would be to investigate how the covariates are related to the dependent variable and maybe predict the price only given the covariates.

In biometrics and epidemiology linear models are often used to account for "confounding variables". Suppose we have two groups and our main goal is to investigate if there is any difference in the level of a specific hormone. If the persons were randomized properly into two groups, we could use a two-sample t-test to detect differences in the mean hormone level. But sometimes it is not possible to randomize. One reason might be that the two groups are naturally given, for instance, by a disease state or type. Assume group one is persons with a type 1-diabetes and group two is persons with type 2-diabetes. These two types of diabetes are very different from a medical point of view (we do not want to elaborate on this). Nevertheless, the typical type1-diabetic is young and the typical type2-diabetic is old. If the hormone level depends on age, the usual two-sample t-test will be misleading, i.e., we over estimate or under estimate the effect of the diabetes status. We need a two-sample test that accounts for the difference in the age structure of the two groups. In this case, age is a "confounding variable" and we want to estimate the effect of the diabetes type on the hormone level "adjusted for" age.

Now, we generate a dataset following

$$Y = 100 - 3.5 \cdot I_{\{\text{diabetes}='\text{Type2}'\}} + 0.1 \cdot \text{age} + \varepsilon,$$

where $\varepsilon \sim N(0, 1)$ that will be analyzed through the current section. Note, the dataset also contains the parameter height, which does not contribute to the hormone level.

```
set.seed(123,kind ="Mersenne-Twister",normal.kind ="Inversion")
hormone_data <-
  data.frame(diabetes = gl(2, 50, labels = c("T1", "T2"))) %>%
  dplyr::mutate(
    age = ifelse(diabetes == "T1",
              rnorm(50, mean = 25, sd = 5),
              rnorm(50, mean = 60, sd = 5)),
    height = rnorm(100, mean = 180, sd = 10),
    hormone = 100 - 3.5 * (diabetes == "T2") +
      0.1 * age + rnorm(100))

head(hormone_data, n = 2)
```

```
##    diabetes        age    height  hormone
## 1         T1 22.19762 172.8959 104.4186
## 2         T1 23.84911 182.5688 103.6973
```

```
tail(hormone_data, n = 2)
```

```
##      diabetes        age    height  hormone
## 99         T2 58.8215 173.8883 102.4031
## 100        T2 54.8679 168.1452 103.2367
```

Looking at Fig. 5.1, it is obvious that age hides the diabetes effect and the t-test will not detect any difference in the hormone level with respect to the diabetes status if age is ignored.

```
ggplot(hormone_data, aes(x=age, y=hormone, color=diabetes)) +
  ylab("hormone level") +
  geom_point()
```

Our data follow a general linear regression model where the hormone levels are given by

$$Y_i = \sum_{q=1}^{p} x_{i,q}\beta_q + \varepsilon_i, \quad 1 \le i \le n, \tag{5.1}$$

and where the *residuals* $\varepsilon_1, \ldots, \varepsilon_n \sim F$ are i.i.d. with $\mathbb{E}(\varepsilon) = 0$ and $\mathrm{VAR}(\varepsilon) = \sigma^2 < \infty$, i.e., *homoscedasticity*. Note, we consider that the model is based on a *fixed design*, i.e., $x_{i,q}$ are not random. Although the generation process in our hormone data sampled age from a normal distribution, $x_{i,q}$ is not considered as random! It is not unusual to consider the covariates as fixed. The results are then interpreted as "given the covariates".

Equation (5.1) can be written in the following compact form:

$$Y(n) = x(n)\beta + \varepsilon(n),$$

where

$$
\begin{aligned}
Y(n) = Y \; &= (Y_1, \ldots, Y_n)^\top && \text{– response vector}\\
x(n) = x \; &= \begin{pmatrix} x_{1,1} & \cdots & x_{1,p} \\ \vdots & & \vdots \\ x_{n,1} & \cdots & x_{n,p} \end{pmatrix} && \text{– design matrix}\\
\varepsilon(n) = \varepsilon \; &= (\varepsilon_1, \ldots, \varepsilon_n)^\top && \text{– vector of residuals}\\
\beta \; &= (\beta_1, \ldots, \beta_p)^\top && \text{– vector of parameters.}
\end{aligned}
$$

If the first column of x has 1 at every place, the model has an intercept.

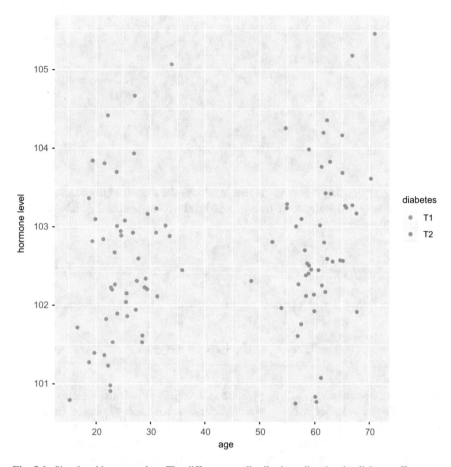

Fig. 5.1 Simulated hormone data. The different age distributions disguise the diabetes effect

Throughout this section we assume maximal rank of $x(n) \equiv x$ so that $x(n)^\top x(n) \equiv x^\top x$ is positive definite and hence invertible. The index n will be omitted for notational convenience.

To estimate the unknown parameter vector β based on the n observations, we take $\hat\beta(n) \equiv \hat\beta$, as the projection of Y onto the vector space $\{z \in \mathbb{R}^n : z = x\gamma, \ \gamma \in \mathbb{R}^p\}$. Thus for all $\gamma \in \mathbb{R}^p$ we have

$$(Y - x\hat\beta) \perp x\gamma \iff \langle Y - x\hat\beta, \ x\gamma \rangle = 0.$$

The right-hand side is equivalent to

$$Y^\top x\gamma = \hat\beta^\top x^\top x\gamma.$$

Since this equality has to hold for all $\gamma \in \mathbb{R}^p$ we get

$$Y^\top x = \hat{\beta}^\top x^\top x.$$

Now multiply both sides with the inverse of $x^\top x$ to get finally after transposing

$$\hat{\beta}(n) \equiv \hat{\beta} = (x^\top x)^{-1} x^\top Y. \tag{5.2}$$

Substitute into this equation the model for Y to get the representation

$$\hat{\beta} = (x^\top x)^{-1} x^\top (x\beta + \varepsilon) = \beta + (x^\top x)^{-1} x^\top \varepsilon, \tag{5.3}$$

which can easily be handled to prove asymptotic results, as we will see in this chapter later on.

Remark 5.1 The estimator (5.2) is known as the *least square estimator* (LSE), because it minimizes the sum of the squared errors, i.e., $\sum_{i=1}^{n}(Y_i - \sum_{q=1}^{p} x_{i,q}\beta_q)^2$.

After the LSE $\hat{\beta}$ is obtained, we can use $\hat{\beta}$ to define the *estimated residuals* given by

$$\hat{\varepsilon} \equiv (\hat{\varepsilon}_1, \ldots, \hat{\varepsilon}_n)^\top = Y - x\hat{\beta} = x(\beta - \hat{\beta}) + \varepsilon \tag{5.4}$$

to get with

$$s_n^2 \equiv \frac{(Y - x\hat{\beta})^\top (Y - x\hat{\beta})}{n} \tag{5.5}$$

a biased estimator for $\sigma^2 = \mathrm{VAR}(\varepsilon)$.

R-Example 5.2 We now calculate the LSE for our hormone data using R standard function `lm`. This function also automatically calculates the intercept and takes care of any coding of non-numerical variables:

```
hormone_fit <- lm(hormone ~ diabetes + age + height,
          data = hormone_data)
coefficients(hormone_fit)
```

```
##    (Intercept)      diabetesT2             age           height
##   1.006844e+02  -2.221115e+00    7.127644e-02    1.698143e-04
```

Exercises 5.86 and 5.87 are dedicated to reproducing the result using other R-functions.

5.1.1 Model-Based Bootstrap

If we want to use the bootstrap for testing, we have already discussed the necessity of a resampling procedure that mimics the null hypothesis. This general resampling principle should also be applied if we want to use bootstrapping for some statistical analysis under model assumptions. To be more precise, the bootstrap data should be drawn under the given model assumptions or at least very close to them.

In this chapter, we focus on the model (5.1), where the residuals are centered random variables. The LSE $\hat{\beta}$ can be used to substitute the true β in our model. Since the residuals are i.i.d. and therefore not depending on x, we can use the edf. of the estimated residuals $\hat{\varepsilon}_1, \ldots, \hat{\varepsilon}_n$ as a base for our resampling. However, we should also address in our resampling approach that the residuals are centered, that is, $\mathbb{E}(\varepsilon) = 0$.

Remark 5.3 If our model (5.1) allows for an intercept, the estimated residuals are always centered, that is, $\sum_{1 \le i \le n} \hat{\varepsilon}_i = 0$. But this is not the case in general when the intercept is excluded!

This remark tells us that the estimated residuals are not centered if our underlying model does not has an intercept. To face this, we use the *centered estimated residuals*

$$\tilde{\varepsilon}_1 = \hat{\varepsilon}_1 - \mu_n, \ldots, \tilde{\varepsilon}_n = \hat{\varepsilon}_n - \mu_n, \tag{5.6}$$

where $\mu_n = 1/n \sum_{1 \le i \le n} \hat{\varepsilon}_i$ as a base for our resampling. Overall, this leads to the following resampling procedure which defines the *model based bootstrap*:

Resampling Scheme 5.4

(A) *Based on the observations*

$$(Y_i, x_i)_{1 \le i \le n} \subset \mathbb{R}^{1+p}$$

calculate the LSE $\hat{\beta}(n)$.

(B) *Determine the estimated residuals $\hat{\varepsilon}_1, \ldots, \hat{\varepsilon}_n$ and denote by $\tilde{F}_n$ the edf. of the centered estimated residuals, i.e., of $\tilde{\varepsilon}_1, \ldots, \tilde{\varepsilon}_n$, where $\tilde{\varepsilon}_i = \hat{\varepsilon}_i - \mu_n$ and $\mu_n = n^{-1} \sum_{i=1}^{n} \hat{\varepsilon}_i$.*

(C) *Draw an i.i.d. sample $\varepsilon_1^*, \ldots, \varepsilon_n^* \sim \tilde{F}_n$ and define*

$$(Y_i^*, x_i)_{1 \le i \le n}, \quad \text{where } Y_i^* = x_i^\top \hat{\beta}(n) + \varepsilon_i^*$$

(D) *Compute the LSE of the bootstrap sample, i.e., determine*

$$\beta^*(n) = (x^\top x)^{-1} x^\top Y^*.$$

In the next example, we apply this approach to a simple model under R.

R-Example 5.5 We now generate 10 bootstrap samples of the coefficient β using the model fit of the preceding section.

```
bootLSE = function(lm_object, R){

  # lm_object - a model fit returned by stats::lm
  # R         - number of MC simulations


  # m is a data.frame containing Y (first column) and all
  # necessary/used covariates
  m <- model.frame(lm_object)

  m[,1] <- fitted.values(lm_object)
  # m[,1] equals now the covariates times estimate of beta

  # Step (B)
  res <- residuals(lm_object)
  centered_res <- res - mean(res)

  getCoef <- function(d, i){
    # note m[,1] directly after entering getCoef() equals
    # fitted.values(lm_object).

    # Step (C)
    # here we add an iid sample of the centered residuals
    m[,1] <- m[,1] + d[i]

    # Step (D)
    # refitting using the same model, but the new locally
    # modified dataset m, that exists in the scope of getCoef()
    coefficients(update(lm_object, data=m))
  }

  ret <- boot::boot(centered_res, getCoef, R=R)$t
  colnames(ret) <- names(coefficients(lm_object))
  ret
}
set.seed(123,kind ="Mersenne-Twister",normal.kind ="Inversion")
bootLSE(hormone_fit, R=10)


  ##       (Intercept) diabetesT2        age        height
  ##  [1,]   102.34053 -2.2475860 0.07826922 -0.010915485
  ##  [2,]    99.71085 -2.2493330 0.07342633  0.005127545
  ##  [3,]    99.59317 -2.6704092 0.08138058  0.004740870
  ##  [4,]    98.49276 -1.7184202 0.06237397  0.013339298
  ##  [5,]   102.25480 -3.5801511 0.10722537 -0.013701580
  ##  [6,]    99.15882 -1.7457254 0.05083991  0.011253981
  ##  [7,]    97.88378 -2.3224875 0.07893495  0.014210316
  ##  [8,]   101.89059 -1.5704854 0.04695695 -0.002841336
  ##  [9,]   101.52333 -0.6861021 0.03155923  0.000668564
  ## [10,]   100.25149 -1.3005371 0.04135630  0.007025591
```

In the rest of this section, we will apply the model-based bootstrap to construct confidence intervals for the single components of β and to test hypotheses about β, asymptotically. This inferential part is based upon the assumption that

$$\sqrt{n}\big(\hat{\beta}(n) - \beta\big), \quad \sqrt{n}\big(\hat{\beta}^*(n) - \hat{\beta}(n)\big) \tag{5.7}$$

both tend to the same multivariate normal distribution. We will prove these asymptotic results later. To get an idea of the variance-covariance structure, recall (5.3) to see that

$$\hat{\beta} - \beta = (x^\top x)^{-1} x^\top \varepsilon.$$

Therefore, the variance-covariance of $\hat{\beta}$ is given by

$$\left((x^\top x)^{-1} x^\top\right) D \left((x^\top x)^{-1} x^\top\right)^\top = \sigma^2 (x^\top x)^{-1} \equiv \Sigma^2(n),$$

where D is a diagonal $p \times p$ matrix with σ^2 as entry in each diagonal component and 0 for all other components. This variance-covariance matrix could be estimated by $s_n^2 (x^\top x)^{-1}$. Asymptotically, the Formula (5.5) to estimate σ^2 is fine but biased. Instead, we will use here

$$\hat{\sigma}_n^2 = \frac{(Y - x\hat{\beta})^\top (Y - x\hat{\beta})}{n - p}, \quad \hat{\sigma}_n^{*2} = \frac{(Y^* - x\hat{\beta}^*)^\top (Y^* - x\hat{\beta}^*)}{n - p}, \tag{5.8}$$

where $n - p$ are the degrees of freedom. Thus

$$\hat{\Sigma}^2(n) = \hat{\sigma}_n^2 (x^\top x)^{-1}, \quad \hat{\Sigma}^{*2}(n) = \hat{\sigma}_n^{*2} (x^\top x)^{-1}$$

will be used here. The diagonal components of these matrices are variance estimates of the corresponding components of $\hat{\beta}$ and $\hat{\beta}^*$, respectively. Denote by

$$\hat{\gamma}_q^2 = \hat{\Sigma}^2(n)_{q,q}, \quad \hat{\gamma}_q^{*2} = \hat{\Sigma}^{*2}(n)_{q,q}$$

the corresponding estimates.

Now we get from (5.7) under proper assumptions that

$$\sup_{t \in \mathbb{R}} \left| \mathbb{P}\big((\hat{\beta}_q - \beta_q)/\hat{\gamma}_q \leq t\big) - \mathbb{P}_n^*\big((\hat{\beta}_q^* - \hat{\beta}_q)/\hat{\gamma}_q^* \leq t\big) \right| \longrightarrow 0, \quad \text{as } n \to \infty$$

and we can proceed as in Sect. 3.1 to construct the confidence intervals for the components of β, see Resampling Scheme 3.3. In the next example, we list the corresponding R-code.

R-Example 5.6 The following R-function is very similar to the one implemented in R-Example 5.5 and returns the confidence interval for β_q, $(q = 1, \dots, p)$.

```
bootLSE_ci = function(lm_object, conf.level=0.95, R=999){

  # lm_object  - a model fit returned by stats::lm
  # conf.level - confidence level for the required interval
  # R          - number of MC simulations

  m <- model.frame(lm_object)
  m[,1] <- fitted.values(lm_object)
  # m[,1] equals now the covariates times estimate of beta

  res <- residuals(lm_object)
  centered_res <- res - mean(res)

  beta_est <- coefficients(lm_object)

  scaled_beta <- function(d, i){
    m[,1] <- m[,1] + d[i]
    fit <- update(lm_object, data=m)
    (beta_est - coefficients(fit)) / sqrt(diag(vcov(fit)))
  }

  boot_scaled_beta <- boot(centered_res, scaled_beta, R=R)$t

  a <- (1 - conf.level) / 2

  # calculate the quantiles for the intercept and the covariates
  # based on the boostrapped (centered and scaled) beta.
  qlu <- apply(boot_scaled_beta, 2, quantile, probs = c(a, 1 - a))

  # calculate the standard deviation for the covariates
  # based on the original data set.
  sigma_est <- sqrt(diag(vcov(lm_object)))

  # return the estimate and the confidence intervals
  # according the formula "est +/- quantile x standard deviation"
  rbind(
    lower    = beta_est - qlu[2,] * sigma_est,
    estimate = beta_est,
    upper    = beta_est - qlu[1,] * sigma_est)
}
```

Finally, we can calculate a 95% confidence intervals for the estimates of our hormone data.

```
set.seed(123,kind ="Mersenne-Twister",normal.kind ="Inversion")
bootLSE_ci(hormone_fit)
```

```
##           (Intercept) diabetesT2        age        height
## lower        96.82218 -3.6652859 0.03130904 -0.0188421761
## estimate    100.68437 -2.2211152 0.07127644  0.0001698143
## upper       104.55555 -0.7184826 0.11285184  0.0210647928
```

In multivariate regression analysis, we often want to know whether a certain component of the model can be neglected or equals a theoretical known value. If we are interested in only a single component, one could simply use the confidence interval for that component. For instance, if the 95% CI for the parameter height contains zero, then, given the other covariates, height can be neglected. But sometimes one has to judge about several components simultaneously. Usually, this is necessary if one of the covariates is ordinal and has more than two categories. For instance, a specific type of diabetes is called LADA-diabetes. Hence, if our dataset would consist of all three types, then, in general, this is coded with two covariates, where the 2-tuple (0,0), (1,0), and (0,1) represents LADA-diabetes, Type1-diabetes, and Type2-diabetes, respectively. Thus, our model would have 4 β's, one parameter for age, one parameter for height, but now also one parameter for Type1-diabetes and one parameter for Type2-diabetes. In this case, the question if the diabetes type is necessary to explain the hormone data refers to two parameters simultaneously. Note, we are not constraint to one variable with more than two categories. Imagine our dataset would contain several parameters from an electrocardiogram. A reasonable question would be if these group of (electro-cardio) parameters are necessary to explain the hormone data. Usually, the likelihood ratio test is used to answer such questions, but a model-based bootstrap can easily be defined.

Resampling Scheme 5.7 *We consider two linear models*

$$(M1) \quad Y_i = \sum_{q=1}^{p} x_{i,q} \beta_q + \varepsilon_i$$

and

$$(M2) \quad Y_i = \sum_{q=1}^{\tilde{p}} x_{i,q} \beta_q + \varepsilon_i,$$

where $i = 1, \ldots, n$ and $\tilde{p} < p$.

(A) *Obtain the LSE, denoted by $\hat{\beta}^{M1}$, under model M1 and calculate the corresponding Mahalanobis distance $d(\hat{\beta}^{M1}, S)$, that is*

$$\sqrt{(\hat{\beta}_{\tilde{p}+1}^{M1}, \ldots, \hat{\beta}_p^{M1})^\top S^{-1} (\hat{\beta}_{\tilde{p}+1}^{M1}, \ldots, \hat{\beta}_p^{M1})},$$

where S is the estimated covariance of $(\hat{\beta}_{\tilde{p}+1}^{M1}, \ldots, \hat{\beta}_p^{M1})$.

(B) *Fit model M2 and generate m bootstrap datasets according to the fitted model M2 using (A)–(C) from Resampling Scheme 5.4.*

(C) *Fit model M1 to each bootstrap dataset and obtain in the k-th fit $(k = 1, \ldots, m)$ the Mahalanobis distance $d(\hat{\beta}_k^{*,M1}, S_k^*)$, where S_k^* is the covariance of $(\hat{\beta}_{k;\tilde{p}+1}^{*,M1}, \ldots, \hat{\beta}_{k;p}^{*,M1})$.*

(D) *Take*

$$\frac{1}{m} \sum_{k=1}^{m} I_{\{d(\hat{\beta}_k^{*,M1}, S_k^*) > d(\hat{\beta}^{M1}, S)\}}$$

as a p-value for comparing model M1 and M2.

Proving that RSS 5.7 works, i.e., can be used to compare the two models is left to the reader, see Exercise 5.88.

R-Example 5.8 Assume we want to test if the age and height are necessary to explain the hormone data, i.e., $H_0 : (\beta_{age}, \beta_{height}) = (0, 0)$ versus $H_1 : (\beta_{age}, \beta_{height}) \neq (0, 0)$. Although height does not influence the hormone level, H_1 is true because age has an effect on the hormone level.

```r
boot_cmp_M1_M2 = function(m1_frml, m2_frml, data, R = 999){
  # M2 must be the smaller model

  # m1_frml - formula for model M1
  # m2_frml - formula for model M2
  # data    - data to be modeled
  # R       - number of MC simulations

  fit_M1 = lm(m1_frml, data = data)
  fit_M2 = lm(m2_frml, data = data)

  # we only need the coefficients that are in M1 an not in M2
  names_extra_coef = setdiff(
    names(coefficients(fit_M1)),
    names(coefficients(fit_M2)))

  # Step (A)
  # coefficients, variances and the Mahalanobis distance
  # for the additional covariates of the larger model M1
  coef_m1 = coefficients(fit_M1)[names_extra_coef]
  S = vcov(fit_M1)[names_extra_coef,names_extra_coef]
  S_inv = solve(S)
  maha_dist = sqrt(t(coef_m1) %*% S_inv %*% coef_m1)[1,1]

  # m is a data.frame containing Y (first column) and all
  # necessary/used covariates
  m = model.frame(fit_M1)

  # Step (B)
  # m[,1] equals covariates times estimate of beta under M2
  m[,1] = fitted.values(fit_M2)
  res = residuals(fit_M2)

  centered_res = res - mean(res)

  get_standardized_beta = function(d, i){
    # This following still belongs to Step (B)
    # here we add an iid sample of the centered residuals, i.e.
    # generating a data set under model M2
    m[,1] = m[,1] + d[i]

    # Step (C)
    # refitting using this new data set under model M1
```

```
      refit = update(fit_M1, data=m)
      coef_refit = coefficients(refit)[names_extra_coef]
      S_boot = vcov(refit)[names_extra_coef,names_extra_coef]
      S_inv_boot = solve(S_boot)

      sqrt(t(coef_refit) %*% S_inv_boot %*% coef_refit)[1,1]
  }
  boot_maha_dist = boot::boot(centered_res, get_standardized_beta,
                              R=R)

  # Step (D)
  c(pvalue = mean(boot_maha_dist$t > maha_dist))
}


set.seed(123,kind ="Mersenne-Twister",normal.kind ="Inversion")
# checking H0: beta(height) = 0, H1: beta(height) != 0
# H0 holds true
boot_cmp_M1_M2(hormone ~ diabetes + age + height,
               hormone ~ diabetes + age, data=hormone_data)



  ##    pvalue
  ## 0.983984

# checking H0: (beta(age), beta(height)) = (0,0),
#            H1: (beta(age), beta(height)) != (0,0)
# H1 holds true
boot_cmp_M1_M2(hormone ~ diabetes + age + height,
               hormone ~ diabetes, data=hormone_data)



  ##      pvalue
  ## 0.005005005
```

5.1.2   LSE Asymptotic

We start this section with an investigation of asymptotic normality of the LSE. In order to apply Cramér-Wold device later on, we provide the following lemma.

Lemma 5.9 *Let* $a^\top = (a_1, \dots, a_p)$ *be a fixed vector. Assume the linear model (5.1) as stated in the introduction. In addition we assume that*

(i) $n^{-1}x^\top x \longrightarrow V$, *for some positive definite* $p \times p$ *matrix* V.

Then, as $n \to \infty$,
$$n^{-1/2}a^\top x^\top \varepsilon \longrightarrow \mathcal{N}(0, \rho^2),$$

where $\rho^2 = \sigma^2 a^\top V a$.

Proof Let $(b_1, \ldots, b_n) = a^\top x^\top$, hence $a^\top x^\top \varepsilon = \sum_{i=1}^n b_i \varepsilon_i$. Since $a^\top x^\top \varepsilon$ is univariate with zero mean, we get by (i) that $\sigma^2 \sum_{i=1}^n b_i^2 = \mathrm{Var}(a^\top x^\top \varepsilon) = \mathbb{E}(a^\top x^\top \varepsilon (a^\top x^\top \varepsilon)^\top) = \sigma^2 a^\top x^\top x a = n\rho^2 + o(n)$. Thus, in order to verify the Lindeberg condition, it suffices to proof

$$\frac{1}{n} \sum_{i=1}^n b_i^2 \int_{\{|\varepsilon_i| > \delta n^{1/2}/|b_i|\}} \varepsilon_i^2 d\mathbb{P} = o(1), \quad \text{for all } \delta > 0.$$

As we have already seen, $n^{-1} \sum_{i=1}^n b_i^2 \to a^\top V a$. This entails, for instance, by contraposition, that $c_n^2 = n^{-1} \max_{i=1,\ldots,n} b_i^2$ converges to zero. Furthermore,

$$\frac{n^{1/2}}{|b_i|} = \frac{1}{n^{-1/2}|b_i|} \geq \frac{1}{c_n} \longrightarrow \infty, \quad \text{as } n \to \infty.$$

Therefore, Lindeberg's condition is fulfilled, since the integrals corresponding to this condition can be bounded by $\mathbb{E}(\varepsilon_1^2 I_{\{|\varepsilon_1| \geq \delta/c_n\}})$ which tends to 0, as $n \to \infty$. This finally completes the proof. □

Theorem 5.10 *Assume the linear model (5.1) as stated in the introduction and that conditions (i) of Lemma 5.9 is fulfilled. Then*

$$n^{1/2}(\hat{\beta}(n) - \beta) \longrightarrow \mathcal{N}(0, \sigma^2 V^{-1}), \quad as \ n \to \infty,$$

in distribution.

Proof Use the representation (5.3) to get

$$n^{1/2}(\hat{\beta}(n) - \beta) = n^{-1/2}(n^{-1}x^\top x)^{-1}x^\top \varepsilon.$$

According to Cramér-Wold device the last lemma implies

$$n^{-1/2}x^\top \varepsilon \longrightarrow \mathcal{N}(0, \sigma^2 V), \quad as \ n \to \infty$$

in distribution. Since $(n^{-1}x^\top x)^{-1} \longrightarrow V^{-1}$, due to (i), we get in summary

$$n^{-1/2}(n^{-1}x^\top x)^{-1}x^\top \varepsilon \longrightarrow \mathcal{N}(0, \sigma^2 V^{-1}) \quad as \ n \to \infty$$

in distribution which completes the proof. □

Theorem 5.11 *Under the assumptions of Theorem 5.10, we get w.p.1*

$$\frac{1}{n}x^\top \varepsilon \longrightarrow 0 \quad and \quad \hat{\beta}(n) \longrightarrow \beta, \quad as \ n \to \infty.$$

Proof Since

$$x^\top \varepsilon = \begin{pmatrix} x_{1,1}\varepsilon_1 + \ldots + x_{n,1}\varepsilon_n \\ \vdots \quad \vdots \quad \vdots \quad \vdots \quad \vdots \\ x_{1,p}\varepsilon_1 + \ldots + x_{n,p}\varepsilon_n \end{pmatrix},$$

we can restrict our considerations to the first coordinate of x and set for notational convenience $x_i \equiv x_{i,1}$. Furthermore, we set

$$S_n = n^{-1} \sum_{i=1}^{n} x_i \varepsilon_i, \quad S_{k,n} = n^{-1} \sum_{i=2^k+1}^{n} x_i \varepsilon_i, \quad \text{for } 2^k < n \leq 2^{k+1},$$

and apply Kolmogorov's inequality to get for $\delta > 0$

$$\mathbb{P}\left(\max_{2^k < n \leq 2^{k+1}} |S_{k,n}| \geq \delta \right) \leq \delta^{-2} 2^{-2k} \sum_{i=2^k+1}^{2^{k+1}} x_i^2 \sigma^2 = O(2^{-k}),$$

since $n^{-1} \sum_{i=1}^{n} x_i^2 \longrightarrow v$ with $v \in \mathbb{R}$.
Similarly,

$$\mathbb{P}\left(|S_{2^k}| \geq \delta \right) = O(2^{-k}).$$

This, together with the Borel-Cantelli Lemma, yields

$$S_{2^k} \longrightarrow 0, \quad \max_{2^k < n \leq 2^{k+1}} |S_{k,n}| \longrightarrow 0$$

w.p.1.
But for $2^k < n \leq 2^{k+1}$ we have

$$|S_n| \leq |S_{k,n}| + |S_{2^k}|$$

which finally proves the first assertion.
For the second assertion use representation (5.3) to get

$$\hat{\beta}(n) - \beta = \left(\frac{1}{n} x^\top x \right)^{-1} n^{-1} x^\top \varepsilon.$$

Application of (i) together with the first part completes the proof.   □

Corollary 5.12 *Under the assumptions of Theorem 5.10 we get w.p.1*

$$s_n^2 \equiv \frac{(Y - x\hat{\beta}(n))^\top (Y - x\hat{\beta}(n))}{n} \xrightarrow[n \to \infty]{} \sigma^2.$$

Proof Note that $\hat{\beta}(n)$ is the LSE and therefore,

$$(Y - x\hat{\beta}(n)) \perp x\gamma$$

for all $\gamma \in \mathbb{R}^p$. Thus

$$
\begin{aligned}
ns_n^2 &= (Y - x\hat{\beta}(n))^\top Y = (Y - x\hat{\beta}(n))^\top (x\beta + \varepsilon) \\
&= (Y - x\hat{\beta}(n))^\top \varepsilon = (x(\beta - \hat{\beta}(n)) + \varepsilon)^\top \varepsilon \\
&= (\beta - \hat{\beta}(n))^\top x^\top \varepsilon + \varepsilon^\top \varepsilon.
\end{aligned}
$$

Now divide both sides by n, use Theorem 5.11 and the SLLN to complete the proof. $\qquad\square$

Next, we consider the vector of the estimated residuals given by

$$\hat{\varepsilon} \equiv (\hat{\varepsilon}_1, \ldots, \hat{\varepsilon}_n)^\top = Y - x\hat{\beta} = x(\beta - \hat{\beta}) + \varepsilon,$$

where we suppressed n of $\hat{\beta}(n)$. Thus,

$$\hat{\varepsilon} - \varepsilon = x(\beta - \hat{\beta})$$

and therefore

$$n^{-1} \sum_{m=1}^{n} (\hat{\varepsilon}_m - \varepsilon_m) = n^{-1} \sum_{m=1}^{n} \sum_{j=1}^{p} x_{m,j} (\beta_j - \hat{\beta}_j).$$

According to assumption (i) of Lemma 5.9 and Cauchy-Schwarz's inequality we get

$$\frac{1}{n} \left| \sum_{m=1}^{n} x_{m,j} \right| \le \left(\frac{1}{n} \sum_{m=1}^{n} x_{m,j}^2 \right)^{1/2} \longrightarrow v_j^{1/2}.$$

Furthermore, $\beta_j - \hat{\beta}_j \longrightarrow 0$ w.p.1 and therefore we obtain

$$\frac{1}{n} \sum_{m=1}^{n} (\hat{\varepsilon}_m - \varepsilon_m) \longrightarrow 0$$

which finally leads to

$$\frac{1}{n} \sum_{m=1}^{n} \hat{\varepsilon}_m \longrightarrow 0 \qquad (5.9)$$

w.p.1.

In summary, Corollary 5.12 together with (5.9) says

Lemma 5.13 *Under the assumptions of Theorem 5.10 let $\hat{F}_n$ be the edf. of the estimated residuals $\hat{\varepsilon}_1, \ldots, \hat{\varepsilon}_n$. Then, w.p.1*

$$\mu_n \equiv \int x\,\hat{F}_n(dx) \longrightarrow 0, \quad s_n^2 = \int x^2\,\hat{F}_n(dx) \longrightarrow \sigma^2.$$

Finally, we want to mention two well-known properties of the LSE.

Lemma 5.14 *Under the assumptions of Theorem 5.10 we have*

$$\mathbb{E}(\hat{\beta}) = \beta, \quad \mathrm{COV}(\hat{\beta}) = \sigma^2(x^\top x)^{-1}.$$

Proof Recall (5.3)

$$\hat{\beta} = \beta + (x^\top x)^{-1}x^\top \varepsilon$$

and take expectation on both sides to get the first equation, since $\mathbb{E}(\varepsilon) = 0$. The second equation we obtain from

$$\mathrm{COV}(\hat{\beta}) = \mathbb{E}\big((\hat{\beta} - \beta)(\hat{\beta} - \beta)^\top\big) = (x^\top x)^{-1}x^\top \mathbb{E}(\varepsilon\varepsilon^\top)x(x^\top x)^{-1}$$
$$= \sigma^2(x^\top x)^{-1},$$

since $\mathbb{E}(\varepsilon\varepsilon^\top) = \sigma^2 I_p$, where I_p denotes the identity matrix of size $p \times p$. □

5.1.3 LSE Bootstrap Asymptotic

In this section, we assume a linear regression model

$$Y(n) = x(n)\beta + \varepsilon(n)$$

such that conditions (i) of Lemma 5.9 are fulfilled. For the bootstrap we use the Resampling Scheme 5.4.

Lemma 5.15 *If the assumptions of Theorem 5.10 are fulfilled we have w.p.1, as* $n \to \infty$,

$$\frac{1}{n}\|\hat{\varepsilon} - \varepsilon\|^2 = \frac{1}{n}\sum_{i=1}^n (\hat{\varepsilon}_i - \varepsilon_i)^2 \longrightarrow 0 \quad \text{and} \quad \frac{1}{n}\|\tilde{\varepsilon} - \varepsilon\|^2 = \frac{1}{n}\sum_{i=1}^n (\tilde{\varepsilon}_i - \varepsilon_i)^2 \longrightarrow 0.$$

Proof Recall from the last section that $\hat{\varepsilon} - \varepsilon = x(\beta - \hat{\beta})$. Thus,

$$\|\hat{\varepsilon} - \varepsilon\|^2 = (\beta - \hat{\beta})^\top x^\top x(\beta - \hat{\beta}).$$

Now, apply Lemma 5.9 and Theorem 5.11 to conclude the first convergence. The second assertion is an immediate consequence of the first part and Lemma 5.13, i.e., $\tilde{\varepsilon}_i - \hat{\varepsilon}_i = \mu_n \to \mathbb{E}(\varepsilon) = 0$ w.p.1. □

Lemma 5.16 *Under the assumptions of Theorem 5.10 we have w.p.1,*

$$\tilde{F}_n \longrightarrow F$$

in distribution, as $n \to \infty$.

Proof Let f be a bounded Lipschitz function, i.e., there exists $0 \le K < \infty$ such that for all $x, y \in \mathbb{R}$:

$$|f(x) - f(y)| \le K|x - y|.$$

It follows

$$\frac{1}{n} \sum_{i=1}^{n} |f(\tilde{\varepsilon}_i) - f(\varepsilon_i)| \le \frac{K}{n} \sum_{i=1}^{n} |\tilde{\varepsilon}_i - \varepsilon_i| \le K \left(\frac{1}{n} \sum_{i=1}^{n} (\tilde{\varepsilon}_i - \varepsilon_i)^2 \right)^{1/2} \longrightarrow 0,$$

as $n \to \infty$, where the last convergence is obtained from Lemma 5.15. Hence

$$\int f(x)\, \tilde{F}_n(\mathrm{d}x) - \int f(x)\, F_n(\mathrm{d}x) \longrightarrow 0, \quad \text{as } n \to \infty,$$

where F_n is the edf. of the true residuals $\varepsilon_1, \ldots, \varepsilon_n$. The assertion follows by applying the SLLN to $\int f(x) F_n(\mathrm{d}x)$. □

In the next theorem, we state the bootstrap version of Theorem 5.10.

Theorem 5.17 *Under the assumption of Theorem 5.10 we have, w.p.1,*

$$n^{1/2}(\beta^*(n) - \hat{\beta}(n)) \longrightarrow \mathcal{N}(0, \sigma^2 V^{-1}), \quad \text{as } n \to \infty.$$

Proof Note first that

$$x^\top x (\beta^*(n) - \hat{\beta}(n)) = x^\top \varepsilon^* = \begin{pmatrix} x_{1,1}\varepsilon_1^* + \ldots + x_{n,1}\varepsilon_n^* \\ \vdots \quad \vdots \quad \vdots \quad \vdots \quad \vdots \\ x_{1,p}\varepsilon_1^* + \ldots + x_{n,p}\varepsilon_n^* \end{pmatrix}.$$

Fix $a \in \mathbb{R}^p$ to obtain, as in the classical situation, i.e., as in the proof of Lemma 5.9,

$$a^\top x^\top \varepsilon^* = \sum_{k=1}^{p} \sum_{m=1}^{n} a_k x_{m,k} \varepsilon_m^* = \sum_{m=1}^{n} \varepsilon_m^* \sum_{k=1}^{p} a_k x_{m,k} = \sum_{m=1}^{n} \varepsilon_m^* b_m.$$

Since $\varepsilon_1^*, \ldots, \varepsilon_n^* \sim \tilde{F}_n$ are i.i.d., the summands on the right-hand side are independent and centered. To prove

$$n^{-1/2} a^\top x^\top \varepsilon^* \longrightarrow \mathcal{N}(0, \rho^2),$$

as $n \to \infty$, where $\rho^2 = \sigma^2 a^\top V a$, we have to verify Lindeberg's condition

$$\frac{1}{n} \sum_{m=1}^{n} b_m^2 \int_{\{|x| \geq \delta n^{1/2}/|b_m|\}} x^2 \, \tilde{F}_n(dx) \longrightarrow 0, \quad \text{as } n \to \infty,$$

for all $\delta > 0$. Compare the proof of Lemma 5.9 to see that it suffices to verify for an arbitrarily chosen fixed δ

$$\int_{\{|x| \geq \delta/c_n\}} x^2 \, \tilde{F}_n(dx) \longrightarrow 0$$

for some $c_n \to 0$. Thus the proof is completed if we can show that

$$\int_{\{|x| \geq K\}} x^2 \, \tilde{F}_n(dx)$$

becomes arbitrarily small if $n \to \infty$ for all constants K large enough. First observe that according to Lemma 5.15 and the SLLN we get

$$\int x^2 \, \tilde{F}_n(dx) \longrightarrow \int x^2 \, F(dx) = \sigma^2, \quad \text{as } n \to \infty,$$

w.p.1. Furthermore, Lemma 5.16 and the continuous mapping theorem (Theorem 5.1, Billingsley (1968)) yields for continuity points K of F that, as $n \to \infty$,

$$\int_{\{|x| < K\}} x^2 \, \tilde{F}_n(dx) \longrightarrow \int_{\{|x| < K\}} x^2 \, F(dx).$$

In summary we therefore conclude that, w.p.1,

$$\int_{\{|x| \geq K\}} x^2 \, \tilde{F}_n(dx) = \int x^2 \, \tilde{F}_n(dx) - \int_{\{|x| < K\}} x^2 \, \tilde{F}_n(dx) \longrightarrow \int_{\{|x| \geq K\}} x^2 \, F(dx),$$

as $n \to \infty$, which completes the proof since the integral on the right-hand side decreases to 0, as $K \to \infty$.   □

5.2 Linear Correlation Model and the Bootstrap

Considering rental prices in Euro, it seems intuitive that rents for small flats differ not as much as rents for very large flats. In such cases, one could assume that the variance of a random variable Y, e.g., rent, depends on the covariate X, e.g., size of the flat in m^2. We now generate a very simple dataset that reflects such a heteroscedasticity using the following structure:

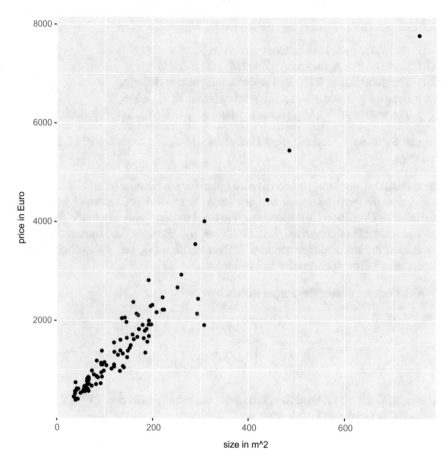

Fig. 5.2 Simulated rent data

$$Y = 10 \cdot \text{size} + \varepsilon(\text{size}),$$

where $\varepsilon(\text{size}) \sim N(0, 4 \cdot \text{size}^2)$.

```
set.seed(123,kind ="Mersenne-Twister",normal.kind ="Inversion")
gen_rents <- function(N = 100){
  data.frame(size = 35 + rexp(n = 100, rate = 1 / 100)) %>%
  dplyr::mutate(price = 100 + 10 * size
  + rnorm(100, mean = 0, sd = 2*size))
}
rents <- gen_rents()
```

Of course, heteroscedasticity may have many faces but the funnel shape as illustrated in Fig. 5.2 is a very typical one.

The following model, compare Stute (1990), allows such a heteroscedastic situation.

Definition 5.18 The linear correlation model fulfills:

(i) $(Y_i, X_i), i \geq 1$, i.i.d. random vectors in $\mathbb{R}^{1+p}$.
(ii) $Y_i = X_i^\top \beta + \varepsilon_i$ for some $\beta^\top = (\beta_1, \ldots, \beta_p) \in \mathbb{R}^p$.
(iii) The matrix $\Sigma = \mathbb{E}(X_i X_i^\top)$ is finite and positive definite.
(iv) For all $i \geq 1$ and $q = 1, \ldots, p$ it holds that $\mathbb{E}(X_{i,q}\varepsilon_i) = 0$.
(v) The matrix $M = (M_{q,s})_{1 \leq q,s \leq p}$, where $M_{qs} = \mathbb{E}(X_{i,q}X_{i,s}\varepsilon_i^2)$ exists.

Remark 5.19 By (i) and (ii) from Definition 5.18 ε_i is a sequence of i.i.d. random variables.

Remark 5.20 Condition (i) and (ii) also holds for the homoscedastic linear regression. Under the fixed design we assumed that $n^{-1}xx^\top \to V$, cf. Lemma 5.9 (i), which is similar to Condition (iii). Moreover, the fixed design implicitly made the covariate and residuals uncorrelated, i.e., Condition (iv). Besides the randomness of the covariates, the major difference now is the condition (v), i.e., we explicitly allow dependency between covariates and residuals.

As before we denote the design matrix by

$$ X = \begin{pmatrix} X_{1,1} & \cdots & X_{1,p} \\ \vdots & \vdots & \vdots \\ X_{n,1} & \cdots & X_{n,p} \end{pmatrix}. $$

Although X_i may be related to ε_i somehow, the usually LSE $\hat{\beta} = (X^\top X)^{-1}X^\top Y$ is a reasonable estimator, i.e., as $n \to \infty$,

$$ \hat{\beta}(n) \to \beta $$

w.p.1 and

$$ n^{1/2}(\hat{\beta}(n) - \beta) \longrightarrow \mathcal{N}(0, \Sigma^{-1}M\Sigma^{-1}), \tag{5.10} $$

in distribution, cf. Sect. 5.2.3. Since X is random, $(X^\top X)^{-1}$ may not exist for fixed n. However, the asymptotic results are not affected by this technical issue. For ease of simplicity, we postpone to address this problem till actually proving the results in the later sections. From the practical point of view, if $(X^\top X)^{-1}$ does not exist for a particular dataset, one could use the Moore-Penrose inverse. It is well known that $\hat{\beta}$ based on the Moore-Penrose inverse minimizes the least square error. However, be aware of the fact that in this case other $\tilde{\beta}$ exist that also minimize the least square error. Hence, interpreting the coefficients is not possible anymore.

Note that the estimator is not unbiased anymore:

$$ \mathbb{E}(\hat{\beta}) = \beta + \mathbb{E}((X^\top X)^{-1}X^\top \varepsilon). \tag{5.11} $$

This bias is technically problematic because the determinant of $(X^{\top}X)^{-1}$ is the inverse of $\det(X^{\top}X)$. Therefore we need that at least the expectation of the inverse of $\det(X^{\top}X)$ exists. For instance, assume that $X^{\top}X = Z$ is a random variable in $\mathbb{R}$ with finite expectation, then $\mathbb{E}(1/Z)$ must not exist. For two dimensions the complexity increases dramatically. Assume that

$$X^{\top}X = \begin{pmatrix} Z_1 & Z_2 \\ Z_2 & Z_3 \end{pmatrix},$$

then we need that $\mathbb{E}\big((Z_1Z_3 - Z_2^2)^{-1}\big)$ must be finite. We will prove, under certain conditions, that $n^{1/2}\mathbb{E}((X^{\top}X)^{-1}X^{\top}\varepsilon) \to 0$, confer to Theorem 5.30. This shows that estimating and bootstrapping the bias is rather an academic exercise than of practical interest. It also allows us to consider the adjusted estimator $\hat{\beta}(n) - \mathbb{E}((X^{\top}X)^{-1}X^{\top}\varepsilon)$, without interfering the asymptotic distribution (5.10).

Unfortunately, Resampling Scheme 5.4 is not appropriate here since it does not reflect the dependence between the error term ε_i and the corresponding X_i. In order to illustrate the inappropriateness of this resampling scheme, i.e., simply resample the residuals, we plot the original generated rent dataset and a dataset that was bootstrapped using Resampling Scheme 5.4, see Fig. 5.3. Especially, the increased variance of the rent for small flats indicates that the bootstrap is not correct. Of course, this results from assigning residuals to small flats that in fact belong to large flats.

```
fit <- lm(price ~ size, data = rents)
rents$type <- "original"
boot_rents <- rents
boot_rents$type <- "residual bootstrap"
boot_rents$price <- fitted(fit) + sample(residuals(fit))
ggplot(data=rbind(rents, boot_rents),
        aes(y = price, x = size, col = type)) +
        xlab("size in m^2") +
        ylab("price in Euro") +
    geom_point() +
    theme(legend.position = "bottom")
```

The following two sections provide resampling schemes that work under the linear correlation model.

5.2.1 Classical Bootstrap

Resampling Scheme 5.4 separates the covariates X_i and the error term ε_i. This is the reason why this scheme, in general, does not work for the linear correlation model, because X_i and ε_i is only uncorrelated, but not independent!

An appropriate resampling scheme is the classical bootstrap that resamples from the set $\{(Y_1, X_1), \ldots, (Y_n, X_n)\}$. This scheme implicitly incorporates the error term.

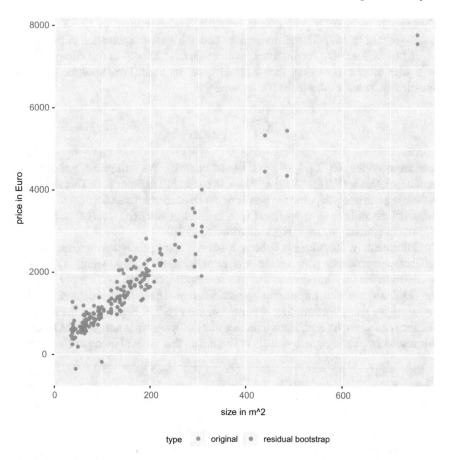

Fig. 5.3 Simulated rent data and a simple bootstrap using only the residuals

Resampling Scheme 5.21

(A) *Based on the observations* $(Y_i, X_i)_{1 \le i \le n}$ *calculate the LSE* $\hat{\beta}$.
(B) *Draw an i.i.d. sample* $(Y_i^*, X_i^*)_{1 \le i \le n}$ *from* $(Y_i, X_i)_{1 \le i \le n}$.
(C) *Compute the LSE of the bootstrap sample, i.e., determine* $\hat{\beta}^* = (X^{*\top} X^*)^{-1}$ $X^{*\top} Y^*$.

Remark 5.22 Although resampling the residuals is not part of the Resampling Scheme 5.21, we want to emphasize that the proof makes explicit usage of resampled residuals defined as $\varepsilon_i^* = Y_i^* - X_i^{*\top} \hat{\beta}$ for $i = 1, \dots, n$.

With the resampled residuals as defined in Remark 5.22 we obtain the usual separation

$$\hat{\beta}^* = (X^{*\top} X^*)^{-1} X^{*\top} Y^* = \hat{\beta} + (X^{*\top} X^*)^{-1} X^{*\top} \varepsilon^*.$$

This presentation is the key to prove Theorem 5.35, i.e.,

$$n^{1/2}(\hat{\beta}^*(n) - \hat{\beta}(n)) \longrightarrow \mathcal{N}(0, \Sigma^{-1} M \Sigma^{-1})$$

in distribution which equals the asymptotic distribution of $n^{1/2}(\hat{\beta}(n) - \beta(n))$. This shows that the classical bootstrap is a reasonable resampling scheme for the linear correlation model. For instance, we have now the theoretical tool to construct confidence intervals or test two models under the Definition 5.18. Taking the covariance matrix for $\hat{\beta}$ stated in this section into account, one can follow the approach we presented for the homoscedastic model, see Sect. 5.1.1.

5.2.1.1 Bias in the Bootstrap World

Looking again at the bias in the bootstrap world, we see that the expectation does not exist, because the probability that all rows of X^* equal the covariate vector of the first sample X_1 is not zero. Therefore, the inverse of $X^{*\top} X^*$ as well as

$$\mathbb{E}_n^*((n^{-1} X^{*\top} X^*)^{-1} n^{-1} X^{*\top} \varepsilon^*)$$

does not exist. An artificial way out could result from the fact that the absolute value of every component of the inverse of $n^{-1} X^{*\top} X^*$ is a ratio of a determinant of sub matrices $n^{-1} X^{*\top} X^*$ and the determinant of $n^{-1} X^{*\top} X^*$. This is based on Cramer's rule for solving linear equations. The determinant of $n^{-1} X^{*\top} X^*$ in the denominator is causing the trouble. Since we know that $\det(n^{-1} X^{*\top} X^*)$ and $\det(n^{-1} X^\top X)$ converge both to the determinant of Σ we could try to substitute the determinant of $n^{-1} X^{*\top} X^*$ in the denominator by the determinant of $n^{-1} X^\top X$ because the last expression is a constant with respect to $\mathbb{E}_n^*$. A more practical way out could be to use the Moore-Penrose pseudo-inverse as an inverse for $X^{*\top} X^*$. A third and more pragmatic option could be to introduce additionally the indicator function that is one if and only if the regular inverse of $n^{-1} X^{*\top} X^*$ exists. In any case one would have to prove at least that

$$n^{1/2} \mathbb{E}_n^*(A_n^{-1} n^{-1} X^{*\top} \varepsilon^*) \to 0$$

w.p. 1, where A_n^{-1} is one of the discussed surrogates for the regular inverse. Otherwise, the bias correction would change the asymptotic distribution.

Under Definition 5.18 for the special case that we have no intercept and only one covariate that is additionally bounded away from zero, the bias can be estimated and used for a correction without disturbing the asymptotic distribution. This can be seen as follows. Note that the assumption $0 < c \leq X_i$ for all i implies that all moments of $\Delta_n = (\sum_{1 \leq i \leq n} X_i^{*2}/n)^{-1} - (\mathbb{E}(X_1^2))^{-1}$ with respect to $\mathbb{E}_n^*$ are finite. For $Z_n^* = \sum_{1 \leq i \leq n} X_i^* \varepsilon_i^*$ we have

$$\left| n^{1/2} \mathbb{E}_n^* \big(\hat{\beta}^*(n) - \hat{\beta}(n) \big) \right| = \left| n^{1/2} \mathbb{E}_n^* \Big(\big(\sum_{1 \le i \le n} X_i^{*2} / n \big)^{-1} n^{-1} Z_n^* \Big) \right|$$

$$= \left| \mathbb{E}_n^* \big((\mathbb{E} X_1^2)^{-1} n^{-1/2} Z_n^* \big) + \mathbb{E}_n^* \big(n^{-1/2} \Delta_n Z_n^* \big) \right|$$

$$= \left| \mathbb{E}_n^* \big(\Delta_n n^{-1/2} Z_n^* \mathbb{I}_{\{|\Delta_n| \le \tau\}} \big) + \mathbb{E}_n^* \big(\Delta_n n^{-1/2} Z_n^* \mathbb{I}_{\{|\Delta_n| > \tau\}} \big) \right|$$

$$\le \tau \, \mathbb{E}_n^* \big(|n^{-1/2} Z_n^*| \big) + \| \Delta_n \|_3^* \cdot \| n^{-1/2} Z_n^* \|_2^* \cdot \| \mathbb{I}_{\{|\Delta_n| > \tau\}} \|_6^*$$

for all $\tau > 0$, where the third equality follows from the fact that $\mathbb{E}_n^*(Z_n^*) = 0$, confer Lemma 5.33 and where $\| \cdot \|_r^*$ denotes the L^r-norm with respect to $\mathbb{E}_n^*$. As we already mentioned $\| \Delta_n \|_3^*$ is bounded. Furthermore, $\| n^{-1/2} Z_n^* \|_2^{*2} = \mathbb{E}_n^*((X_1^* \varepsilon_1^*)^2) \to \mathbb{E}((X_1 \varepsilon_1)^2)$ is also bounded w.p.1. Finally, w.p.1 we have $\mathbb{P}_n^*(|\Delta_n| > \tau) \to 0$ by the WLLN for $n^{-1} \sum_{1 \le i \le n} X_i^{*2}$. Altogether we can conclude that the right-hand side converges to zero.

Interestingly, the next section (much easier) reveals that the bias in the bootstrap world applying the wild bootstrap is zero.

5.2.2 Wild Bootstrap

The backbone for all resampling schemes so far is drawing with replacement directly from the observations or from the estimated residuals. The *wild bootstrap* introduced in this section has a complete different concept. As we already know, we are not allowed to separate the error term and covariates. Therefore, we leave the estimated residuals $\hat{\varepsilon}_i$ and the corresponding covariates X_i together and introduce randomness by multiplying $\hat{\varepsilon}_i$ with a standardized random variable τ. This idea goes back to Wu (1986). For our investigations, we only consider *Rademacher* random variables, i.e., $\tau = -1$ or $\tau = 1$, where both events have probability 1/2.

Resampling Scheme 5.23

(A) *Based on the observations $(Y_i, X_i)_{1 \le i \le n} \subset \mathbb{R}^{1+p}$ calculate the LSE $\hat{\beta}(n)$.*
(B) *Determine the estimated residuals $\hat{\varepsilon}_i = Y_i - X_i^\top \hat{\beta}$.*
(C) *Define the wild bootstrap residuals by $\varepsilon_i^* = \hat{\varepsilon}_i \cdot \tau_i$, where $\tau_1, \ldots, \tau_n$ is an i.i.d. sequence of Rademacher rvs. which is also independent of $(X_1, \varepsilon_1), \ldots, (X_n, \varepsilon_n)$.*
(D) *Set $X_i^* = X_i$, $Y_i^* = X_i^{*\top} \hat{\beta} + \varepsilon_i^*$.*
(E) *Compute $\beta^*(n) = (X^{*\top} X^*)^{-1} X^{*\top} Y^*$, the LSE of the bootstrap sample.*

Of course, other distributions for τ are also possible, but they should have zero mean and variance one. For instance, under certain models the third moments of $n^{1/2}(\hat{\beta} - \beta)$ can be estimated by the bootstrap if $\mathbb{E}^*(\tau^3) = 1$ holds, see Liu (1988).

Changing the way how we resample the data is also reflected by changing from $\mathbb{P}_n^*$ to $\mathbb{P}^*$. $\mathbb{P}_n^*$ was the measure that puts equal mass on all observed data points, whereas $\mathbb{P}^*$ or $\mathbb{E}^*$ consider anything beside the random variables τ_i as constants! For instance, $\mathbb{E}^*(\varepsilon_i^*) = \int \hat{\varepsilon}_i \tau \mathbb{P}^*(d\tau) = \hat{\varepsilon}_i 1/2 - \hat{\varepsilon}_i 1/2 = 0$.

Remark 5.24 It is important to note that $X^*_{i,q}$ and ε^*_i are independent with respect to $\mathbb{P}^*$ for all $q = 1, \ldots, p$. In Definition 5.18 it is only assumed that $X_{i,q}$ and ε_i are uncorrelated for all $q = 1, \ldots, p$.

The implementation of the wild bootstrap is rather simple.

```
WB = function(lm_object){

  # lm_object - a model fit returned by stats::lm

  # Step (B)
  res <- residuals(lm_object)

  # Step (C)
  e = 2 * rbinom(length(res), 1, prob = 0.5) - 1
  res <- res * e

  # Step (D)
  # m is a data.frame containing Y (first column) and all
  # necessary/used covariates
  m <- model.frame(lm_object)
  m[,1] <- fitted.values(lm_object) + res
  # m[,1] equals now the covariates times estimate of beta plus
  # the wild-boostrap-residual

  m
}
```

Applying this algorithm to the rent data is visualized in Fig. 5.4. Clearly the wild bootstrap introduces variation into the dataset and does not change the funnel shape of the original dataset in contrast to the simple algorithm that draws directly from the residuals, see Fig. 5.3. But the bias of least square estimator $\hat{\beta}$, see Eq. (5.11), vanishes for the estimator $\hat{\beta}^*$ when the wild bootstrap is applied. This can be seen as follows. As usual we have $\hat{\beta}^*(n) - \hat{\beta}(n) = (X^{*\top}X^*)^{-1}X^{*\top}\varepsilon^*$. Due to the Resampling Scheme 5.23 we have $X^*_i = X_i$ and

$$\mathbb{E}^*((X^{*\top}X^*)^{-1}X^{*\top}\varepsilon^*) = (X^\top X)^{-1}X^\top \mathbb{E}^*(\varepsilon^*),$$

where the expectation on the right-hand side is zero. Despite of the departure from the original model and the changed properties of the least square estimator, it is shown in Theorem 5.41 that the wild bootstrap can be used to approximate the asymptotic distribution of $\hat{\beta}$, i.e., w.p.1

$$n^{1/2}(\hat{\beta}^*(n) - \hat{\beta}(n)) \longrightarrow \mathcal{N}(0, \Sigma^{-1}M\Sigma^{-1}), \quad \text{as } n \to \infty,$$

in distribution with respect to $\mathbb{P}^*$.

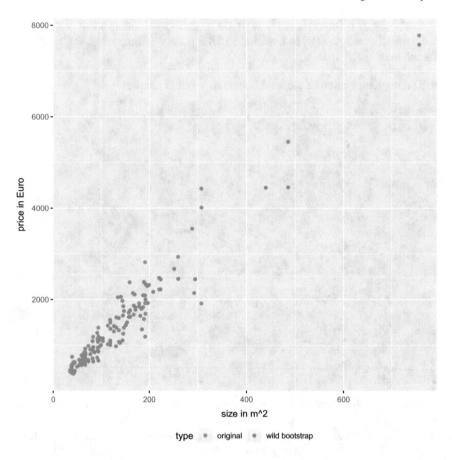

type ● original ● wild bootstrap

Fig. 5.4 Simulated rent data with a dataset obtained by the wild bootstrap

```
set.seed(123,kind ="Mersenne-Twister",normal.kind ="Inversion")
fit <- lm(price ~ size, data = rents)
rents$type <- "original"
wb_rents <-
  fit %>%
  WB %>%
  dplyr::mutate(type = "wild bootstrap")
ggplot(data=rbind(rents, wb_rents),
       aes(y = price, x = size, col = type)) +
       xlab("size in m^2") +
       ylab("price in Euro") +
  geom_point() +
  theme(legend.position = "bottom")
```

Finally, we want to remark that the classical bootstrap and the wild bootstrap can yield under certain circumstances very different bootstrap distributions, see Exercise 5.85.

5.2.3 Mathematical Framework of LSE

As in the regression model, the LSE of β, denoted again by $\hat{\beta}(n) \equiv \hat{\beta}$, equals

$$\hat{\beta} = (X^\top X)^{-1} X^\top Y, \tag{5.12}$$

where we use the Moore-Penrose inverse if $\det(X^\top X)$ equals zero. Within asymptotic considerations this is negligible because

$$n^{-1} X^\top X = n^{-1} \begin{pmatrix} \sum_{i=1}^{n} X_{i,1} X_{i,1} & \cdots & \sum_{i=1}^{n} X_{i,1} X_{i,p} \\ \vdots & \vdots & \vdots \\ \sum_{i=1}^{n} X_{i,p} X_{i,1} & \cdots & \sum_{i=1}^{n} X_{i,p} X_{i,p} \end{pmatrix}$$

and applying the SLLN gives

Lemma 5.25 *Under the assumptions (i) and (iii) of Definition 5.18 it holds w.p.1 that*

$$n^{-1} X^\top X \longrightarrow \Sigma, \quad as\ n \to \infty.$$

Since Σ is positive definite, w.p.1 there exists a $N = N(\omega)$ such that $\det(X^\top X) > \det(\Sigma)/2 > 0$ for all $n > N$. This means that the Moore-Penrose inverse is used at most N times.

Furthermore, we have

$$(X^\top X)(\hat{\beta} - \beta) = X^\top X\big((X^\top X)^{-1} X^\top Y - \beta\big)$$

$$= X^\top \varepsilon = \Big(\sum_{i=1}^{n} X_{i,1} \varepsilon_i, \ldots, \sum_{i=1}^{n} X_{i,p} \varepsilon_i \Big)^\top \tag{5.13}$$

and we can apply the multivariate CLT to obtain

Lemma 5.26 *Under the assumptions in Definition 5.18 it holds that, as $n \to \infty$,*

$$n^{-1/2} (X^\top X)(\hat{\beta} - \beta) = n^{-1/2} X^\top \varepsilon \longrightarrow \mathcal{N}(0, M)$$

in distribution.

Combining the last two lemmas we get from a well-known result of Cramér.

Theorem 5.27 *Under the assumptions in Definition 5.18 it holds that, as $n \to \infty$,*

$$n^{1/2}(\hat{\beta}(n) - \beta) \longrightarrow \mathcal{N}(0, \Sigma^{-1} M \Sigma^{-1})$$

in distribution.

Finally, we have

Theorem 5.28 *Under the assumptions $(i) - (iv)$ in Definition 5.18 it holds w.p.1 that*

$$\hat{\beta}(n) \longrightarrow \beta, \quad as\ n \to \infty.$$

Proof Note that

$$\hat{\beta}(n) = (X^\top X)^{-1} X^\top Y = \beta + (X^\top X)^{-1} X^\top \varepsilon = \beta + (n^{-1} X^\top X)^{-1}(n^{-1} X^\top \varepsilon).$$

Apply Lemma 5.25 and the SLLN, upon observing that $\mathbb{E}(X_{i,j}\varepsilon_i) = 0$, to complete the proof. $\square$

Lemma 5.26 already provided information about the asymptotic distribution of $n^{-1/2} X^\top \varepsilon$, but we even have L^2-convergence.

Lemma 5.29 *Under the assumptions (i)–(iii) and (v) of Definition 5.18 the random variable $n^{-1/2} X^\top \varepsilon$ converge in L^2.*

Proof Consider the q−th component of $n^{-1/2} X^\top \varepsilon$. According to Remark 5.19 and assumption (i) $\{X_{i,q}\varepsilon_i\}_i$ is a sequence of i.i.d. random variables. Therefore we have

$$\mathbb{E}(n^{-1/2} \sum_{i=1}^{n} X_{i,q}\varepsilon_i)^2 = \mathbb{E}(X_{1,q}^2 \varepsilon_1^2) = M_{q,q}.$$

The results follow directly from Vitali's Theorem, see (18) of Theorem 5.5 in Shorack (2000). $\square$

Theorem 5.30 *Denote by $S_{qr}(n)$ the component in the q−th row and r−th column of $(n^{-1} X^\top X)^{-1}$. Assume that $\mathbb{E}(S_{qr}^2(n)) < K < \infty$ for all $1 \le q, r \le p$. Under the Definition 5.18 it holds that $n^{1/2}\mathbb{E}(\hat{\beta}(n) - \beta) \to 0$, as $n \to \infty$.*

Proof We have

$$n^{1/2}\mathbb{E}(\hat{\beta}(n) - \beta) = \mathbb{E}((n^{-1} X^\top X)^{-1} n^{-1/2} X^\top \varepsilon).$$

For notational convenience denote by Z_{nr} the r−th component of $n^{-1/2} X^\top \varepsilon$. The q-th component of $n^{1/2}\mathbb{E}(\hat{\beta}(n) - \beta)$ equals then

$$\mathbb{E}\Big(\sum_{r=1}^{p} S_{qr}(n) Z_{nr}\Big) = \sum_{r=1}^{p} \mathbb{E}(S_{qr}(n) Z_{nr}).$$

The result follows if we show that $\mathbb{E}(S_{qr}(n) Z_{nr})$ converges to zero. According to Lemma 5.25 we have that $S_{qr}(n)$ converges a.s. to some $s \in \mathbb{R}$. Therefore $a_n = S_{qr}(n) - s$ defines a random variable that converges a.s. to zero. Note, by assumption (iv) we have $\mathbb{E}(s Z_{nr}) = 0$. Choosing $\delta > 0$ gives

$$
\begin{aligned}
|\mathbb{E}(S_{qr}(n) Z_{nr})| &= |0 + \mathbb{E}(a_n Z_{nr})| \\
&= \big|\mathbb{E}\big(a_n Z_{nr} I_{\{|a_n| \le \delta\}}\big) + \mathbb{E}\big(a_n Z_{nr} I_{\{|a_n| > \delta\}}\big)\big| \\
&\le \delta \mathbb{E}(|Z_{nr}|) + \big[\mathbb{E}(a_n^2)\, \mathbb{E}\big(Z_{nr}^2 I_{\{|a_n| > \delta\}}\big)\big]^{1/2} \\
&\le \delta \mathbb{E}(Z_{nr}^2)^{1/2} + \big[(K + 2|s| K^{1/2} + s^2)\mathbb{E}\big(Z_{nr}^2 I_{\{|a_n| > \delta\}}\big)\big]^{1/2}.
\end{aligned}
$$

By the Lemma of Pratt, we have that $\mathbb{E}(Z_{nr}^2 I_{\{|a_n| > \delta\}})$ converges to zero because $Z_{nr}^2 I_{\{|a_n| > \delta\}}$ converges a.s. to zero and is bounded by the Z_{nr}^2 which converges in L^2. Since $\delta > 0$ can chosen arbitrarily small and $\mathbb{E}(Z_{nr}^2)$ is constant in n, we obtain altogether that $\mathbb{E}(S_{qr}(n) Z_{nr})$ converges to zero. □

5.2.4 Mathematical Framework of Classical Bootstrapped LSE

As already indicated in the introduction, the resampling procedure for the correlation model cannot be the same as the one stated for the regression model, since the error terms may be correlated to the corresponding design points and therefore it makes no sense to tear them apart.

In the classical bootstrap approach the resampling is done according to F_n, the edf. of the observations. To be precise:

Resampling Scheme 5.31

(A) *Based on the i.i.d. observations $(Y_1, X_1), \ldots, (Y_n, X_n)$ determine the LSE $\hat{\beta}$ and denote with F_n the edf. of the observations. Note that F_n now is a $(p + 1)$−variate edf.*

(B) *Draw the classical bootstrap sample as i.i.d. sample $(Y_1^*, X_1^*), \ldots, (Y_n^*, X_n^*)$ according to F_n and denote with $X^* = X^*(n)$ the corresponding design matrix, precisely*

$$
X^* = \begin{pmatrix} X_{1,1}^* & \cdots & X_{1,p}^* \\ \vdots & \vdots & \vdots \\ X_{n,1}^* & \cdots & X_{n,p}^* \end{pmatrix}.
$$

(C) *Calculate the LSE of the bootstrap sample according to equation (5.12), i.e.,*

$$\hat{\beta}^*(n) = \hat{\beta}^* = (X^{*\top}X^*)^{-1}X^{*\top}Y^*$$

and set

$$\varepsilon_i^* = Y_i^* - X_i^{*\top}\hat{\beta}, \quad for\ 1 \leq i \leq n.$$

Since the calculation of the LSE is not new and due to the simplicity of step (B), we omit the implementation of this resampling scheme.

To prove that the bootstrap approximation holds, we follow the approach Stute (1990) and mimic the proof given in the section above.

Lemma 5.32 *Under the assumptions (i) and (iii) of Definition 5.18 it holds w.p.1 for Resampling Scheme 5.31 that, as $n \to \infty$,*

$$\mathbb{P}_n^*\left(\|\,n^{-1}X^{*\top}X^* - \Sigma\,\| > \varepsilon\right) \longrightarrow 0, \qquad for\ each\ \varepsilon > 0.$$

Proof Note that

$$n^{-1}X^{*\top}X^* = n^{-1}\begin{pmatrix} \sum\limits_{i=1}^{n} X_{i,1}^* X_{i,1}^* & \cdots & \sum\limits_{i=1}^{n} X_{i,1}^* X_{i,p}^* \\ \vdots & \vdots & \vdots \\ \sum\limits_{i=1}^{n} X_{i,p}^* X_{i,1}^* & \cdots & \sum\limits_{i=1}^{n} X_{i,p}^* X_{i,p}^* \end{pmatrix},$$

where each component of the matrix is an i.i.d. sum with finite first moment given by the corresponding component of Σ. Thus, we can apply WLLN (Theorem 3.7) to complete the proof. $\qquad\square$

Lemma 5.33 *Under the assumptions (i) and (ii) of Definition 5.18 and Resampling Scheme 5.31 it holds w.p.1 for all $1 \leq q \leq p$ and $1 \leq i \leq n$ that*

$$\mathbb{E}_n^*(X_{i,q}^* \varepsilon_i^*) = 0.$$

Proof Due to the given Resampling Scheme 5.31 we get

$$\mathbb{E}_n^*(X_{i,q}^* \varepsilon_i^*) = n^{-1}\sum_{k=1}^{n} X_{k,q}(Y_k - X_k^\top \hat{\beta}).$$

But $\hat{\beta}$ is by definition chosen such that $X\hat{\beta}$ is the projection of Y onto the space spanned by the columns of X. Thus, if we take column q of X it has to be perpendicular to $Y - X\hat{\beta}$. Since the sum on the right-hand side equals the inner product of column q of X with $Y - X\hat{\beta}$, this sum has to be 0. $\qquad\square$

Lemma 5.34 *Under Definition 5.18 it holds for the Resampling Scheme 5.31 w.p.1 that*

$$n^{-1/2} X^{*\top} \varepsilon^* \longrightarrow \mathcal{N}(0, M), \quad as \ n \to \infty,$$

in distribution with respect to $\mathbb{P}_n^*$.

Proof To prove the Lemma we will use the Cramér-Wold device, i.e., we have to show that w.p.1

$$n^{-1/2} a^\top X^{*\top} \varepsilon^* \longrightarrow \mathcal{N}(0, a^\top M a), \quad as \ n \to \infty,$$

for all $0 \neq a \in \mathbb{R}^p$.
According to the resampling scheme and the definition of ε^* we get that

$$X^{*\top} \varepsilon^* = \sum_{k=1}^n \begin{pmatrix} X_{k,1}^* \varepsilon_k^* \\ \vdots \\ X_{k,p}^* \varepsilon_k^* \end{pmatrix}$$

is a sum of i.i.d. random vectors which are centered as we have seen in Lemma 5.33. Now, for an arbitrarily chosen $0 \neq a \in \mathbb{R}^p$ we set

$$Z_n^* = n^{-1/2} a^\top X^{*\top} \varepsilon^* = n^{-1/2} \sum_{k=1}^n \sum_{q=1}^p a_q X_{k,q}^* \varepsilon_k^*$$

which consists, for a given n, of the i.i.d. rvs. $(\sum_{q=1}^p a_q X_{k,q}^* \varepsilon_k^*)_{1 \leq k \leq n}$. Since $X_{k,q}^* \varepsilon_k^*$ is centered, see Lemma 5.33, we obtain

$$\mathrm{VAR}_n^*(Z_n^*) = \mathbb{E}_n^* \Big(\Big(\sum_{q=1}^p a_q X_{1,q}^* \varepsilon_1^* \Big)^2 \Big) = \sum_{q=1}^p \sum_{r=1}^p a_q a_r \mathbb{E}_n^* \big(X_{1,q}^* \varepsilon_1^* X_{1,r}^* \varepsilon_1^* \big)$$

$$= \sum_{q=1}^p \sum_{r=1}^p a_q a_r \Big(n^{-1} \sum_{i=1}^n X_{i,q} X_{i,r} (Y_i - X_i^\top \hat{\beta})^2 \Big).$$

From $\hat{\beta} \to \beta$ w.p.1, see Theorem 5.28, we get w.p.1 from the SLLN

$$\mathrm{VAR}_n^*(Z_n^*) \longrightarrow \sum_{q=1}^p \sum_{r=1}^p a_q a_r M_{q,r} = a^\top M a, \quad as \ n \to \infty.$$

Thus, it remains to show that Lindeberg's condition holds, i.e., w.p.1 for every $\delta > 0$

$$\int_{\{|\sum_{q=1}^p a_q X_{1,q}^* \varepsilon_1^*| \geq \delta n^{1/2}\}} \Big(\sum_{q=1}^p a_q X_{1,q}^* \varepsilon_1^* \Big)^2 \, d\mathbb{P}_n^* \longrightarrow 0 \quad as \ n \to \infty.$$

Replace $\delta n^{1/2}$ by a constant $K > 0$. Then, we obtain from the SLLN and Theorem 5.28 that w.p.1

$$
\int_{\{|\sum_{q=1}^{p} a_q X_{1,q}^* \varepsilon_1^*| \geq K\}} \Big(\sum_{q=1}^{p} a_q X_{1,q}^* \varepsilon_1^*\Big)^2 \, d\mathbb{P}_n^* \longrightarrow \int_{\{|\sum_{q=1}^{p} a_q X_{1,q} \varepsilon_1| \geq K\}} \Big(\sum_{q=1}^{p} a_q X_{1,q} \varepsilon_1\Big)^2 \, d\mathbb{P}
$$

which can be made arbitrarily small if $K \to \infty$. This finally proves the lemma. □

Our final theorem of this chapter together with Theorem 5.27 shows that the bootstrap approximation based on the Resampling Scheme 5.31 works.

Theorem 5.35 *Under Definition 5.18 it holds for the Resampling Scheme 5.31 w.p.1 that*

$$
n^{1/2}(\hat{\beta}^*(n) - \hat{\beta}(n)) \longrightarrow \mathcal{N}(0, \Sigma^{-1} M \Sigma^{-1}), \quad as\ n \to \infty,
$$

in distribution with respect to $\mathbb{P}_n^*$.

Proof First note that due to Lemma 5.32,

$$
I_{\{\det(X^{*\top} X^*)=0\}} = o_{\mathbb{P}_n^*}(1).
$$

Recall the definition of $\hat{\beta}^*$ to verify

$$
\begin{aligned}
n^{1/2}(\hat{\beta}^*(n) - \hat{\beta}(n)) &= I_{\{\det(X^{*\top} X^*)\neq 0\}} n^{1/2}(\hat{\beta}^*(n) - \hat{\beta}(n)) + o_{\mathbb{P}_n^*}(1) \\
&= I_{\{\det(X^{*\top} X^*)\neq 0\}} n^{1/2}\big((X^{*\top} X^*)^{-1} X^{*\top}(X^* \hat{\beta} + \varepsilon^*) - \hat{\beta}\big) + o_{\mathbb{P}_n^*}(1) \\
&= I_{\{\det(X^{*\top} X^*)\neq 0\}} n^{1/2}(X^{*\top} X^*)^{-1} X^{*\top} \varepsilon^* + o_{\mathbb{P}_n^*}(1) \\
&= I_{\{\det(X^{*\top} X^*)\neq 0\}} (n^{-1} X^{*\top} X^*)^{-1} (n^{-1/2} X^{*\top} \varepsilon^*) + o_{\mathbb{P}_n^*}(1).
\end{aligned}
$$

Now, apply Lemma 5.32 and Lemma 5.34 to complete the proof. □

5.2.5   Mathematical Framework of Wild Bootstrapped LSE

Recall that the resampling scheme of the wild bootstrap, RSS 5.23, introduces variability by generating an i.i.d. sequence, $(\tau_i)_{i\geq 1}$, of Rademacher rvs. that is additionally independent of the data we want to analyze. Consequently, $\mathbb{P}^*$ or $\mathbb{E}^*$ consider anything beside the (wild bootstrap) random variables τ_i as constants! For instance, $\mathbb{E}^*(\varepsilon_i^*) = \int \hat{\varepsilon}_i \tau \, \mathbb{P}^*(d\tau) = \hat{\varepsilon}_i 1/2 - \hat{\varepsilon}_i 1/2 = 0$. Furthermore, due to the resampling scheme, $X^{*\top} X^* = X^\top X$, which implies w.p.1 that it is not invertible at most a finite number of times, see Sect. 5.2.3.

Remark 5.36 We want to remark that the classical boostrap and the wild bootstrap can yield under certain circumstances very different boostrap distributions and therefore also very different confidence intervals, see Exercise 5.85

Lemma 5.37 *Under Assumption (i) and (iii) of Definition 5.18 using Resampling Scheme 5.23 it holds w.p.1 that*

$$\mathbb{P}^*\left(\| n^{-1}X^{*\top}X^* - \Sigma \| > \varepsilon\right) \longrightarrow 0, \quad as \; n \to \infty,$$

for each $\varepsilon > 0$.

The proof is left to the reader in Exercise 5.89.

Lemma 5.38 *Under assumption (i) and (iii) of Definition 5.18 using Resampling Scheme 5.23 it holds w.p.1 for all $1 \leq q \leq p$ and $1 \leq i \leq n$ w.p.1 that*

$$\mathbb{E}^*(X_{i,q}^* \varepsilon_i^*) = 0.$$

The proof is left to the reader in Exercise 5.90.

Remark 5.39 Note that Lemma 5.38 holds even if the covariates and residuals are correlated. This means that the wild bootstrap in any case forces the covariates and residuals to be uncorrelated. In fact, we even have that the covariates and the residuals are independent!

Lemma 5.40 *Under Definition 5.18 using Resampling Scheme 5.23 it holds w.p.1 that*
$$n^{-1/2}X^{*\top}\varepsilon^* \longrightarrow \mathcal{N}(0, M), \quad as \; n \to \infty,$$

in distribution with respect to $\mathbb{P}^*$.

Proof Due to the Cramér-Wold device it suffices to show

$$n^{-1/2}a^\top X^{*\top}\varepsilon^* \longrightarrow \mathcal{N}(0, a^\top Ma).$$

According to Lemma 5.40 $n^{-1/2}a^\top X^{*\top}\varepsilon^*$ is centered. We will now verify the Lindeberg condition. Let $Z_{ni} = \sum_{q=1}^{p} n^{-1/2}a_q X_{i,q}\hat{\varepsilon}_i \tau_i$, then $n^{-1/2}a^\top X^{*\top}\varepsilon^* = \sum_{i=1}^{n} Z_{ni}$. Setting $s_n^2 = \sum_{i=1}^{n} \text{VAR}^*(Z_{ni})$, we have to prove that, w.p.1

$$\frac{1}{s_n^2}\sum_{i=1}^{n}\int_{|Z_{ni}|>\varepsilon s_n} Z_{ni}^2 d\mathbb{P}^* \longrightarrow 0, \quad as \; n \to \infty,$$

holds for all $\varepsilon > 0$.
We first show, that $s_n^2 \to a^\top Ma$.

$$s_n^2 = \sum_{i=1}^n \text{VAR}^*(Z_{ni}) = \sum_{i=1}^n \text{VAR}^* \Big(\sum_{q=1}^p n^{-1/2} a_q X_{i,q} \hat{\varepsilon}_i \tau_i \Big)$$

$$= n^{-1} \sum_{i=1}^n \sum_{q,s=1}^p a_q a_s X_{i,q} X_{i,s} \hat{\varepsilon}_i^2 \text{VAR}^*(\tau_i)$$

$$= \sum_{q,s=1}^p n^{-1} \sum_{i=1}^n a_q a_s X_{i,q} X_{i,s} (Y_i - X_i^\top \hat{\beta})^2.$$

From $\hat{\beta} \to \beta$ w.p.1, see Theorem 5.28, we get w.p.1 from the SLLN that $s_n^2 \to a^\top M a$. We focus now on the sum of the Lindeberg condition. Due to the very simple structure of $\mathbb{P}^*$ we can easily integrate with respect to $\mathbb{P}^*$, i.e.,

$$\sum_{i=1}^n \int_{|Z_{ni}|>\varepsilon s_n} Z_{ni}^2 d\mathbb{P}^* = \sum_{i=1}^n \Big(\sum_{q=1}^p n^{-1/2} a_q X_{i,q} \hat{\varepsilon}_i \Big)^2 \mathbb{I}_{\{|\sum_{q=1}^p n^{-1/2} a_q X_{i,q} \hat{\varepsilon}_i | > \varepsilon s_n \}}$$

$$= n^{-1} \sum_{i=1}^n \Big(\sum_{q=1}^p a_q X_{i,q} \hat{\varepsilon}_i \Big)^2 \mathbb{I}_{\{|\sum_{q=1}^p a_q X_{i,q} \hat{\varepsilon}_i | > n^{1/2} \varepsilon s_n \}}.$$

As we have just seen $n^{-1} \sum_{i=1}^n (\sum_{q=1}^p a_q X_{i,q} \hat{\varepsilon}_i)^2 \to a^\top M a$ w.p.1. Therefore,

$$\sum_{i=1}^n \int_{|Z_{ni}|>\varepsilon s_n} Z_{ni}^2 d\mathbb{P}^* \to 0, \quad \text{as } n \to \infty,$$

w.p.1, which verifies the Lindeberg condition and finishes the proof.   □

Finally, we show that $\hat{\beta}^*$ from Resampling Scheme 5.23 has asymptotically the same distribution as $\hat{\beta}$ under the linear correlation model, see Theorem 5.27. Using Lemma 5.37 and Lemma 5.40 we can follow the proof of Theorem 5.35 to obtain the following.

Theorem 5.41 *Under Definition 5.18 using Resampling Scheme 5.23 it holds w.p.1 that*

$$n^{1/2}(\hat{\beta}^*(n) - \hat{\beta}(n)) \longrightarrow \mathcal{N}(0, \Sigma^{-1} M \Sigma^{-1}), \quad \text{as } n \to \infty,$$

in distribution with respect to $\mathbb{P}^*$.

5.3 Generalized Linear Model (Parametric)

In order to motivate the generalized linear model assume we have n independent univariate outcomes $Y_1, \ldots, Y_n$ with n corresponding p-dimensional covariate vectors $x_1, \ldots, x_n$. Within the framework of a classical linear model it is assumed that there exists a vector $\beta = (\beta_1, \ldots, \beta_p)^\top$ such that $Y_i = \beta^\top x_i + \varepsilon_i$ with normal distributed error terms ε_i. A different way to represent this situation is to say that the regression function $\mathbb{E}(Y|X = x) = \beta^\top x$ holds and Y given X follows a normal distribution. In a parametric generalized linear model other distributions beside the normal distributions are allowed. Depending on the distribution, $\mathbb{E}(Y|X = x)$ may be bounded, e.g., $\mathbb{E}(Y|X = x) \in [0, 1]$ if Y given X is Bernoulli distributed. Since $\beta^\top x$ is unbounded, a so-called link function g ensures that the expectation and the covariates are related in an appropriate way, i.e., $g(\mathbb{E}(Y|X = x)) = \beta^\top x$. The most common distributions used are binomial-, Poisson-, negative-binomial-, Gaussian-, gamma- and inverse gamma-distribution, which all belong to the larger family of exponential distributions with dispersion, see Sect. 5.3.1 for the definition. In general, an additional parameter ϕ, the "dispersion" parameter, is necessary to fully specify the distribution of Y. For instance, $\phi = \sigma^2$ for the Gaussian-distribution. For this introduction, let $F(y|x, \beta, \phi)$ denote the distribution function of Y given x, β and ϕ.

After fitting the model using the maximum likelihood approach the (estimated) distribution of Y is fully specified and can be used to generate new observations. This is the backbone of the resampling scheme that we formulate now.

Resampling Scheme 5.42

(A) Calculate the MLE $\hat{\beta}_n$ (and if unknown $\hat{\phi}_n$) for $(Y_1, X_1), \ldots, (Y_n, X_n)$. Note, if ϕ is known, for instance in the binomial model, still denote the parameter by $\hat{\phi}_n$.

(B) Set $X_{k;i}^* = X_i$ for all $i = 1, \ldots, n$ and all $k = 1, \ldots, m$.

(C) Generate $Y_{k;i}^*$ (independent) according to the distribution $F(y|X_{k;i}^*, \hat{\beta}_n, \hat{\phi}_n)$ for all $i = 1, \ldots, n$ and all $k = 1, \ldots, m$.

(D) Calculate the MLE $\hat{\beta}_{k;n}^*$ for $(Y_{k;1}^*, X_{k;1}^*), \ldots, (Y_{k;n}^*, X_{k;n}^*)$ for all $k = 1, \ldots, m$.

Fortunately, R provides a method to generate Y's from a model fit. This makes the implementation of this resampling scheme very easy.

```
model_parametric_boot <- function(model, data, B = 1000) {

  # Step A
  # was already performed and the result is passed
  # to this function via the parameter 'model'
  data_boot <- data

  # get the name of the dependent variable
  y_name <- all.vars(formula(model), max.names = 1)

  ret <- sapply(seq_len(B), function(i) {
    # Step C
    data_boot[[y_name]] <- simulate(model)[,1]

    # Step D
    m_boot <- update(model, formula. = formula(model),
                     data = data_boot)
    coefficients(m_boot)
  })
```

```
    ret
}
```

R-Example 5.43   Theorem 5.60 shows that the sampling distribution of $\hat{\beta}_n$ (see Theorem 5.55) can be approximated by the sampling distribution of $\hat{\beta}_n^*$. We already implemented the Resampling Scheme 5.42 after its definition and reuse it now to calculate a bootstrap confidence intervals for $\hat{\beta}_n$.

```
fit = glm(hormone ~ age + diabetes, data = hormone_data,
          family = gaussian())
set.seed(123,kind ="Mersenne-Twister",normal.kind ="Inversion")
beta.boot = model_parametric_boot(fit, hormone_data, B = 1000)
```

For the confidence intervals, we simply calculate the 2.5% and 97.5% quantiles of each component of $\hat{\beta}_{k;n}^*$, $k = 1, \ldots, 1000$.

```
apply(beta.boot, 1, quantile, c(0.025, 0.975)) %>% t
```

```
##                     2.5%        97.5%
## (Intercept) 99.62433768 101.7633860
## age          0.03263374   0.1124009
## diabetesT2  -3.67543183  -0.7334442
```

For plausibility purpose, we use the functions R provides to calculate another confidence interval for the components of $\hat{\beta}_n$. According to the documentation this confidence interval is based on the profile (likelihood).

```
confint(fit)
```

```
## Waiting for profiling to be done...
```

```
##                    2.5 %       97.5 %
## (Intercept) 99.65765055 101.7724396
## age          0.03054754   0.1119628
## diabetesT2  -3.71372111  -0.7260019
```

Obviously, the two methods yield quite similar confidence intervals.

Example 5.44 **Bike sharing data, part 1.**   The following analysis is a bit more elaborated and we will reuse it in the next chapter to illustrate goodness-of-fit (GOF) testing for generalized linear models. It is a real-world dataset,[1] see Fanaee-T and Gama (2013), that can be downloaded from the Machine Learning Repository at the University of California, Irvine, see Dua and Graff (2017). The downloaded files contain information about ridership of registered and casual users in Washington D.C.

---

[1] https://archive.ics.uci.edu/ml/datasets/Bike+Sharing+Dataset

on an hourly and daily basis. For our analysis, we focus on the information per day
and on the ridership of the registered users only. Beside the number of rented bikes
the dataset provides further important information. For instance, it was recorded if
a particular date was a holiday or a working day and various information about the
weather is provided. This is the variable description from the website

instant:	record index
dteday:	date
season:	season (1:springer, 2:summer, 3:fall, 4:winter)
yr:	year (0: 2011, 1:2012)
mnth:	month (1 to 12)
hr:	hour (0 to 23)
holiday:	whether day is holiday or not
	(extracted from https://dchr.dc.gov/page/holiday-schedule)
weekday:	day of the week
workingday:	if day is neither weekend nor holiday is 1, otherwise is 0.
weathersit:	1:= Clear, Few clouds, Partly cloudy, Partly cloudy
	2:= Mist + Cloudy, Mist + Broken clouds, Mist + Few clouds, Mist
	3:= Light Snow, Light Rain + Thunderstorm + Scattered clouds, Light Rain + Scattered clouds
	4:= Heavy Rain + Ice Pallets + Thunderstorm + Mist, Snow + Fog
temp:	Normalized temperature in Celsius. The values are derived via $(t - t_{min})/(t_{max} - t_{min})$, $t_{min} = -8$, $t_{max} = +39$ (only in hourly scale)
atemp:	Normalized feeling temperature in Celsius. The values are derived via $(t - t_{min})/(t_{max} - t_{min})$, $t_{min} = -16$, $t_{max} = +50$ (only in hourly scale)
hum:	Normalized humidity. The values are divided to 100 (max)
windspeed:	Normalized wind speed. The values are divided to 67 (max)
casual:	count of casual users
registered:	count of registered users
cnt:	count of total rental bikes including both casual and registered

First, we create some model candidates. Since it is a real dataset, a bit of data
wrangling is necessary before we can model the dataset. For instance, one entry
for humidity is zero. We create a new variable *hum_imp* that replaces this particular
entry by the average humidity for the corresponding month. Furthermore, the feeling
temperature shows a very unusual value of 0.24. From a univariate point of view a
value of 0.24 is not very unusual, but in the context of the other variables, a warm day
in August, that measurement seems to be far too low, see Fig. 5.5. It is reasonable that
the feeling temperature is an important factor for ridership. Fortunately, the feeling
temperature is highly correlated with the variable *temp*. Therefore, we can easily
restrict the model activities in this initial phase to *temp*. Renting a bike is probably
less likely if it is too cold or too hot. The same is probably true for humidity, i.e.,
too damp or too dry, therefore quadratic terms may improve the model. The dataset

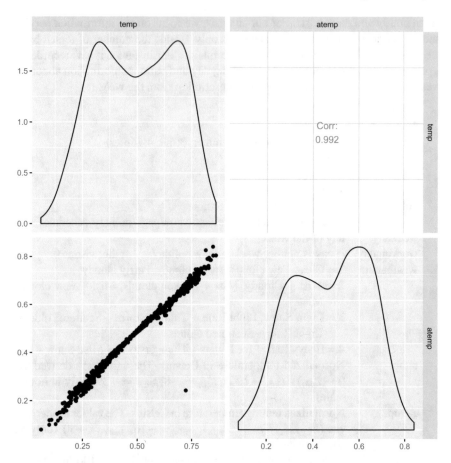

Fig. 5.5 Scatterplot and correlation of normalized temperature and normalized feeling temperature. The scatterplot reveals a very unexpected point

already provides a variable that is one for holidays. But people tend to take a vacation on bridge days or take a vacation for certain periods like the days between christmas and new year. If we assume that most of the registered riders rent bikes on their workdays a further variable that is one for such days may also improve the model. In order to keep it simple, only a variable christmas is created that is one for days between christmas and new year. We now import and preprocess the data

```
data_preprocess <- function(dt){
  dt %>%
    dplyr::mutate_at(
      as.factor,    # adapt the data-type of various variables
      .vars = dplyr::vars(season, yr, mnth, holiday, weekday,
                          workingday, weathersit)) %>%
    dplyr::mutate(
```

```
    # set humidity of 0 to missing
    hum = ifelse(hum == 0, NA, hum),
    christmas = as.factor(
    # one between chritmas and new year, zero otherwise
        lubridate::month(dteday) == 12 &
            dplyr::between(lubridate::day(dteday), 24, 31)')) %>%
    dplyr::group_by(yr, mnth) %>%
    # replace missing humidity with the
    # average for that particular year and month
    dplyr::mutate(
      hum_imp = ifelse(is.na(hum),
                        mean(hum, na.rm = TRUE),
                        hum)) %>%
    dplyr::ungroup() %>%
    # rename dependent variable to 'y'
    dplyr::rename(y = registered) %>%
    dplyr::select(-instant, -casual, -cnt)
}

ridership <- readr::read_csv("day.csv") %>%
  data_preprocess()

## Parsed with column specification:
## cols(
##   instant = col_double(),
##   dteday = col_date(format = ""),
##   season = col_double(),
##   yr = col_double(),
##   mnth = col_double(),
##   holiday = col_double(),
##   weekday = col_double(),
##   workingday = col_double(),
##   weathersit = col_double(),
##   temp = col_double(),
##   atemp = col_double(),
##   hum = col_double(),
##   windspeed = col_double(),
##   casual = col_double(),
##   registered = col_double(),
##   cnt = col_double()
## )
```

Plotting ridership against time reveals (as expected) a seasonal effect but also that ridership is constantly increasing (taking the season into account), see Fig. 5.6. This could be a result of growing business, where the bike sharing system started around 2011 and getting more popular until the end of 2012.

```
ridership %>%
  ggplot(aes(x = dteday, y = y)) +
  geom_point(aes(color = season)) +
  geom_vline(xintercept = lubridate::ymd("2012-10-29"))
```

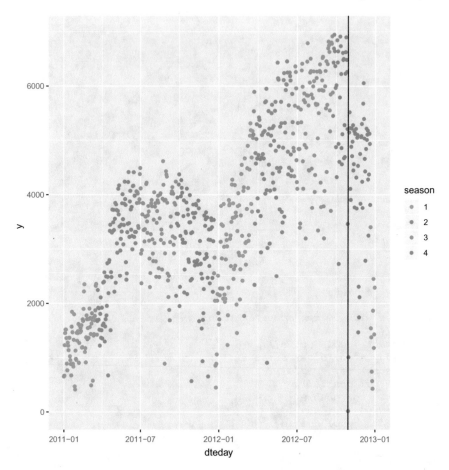

Fig. 5.6 Ridership versus time. Colored according to the seasons. The vertical line shows the date 2012-10-29, when Hurricane Sandy hits the east coast

Therefore an interaction term between *yr* and *season* might be helpful. We also see that a few time points (also left of the vertical line) show unusual low rider ships. Actually, one should check if those dates are related to certain events in or around Washington, DC like concerts, sport events, alerts, etc. Instead of checking all of them we restrict our investigations to the observation with nearly zero ridership. Furthermore, the vertical line indicates that after this observation the ridership recovers only partly. Of course, one must be careful to not over-interpret such patterns. However, looking at that odd observation via

```
ridership %>%
  dplyr::filter(y == 20) %>%
  t()
```

```
##                    [,1]
## dteday        "2012-10-29"
## season        "4"
## yr            "1"
## mnth          "10"
## holiday       "0"
## weekday       "1"
## workingday    "1"
## weathersit    "3"
## temp          "0.44"
## atemp         "0.4394"
## hum           "0.88"
## windspeed     "0.3582"
## y             "20"
## christmas     "FALSE"
## hum_imp       "0.88"
```

The most striking is *weathersit*= 3 and searching the internet for date 2012-10-29 quickly reveals that hurricane "Sandy" hit the east coast and according to Homeland Security and Emergency Management Agency, the Mayor of Washington, DC declared the "state of emergency" on 2012-10-26. This explains the large drop and of course the effect of this incident lasts at least for few days. But that the ridership did not recover fully is a bit unexpected. One explanation could be that the infrastructure of the bike sharing service was partly destroyed so that it was not possible to rent a bike at a certain places or simple a fraction of the bikes were destroyed during the hurricane. In order to make a reasonable model even for the time after hurricane "Sandy" it would be helpful to have a discussion with the people maintaining the bike sharing system. Anyway, we choose the simple approach and consider only ridership till hurricane "Sandy".

```
ridership <-
  ridership %>%
  dplyr::filter(dteday < lubridate::ymd("2012-10-29"))
```

Since ridership is count data, the Poisson- or negative-binomial-distribution are natural candidates. The univariate distribution of ridership is more or less symmetric. Hence, we also try the normal distribution as a potential candidate. It is also a common practice to model the logarithm of the dependent variable. Though this is usually done if the dependent variable is skewed, we want to do it anyway, especially for the GOF test in the next chapter. Therefore, we also try the normal distribution for the log-transformed ridership data. The above considerations about the ridership are forged into a formula that is used for the different models:

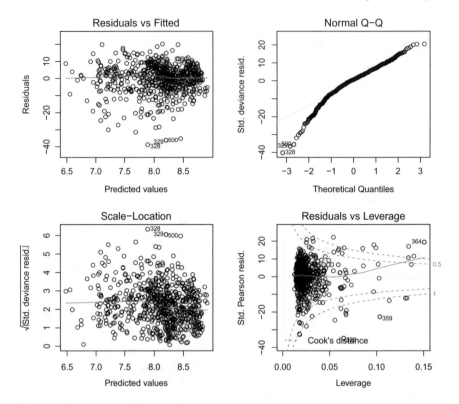

Fig. 5.7 Diagnostic plots for the Poisson model of the ridership

```
frml <- y ~ temp + I(temp^2) + hum_imp + I(hum_imp^2) +
  windspeed + yr*season + workingday +
  weathersit + holiday + christmas
```

For instance, the quadratic term reflects that the ridership is low if it is to damp/dry
or hot/cold. We start with the Poisson model

```
fit_poi <- glm(frml, data = ridership, family = poisson())
summary(fit_poi)
```

```
##
## Call:
## glm(formula = frml, family = poisson(), data = ridership)
##
## Deviance Residuals:
##      Min       1Q    Median       3Q      Max
## -38.828   -4.156    0.631    4.981   20.098
##
```

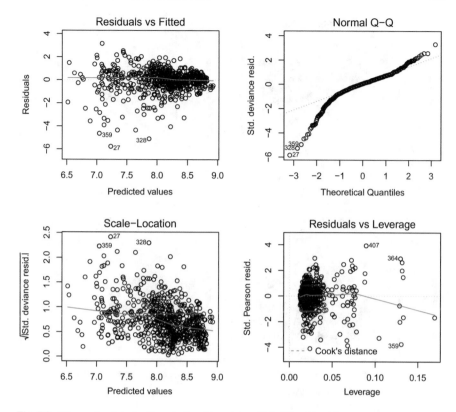

Fig. 5.8 Diagnostic plots for the negative-binomial-model of the ridership

```
## Coefficients:
##
##                Estimate Std. Error   z value  Pr(>|z|)
## (Intercept)    6.045130   0.013906   434.728  < 2e-16 ***
## temp           4.624398   0.030017   154.057  < 2e-16 ***
## I(temp^2)     -3.731145   0.028160  -132.498  < 2e-16 ***
## hum_imp        1.204983   0.040369    29.849  < 2e-16 ***
## I(hum_imp^2)  -1.306540   0.032813   -39.818  < 2e-16 ***
## windspeed     -0.577589   0.009566   -60.376  < 2e-16 ***
## yr1            0.682619   0.003612   188.972  < 2e-16 ***
## season2        0.357664   0.004114    86.941  < 2e-16 ***
## season3        0.437418   0.004495    97.318  < 2e-16 ***
## season4        0.508134   0.003875   131.117  < 2e-16 ***
## workingday1    0.263993   0.001525   173.068  < 2e-16 ***
## weathersit2   -0.077092   0.001796   -42.920  < 2e-16 ***
## weathersit3   -0.483941   0.006381   -75.840  < 2e-16 ***
## holiday1      -0.040959   0.004735    -8.650  < 2e-16 ***
```

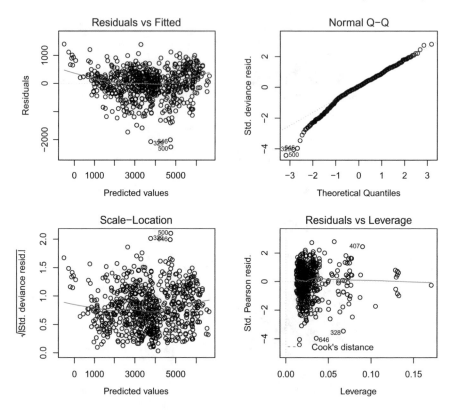

Fig. 5.9 Diagnostic plots for the Gaussian model of the ridership

```
## christmasTRUE  -0.076190     0.009709    -7.847  4.25e-15  ***
## yr1:season2     -0.255720     0.004329   -59.067   < 2e-16  ***
## yr1:season3     -0.252835     0.004255   -59.416   < 2e-16  ***
## yr1:season4     -0.222000     0.004605   -48.214   < 2e-16  ***
## ---
## Signif. codes:
## 0 '***' 0.001 '**' 0.01 '*' 0.05 '.' 0.1 ' ' 1
##
## (Dispersion parameter for poisson family taken to be 1)
##
##     Null deviance: 473082  on 666  degrees of freedom
## Residual deviance:  46065  on 649  degrees of freedom
## AIC: 52718
##
## Number of Fisher Scoring iterations: 4
```

The fitted negative-binomial model is

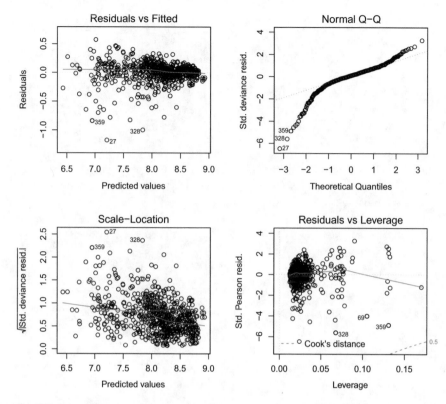

Fig. 5.10 Diagnostic plots for the Gaussian model of the log-transformed ridership

```
fit_nb <- MASS::glm.nb(frml, data = ridership)
summary(fit_nb)
```

```
##
## Call:
## MASS::glm.nb(formula = frml, data = ridership, init.theta =
## 34.38042658,
##     link = log)
##
## Deviance Residuals:
##     Min       1Q    Median       3Q       Max
## -5.7714  -0.4465    0.0596   0.5007    3.1589
##
## Coefficients:
##             Estimate Std. Error z value Pr(>|z|)
## (Intercept)  6.16439    0.12836  48.024  < 2e-16 ***
```

```
## temp             4.19282     0.25926  16.172  < 2e-16 ***
## I(temp^2)        -3.29091    0.25822 -12.745  < 2e-16 ***
## hum_imp           1.17952    0.38049   3.100  0.00194 **
## I(hum_imp^2)     -1.32915    0.30569  -4.348 1.37e-05 ***
## windspeed        -0.69844    0.09660  -7.230 4.81e-13 ***
## yr1               0.70208    0.02790  25.164  < 2e-16 ***
## season2           0.36842    0.03263  11.292  < 2e-16 ***
## season3           0.44199    0.03903  11.324  < 2e-16 ***
## season4           0.53353    0.03066  17.403  < 2e-16 ***
## workingday1       0.27441    0.01486  18.472  < 2e-16 ***
## weathersit2      -0.07076    0.01840  -3.846  0.00012 ***
## weathersit3      -0.50100    0.05033  -9.955  < 2e-16 ***
## holiday1         -0.06676    0.04260  -1.567  0.11706
## christmasTRUE    -0.10342    0.06484  -1.595  0.11072
## yr1:season2      -0.27139    0.03737  -7.261 3.83e-13 ***
## yr1:season3      -0.27468    0.03749  -7.326 2.37e-13 ***
## yr1:season4      -0.24014    0.04379  -5.484 4.15e-08 ***
## ---
## Signif. codes:
## 0 '***' 0.001 '**' 0.01 '*' 0.05 '.' 0.1 ' ' 1
##
## (Dispersion parameter for Negative Binomial(34.3804) family
## taken to be 1)
##
##     Null deviance: 5267.19  on 666  degrees of freedom
## Residual deviance:  675.41  on 649  degrees of freedom
## AIC: 10373
##
## Number of Fisher Scoring iterations: 1
##
##
##             Theta:  34.38
##         Std. Err.:   1.91
##
##  2 x log-likelihood:  -10334.58
```

The large *Theta* $\approx$ 34.38 is quite striking and indicates that we have overdispersed data. It is also a bit surprising that holiday and Christmas are not significant in the negative-binomial model compared to the Poisson model. One reason for that is the strong over-dispersion. Therefore, confidence intervals derived from the negative-binomial model will be much wider compared to confidence intervals derived from the Poisson model.

Finally, we fit the Gaussian model,

```
fit_norm <- glm(frml, data = ridership, family = gaussian())
summary(fit_norm)
```

```
##
## Call:
## glm(formula = frml, family = gaussian(), data = ridership)
##
## Deviance Residuals:
##       Min        1Q    Median        3Q       Max
## -2260.79   -258.21     36.69    321.36   1401.59
##
## Coefficients:
##                 Estimate Std. Error t value Pr(>|t|)
## (Intercept)     -1643.02     385.07  -4.267 2.28e-05 ***
## temp            11309.89     776.78  14.560  < 2e-16 ***
## I(temp^2)       -8984.86     774.45 -11.602  < 2e-16 ***
## hum_imp          3674.60    1141.77   3.218 0.001354 **
## I(hum_imp^2)    -3908.94     917.12  -4.262 2.32e-05 ***
## windspeed       -2048.80     290.18  -7.060 4.28e-12 ***
## yr1              1502.10      83.58  17.972  < 2e-16 ***
## season2           572.10      97.76   5.852 7.72e-09 ***
## season3           785.56     117.13   6.707 4.34e-11 ***
## season4           964.84      91.87  10.502  < 2e-16 ***
## workingday1       925.47      44.61  20.745  < 2e-16 ***
## weathersit2      -322.56      55.28  -5.835 8.49e-09 ***
## weathersit3     -1174.80     150.62  -7.800 2.49e-14 ***
## holiday1         -128.81     127.77  -1.008 0.313762
## christmasTRUE    -295.45     193.66  -1.526 0.127582
## yr1:season2       168.14     112.16   1.499 0.134343
## yr1:season3       402.05     112.56   3.572 0.000381 ***
## yr1:season4       732.16     131.57   5.565 3.84e-08 ***
## ---
## Signif. codes:
## 0 '***' 0.001 '**' 0.01 '*' 0.05 '.' 0.1 ' ' 1
##
## (Dispersion parameter for gaussian family taken to be
## 265754.5)
##
##     Null deviance: 1614240514  on 666  degrees of freedom
## Residual deviance:  172474646  on 649  degrees of freedom
## AIC: 10244
##
## Number of Fisher Scoring iterations: 2
```

and the Gaussian model but with a log-transformed dependent variable,

```
fit_lognorm <-
  ridership %>%
  dplyr::mutate(y = log(y)) %>%
  glm(frml, data = ., family = gaussian())
summary(fit_lognorm)
```

```
##
## Call:
## glm(formula = frml, family = gaussian(), data = .)
##
## Deviance Residuals:
##       Min         1Q     Median         3Q        Max
## -1.17838   -0.06295    0.01873    0.09874    0.57513
##
## Coefficients:
##                  Estimate Std. Error t value Pr(>|t|)
## (Intercept)       6.14970    0.13762  44.685  < 2e-16 ***
## temp              4.22762    0.27762  15.228  < 2e-16 ***
## I(temp^2)        -3.29088    0.27679 -11.889  < 2e-16 ***
## hum_imp           1.16735    0.40807   2.861 0.004364 **
## I(hum_imp^2)     -1.35617    0.32778  -4.137 3.97e-05 ***
## windspeed        -0.73103    0.10371  -7.049 4.63e-12 ***
## yr1               0.71454    0.02987  23.920  < 2e-16 ***
## season2           0.36643    0.03494  10.487  < 2e-16 ***
## season3           0.44603    0.04186  10.655  < 2e-16 ***
## season4           0.54104    0.03283  16.478  < 2e-16 ***
## workingday1       0.28179    0.01594  17.673  < 2e-16 ***
## weathersit2      -0.07235    0.01976  -3.662 0.000271 ***
## weathersit3      -0.54895    0.05383 -10.197  < 2e-16 ***
## holiday1         -0.08229    0.04567  -1.802 0.071993 .
## christmasTRUE    -0.16609    0.06921  -2.400 0.016691 *
## yr1:season2      -0.27502    0.04009  -6.861 1.60e-11 ***
## yr1:season3      -0.28757    0.04023  -7.148 2.37e-12 ***
## yr1:season4      -0.24809    0.04702  -5.276 1.80e-07 ***
## ---
## Signif. codes:
## 0 '***' 0.001 '**' 0.01 '*' 0.05 '.' 0.1 ' ' 1
##
## (Dispersion parameter for gaussian family taken to be
## 0.03394651)
##
##     Null deviance: 184.681  on 666  degrees of freedom
## Residual deviance:  22.031  on 649  degrees of freedom
```

```
## AIC: -343.82
##
## Number of Fisher Scoring iterations: 2
```

The large coefficients of the first Gaussian model result from the fact that we model ridership on the original scale, while the other models directly transformed ridership to the log-scale or used a log-link.

In general it is recommended to inspect the models. Usually one starts with some diagnostic plots. We now present the four standard diagnostic plots produced by R for all four models, see Fig. 5.7, 5.8, 5.9, and 5.10, and discuss them afterward. Obviously, the Q–Q-plots show that all models have problems with very small observations. We could expect this a bit because we did not investigate the unusual low ridership for a pattern that they might have in common, for instance, some kind of events like football games, concerts, and so on. Anyway, surprisingly the Gaussian model looks best with respect to the Q–Q-plot, though the residual plot shows quadratic behavior. Whereas the residual plots of the models using the log-link or log-transformation do not reveal strong non-constant behavior. At this point one could try to exclude models and try to improve the remaining ones. In the next chapter, we will come back to this dataset and the model fits and presents a goodness-of-fit test based on the results of this chapter which provides an additional tool for excluding/rejecting models.

5.3.1 Mathematical Framework of MLE

Suppose we have n independent univariate outcomes $Y_1, \ldots, Y_n$ with n corresponding non-random p-dimensional covariate vectors $X_1, \ldots, X_n$ such that

$$g(\mathbb{E}(Y_i)) = \beta^\top X_i \qquad (5.14)$$

and assuming that Y_i has a density function

$$f(y|\theta_i, \phi) = \exp\left(\frac{\theta_i y - \zeta(\theta_i)}{\phi}\right) h(y, \phi) \qquad (5.15)$$

with respect to the dominating σ-finite measure ν, we obtain the GLM, where g, ζ and h are known functions and g is invertible. Furthermore, it is assumed that $\phi > 0$ and ζ is twice continuously differentiable with $\zeta''(\theta) > 0$ for all θ such that (5.15) is a proper density function. Note, every Y_i may have its own parameter θ_i. It should also be noted that the class of all densities of type (5.15) is called an *exponential family with dispersion parameter* ϕ with respect to the dominating measure ν.

Calculating the moment generating function for a random variable with density (5.15) is easy:

$$\mathbb{E}\big(\exp(uY)\big) = \int \exp\left(uy + \frac{\theta_i y - \zeta(\theta_i)}{\phi}\right) h(y, \phi) v(\mathrm{d}y)$$

$$= \int \exp\left(\frac{\zeta(u\phi + \theta_i) - \zeta(\theta_i)}{\phi}\right) f(y|u\phi + \theta_i, \phi) h(y, \phi) v(\mathrm{d}y)$$

$$= \exp\left(\frac{\zeta(u\phi + \theta_i) - \zeta(\theta_i)}{\phi}\right). \tag{5.16}$$

The first and second derivative of this moment generating function with respect to u at $u = 0$ gives the first and second moment of Y. Obviously, this entails

$$\mathbb{E}(Y_i) = \zeta'(\theta_i), \quad \mathrm{VAR}(Y_i) = \phi\zeta''(\theta_i). \tag{5.17}$$

Thus, the assumptions on ϕ and ζ'' assure that the variance is not zero. A natural choice for g is the inverse of ζ' because then by (5.14) and (5.17) it holds that

$$\beta^\top X_i = g(\mathbb{E}(Y_i)) = \theta_i.$$

Such a g is usually called the canonical link function.

Classical text books on statistics assume that the covariate vectors $X_1, \ldots, X_n$ are non-random or the analysis is conducted "conditioned" on $X_1, \ldots, X_n$. However, in most scientific fields the covariates are random variables. Hence, we assume that the covariate vector has distribution function H. In order to emphasize that θ_i is actually a function of x and β we use the notation $\theta_x(\beta)$ to get

$$\mathbb{P}(Y \in A, X \in B) = \int_B \int_A f(y|\theta_x(\beta), \phi) v(\mathrm{d}y) H(\mathrm{d}x). \tag{5.18}$$

By (5.18) the conditional density of Y given $X = x$ is $f(y|\theta_x(\beta), \phi)$ and according to Shorack (2000, Example 8.5.1) we obtain

$$\mathbb{E}(\exp(uY)|X = x) = \int \exp(uy) f(y|\theta_x, \phi) v(\mathrm{d}y)$$

$$= \exp\left(\frac{\zeta(u\phi + \theta_x(\beta)) - \zeta(\theta_x(\beta))}{\phi}\right)$$

by applying the same steps that were used to derive the moment generating function in the classical situation, that is non-random covariates, see (5.16). Again calculating the first and second derivative of this moment generating function gives

$$\mathbb{E}(Y|X = x) = \zeta'(\theta_x(\beta)) \quad \text{and} \quad \mathbb{E}(Y^2|X = x) = \zeta'(\theta_x(\beta)) + \phi\zeta''(\theta_x(\beta)).$$

This easily leads to

$$\mathbb{E}(Y|X) = \zeta'(\theta_X(\beta)), \quad \mathrm{VAR}(Y|X) = \mathbb{E}\left([Y - \mathbb{E}(Y|X)]^2|X\right) = \phi\zeta''(\theta_X(\beta)). \tag{5.19}$$

Assuming that

$$g(\mathbb{E}(Y|X = x)) = \beta^\top x \tag{5.20}$$

we directly obtain the relation

$$g(\zeta'(\theta_x(\beta))) = \beta^\top x.$$

That the second derivative of ζ is greater than zero for all θ implies that ζ' is invertible and therefore $\theta_x(\beta) = (g \circ \zeta')^{-1}(\beta^\top x)$. In order to have a more compact notation we define

$$\vartheta = (\beta, \phi)$$

and denote the true parameters by $\vartheta_0 = (\beta_0, \phi_0)$. For the whole section we assume that ϑ_0 lies in the interior of

$$\Xi = \{\vartheta | \int \int f(y|\theta_x(\beta), \phi)v(dy)H(dx) < \infty\}.$$

In summary, this results in

Definition 5.45 Let $\mathscr{D} = \big(f(\cdot, \theta, \phi)\big)_{(\theta,\phi)\in\Theta\times(0,\infty)}$ be an exponential family with dispersion parameter $\phi > 0$ and densities with respect to a σ−finite measure v given by

$$f(y, \theta, \phi) = \exp\left(\frac{\theta y - \zeta(\theta)}{\phi}\right)h(y, \phi),$$

such that ζ is twice continuously differentiable with $\zeta''(\cdot) > 0$. For $(Y, X) \in \mathbb{R}^{1+p}$ let $g : \mathbb{R} \to \mathbb{R}$ be an invertible link function and set $\theta_x(\beta) = (g \circ \zeta')^{-1}(\beta^\top x)$. Assume that there exists a $(\beta_0, \phi_0) \in \Xi$ such that the conditional distribution of Y given $X = x$ has v−density

$$f(y|\theta_x(\beta_0), \phi_0) \equiv f(y, \beta_0, \phi_0, x) = f(y, \theta_x(\beta_0), \phi_0),$$

then (Y, X) follows a *parametric generalized linear model* with link function g with respect to the class $\mathscr{D}$.

The mainframe for the following proofs of the almost sure convergence of the maximum likelihood estimator is based on Perlman (1972) and the central tool is the Kullback-Leibler information.

Definition 5.46 Suppose F and G are probability measures with strict positive densities f and g with respect to a σ−finite measure v on a measurable space $(X, \mathscr{B})$. Then

$$I_{KL}(F : G) = \int \log(f/g) f \, dv$$

defines the *Kullback-Leibler information*.

We only need the following two properties of the Kullback-Leibler information.

Lemma 5.47 *Suppose F and G are probability measures that are both dominated by a σ−finite measure v on a measurable space $(X, \mathcal{B})$ such that the corresponding v−densities f and g are strict positive. Then*

(i) $I_{KL}(F : G) \in [0, \infty]$
(ii) $I_{KL}(F : G) = 0$ *if and only if $F = G$.*

Proof Both assertions follow from Jensen's inequality, see Shorack (2000, Inequality 4.10). Denote by f and g the densities of F and G with respect to v. Since the negative of the logarithm is convex, Jensen's inequality provides

$$I_{KL}(F : G) = \int -\log(g/f) f dv \geq -\log\left(\int (g/f) f dv\right) = -\log\left(\int g dv\right) = 0.$$

According to the addendum to Jensen inequality Shorack (2000, Inequality 4.10), equality holds if and only if $g/f = \int (g/f) f dv$, F−a.e. Since $\int (g/f) f dv = 1$, this implies that $\int I_{\{A\}} f \, dv = 0$, where $A = \{x : f(x) \neq g(x)\}$. Furthermore, since f is strict positive, we have

$$v(A) = \int I_{\{A\}} \frac{1}{f} f \, dv = 0.$$

Denote by A^c the complement of A in X. For an arbitrarily chosen $B \in \mathcal{B}$ we get

$$G(B) = \int I_{\{B\}} g \, dv = \int I_{\{B\}} I_{\{A^c\}} g \, dv = \int I_{\{B\}} I_{\{A^c\}} f \, dv = F(B)$$

which shows that $F = G$. This completes the proof.   □

For our purposes, we need to modify the Kullback-Leibler information as follows.

Definition 5.48 Let $\vartheta_1, \vartheta_2 \in \Xi$, then

$$K_H(\vartheta_1, \vartheta_2) = \int I_{KL}(F_{\theta_x(\beta_1), \phi_1} : F_{\theta_x(\beta_2), \phi_2}) H(dx)$$

defines the *modified Kullback-Leibler information* with respect to H, the df. of the covariate vector X, where $F_{\theta_x(\beta), \phi}$ denotes the conditional distribution of Y given $X = x$.

Remark 5.49 Due to the inner product of β and x it may happen that $\theta_x(\beta_1) = \theta_x(\beta_2)$, which imply $F_{\theta_x(\beta_1), \phi} = F_{\theta_x(\beta_2), \phi}$. Therefore, if $\mathbb{P}(\beta_1^\top X = \beta_2^\top X) = 1$ we have no chance to distinguish β_1 and β_2, because the (conditional) distribution of Y does not change.

We now establish similar results for the modified Kullback-Leibler information as we did in Lemma 5.47 for the Kullback-Leibler information.

Lemma 5.50 *Let $\vartheta_1, \vartheta_2 \in \Xi$, then*

(i) $K_H(\vartheta_1, \vartheta_2) \in [0, \infty]$.
(ii) $K_H(\vartheta_1, \vartheta_2) = 0$ if and only if $\int I_{\{\phi_1 = \phi_2, \theta_x(\beta_1) = \theta_x(\beta_2)\}} H(dx) = 1$.

Proof The first assertion follows directly from the definition of the modified Kullback-Leibler information and from (i) of Lemma 5.47.
If $\int I_{\{\phi_1 = \phi_2, \theta_x(\beta_1) = \theta_x(\beta_2)\}} H(dx) = 1$, we easily verify that $K_H(\vartheta_1, \vartheta_2) = 0$ holds true. Finally, assume $K_H(\vartheta_1, \vartheta_2) = 0$, then

$$
\begin{aligned}
0 &= K_H(\vartheta_1, \vartheta_2) \\
&= \int I_{KL}(F_{\theta_x(\beta_1), \phi_1} : F_{\theta_x(\beta_2), \phi_2}) \, H(dx) \\
&= \int I_{KL}(F_{\theta_x(\beta_1), \phi_1} : F_{\theta_x(\beta_2), \phi_2}) I_{\{\phi_1 = \phi_2, \theta_x(\beta_1) = \theta_x(\beta_2)\}} \, H(dx) \\
&\quad + \int I_{KL}(F_{\theta_x(\beta_1), \phi_1} : F_{\theta_x(\beta_2), \phi_2})(1 - I_{\{\phi_1 = \phi_2, \theta_x(\beta_1) = \theta_x(\beta_2)\}}) \, H(dx) \\
&= \int I_{KL}(F_{\theta_x(\beta_1), \phi_1} : F_{\theta_x(\beta_2), \phi_2})(1 - I_{\{\phi_1 = \phi_2, \theta_x(\beta_1) = \theta_x(\beta_2)\}}) \, H(dx),
\end{aligned}
$$

where the last equality holds by (ii) of Lemma 5.47. Again, by (ii) of Lemma 5.47 we have that $0 < I_{KL}(F_{\theta_x(\beta_1), \phi_1} : F_{\theta_x(\beta_2), \phi_2})$ on the complement of $\{\phi_1 = \phi_2, \theta_x(\beta_1) = \theta_x(\beta_2)\}$, therefore $1 - I_{\{\phi_1 = \phi_2, \theta_x(\beta_1) = \theta_x(\beta_2)\}} = 0$ holds true almost surely with respect to H. $\qquad\square$

The log likelihood of an i.i.d. sequence $(Y_1, X_1), \ldots, (Y_n, X_n)$ is

$$
\begin{aligned}
\ell_n(\vartheta) &= \ell_n(\beta, \phi) \\
&= \sum_{i=1}^{n} \log(f(y_i | \theta_{x_i}(\beta), \phi)) \\
&= \sum_{i=1}^{n} \frac{\theta_{x_i}(\beta) y_i - \zeta(\theta_{x_i}(\beta))}{\phi} + \log(h(y_i, \phi)).
\end{aligned}
$$

According to SLLN

$$
\begin{aligned}
\lim_{n \to \infty} n^{-1} \ell_n(\vartheta) &= \mathbb{E}_{\vartheta_0}(\ell_1(\vartheta)) \\
&= \int \int \log(f(y | \theta_x(\beta), \phi)) f(y | \theta_x(\beta_0), \phi_0) \nu(dy) H(dx) \\
&=: L_H(\vartheta_0, \vartheta),
\end{aligned}
$$

if $\mathbb{E}_{\vartheta_0}(\ell_1(\vartheta))$ exists. We will now study $L_H(\vartheta_0, \cdot)$. The SLLN will allow us to carry over the results to the corresponding expressions in terms of ℓ_n. First, we investigate when $L_H(\vartheta_0, \cdot)$ has a unique maximum.

Lemma 5.51 *Assume that*

(i) $L_H(\vartheta_0, \vartheta_0) < \infty$
(ii) *for all* $\vartheta \in \Xi \backslash \{\vartheta_0\}$ *it holds that* $\int I_{\{\phi_0 = \phi, \theta_x(\beta_0) = \theta_x(\beta)\}} H(dx) < 1$

then $L_H(\vartheta_0, \cdot)$ *has a unique maximum at* ϑ_0.

Proof Due to assumption (ii) and Lemma 5.50 (ii) we obtain

$$
0 < K_H(\vartheta_0, \vartheta)
$$

$$
= \int I_{KL}(F_{\theta_x(\beta_0), \phi_0} : F_{\theta_x(\beta), \phi}) H(dx)
$$

$$
= \int \int \log \left(\frac{f(y|\theta_x(\beta_0), \phi_0)}{f(y|\theta_x(\beta), \phi)} \right) f(y|\theta_x(\beta_0), \phi_0) \nu(dy) H(dx)
$$

$$
= L_H(\vartheta_0, \vartheta_0) - L_H(\vartheta_0, \vartheta).
$$

Note that assumption (i) is necessary to guarantee the last equality, i.e., it prevents $\infty - \infty$. Altogether, this shows the assertion. $\square$

Theorem 5.52 *Assume that Ξ is compact and*

(i) *for all $\vartheta^* \in \Xi$ exists an open neighborhood $V^* = V(\vartheta^*)$ of ϑ^* such that*

$$
\mathbb{E} \left(\sup_{\vartheta \in V^*} \log f(Y|\theta_X(\beta), \phi) \right) < \infty.
$$

Under the assumption of Lemma 5.51 it holds that $\hat{\vartheta}_n \to \vartheta_0$, as $n \to \infty$, w.p.1, where $\hat{\vartheta}_n$ is the maximum of $\ell_n(\cdot)$.

Proof The continuity of the density functions and the compactness of Ξ assure the existence of $\hat{\vartheta}_n \in \Xi$. Denote by V an arbitrary open neighborhood of ϑ_0. Let $U = \Xi \backslash V$. If $\limsup_{n \to \infty} \sup_{\vartheta \in U} \ell_n(\vartheta) - \ell_n(\vartheta_0) < 0$, we can find an $N \in \mathbb{N}$ such that $\sup_{\vartheta \in U} \ell_n(\vartheta) < \ell_n(\vartheta_0)$ for all $n > N$. Hence, $\hat{\vartheta}_n \in V$ for all $n > N$. Therefore, it is sufficient to prove

$$
\mathbb{P}(\limsup_{n \to \infty} \sup_{\vartheta \in U} \ell_n(\vartheta) - \ell_n(\vartheta_0) < 0) = 1. \tag{5.21}
$$

Note that we might have measurability issues because U is uncountable. In this case we would use the inner probability measure.

We will now find a finite cover $V_1, \ldots, V_m$ for U, where every V_i will have the property (5.21). Choose $\vartheta^* \in U$ arbitrary and denote by $V_\varepsilon(\vartheta^*)$ open neighborhoods of ϑ^* with

$$
\bigcap_{\varepsilon > 0} V_\varepsilon(\vartheta^*) = \{\vartheta^*\}.
$$

Choosing $\varepsilon > 0$ such that $V_\varepsilon(\vartheta^*) \subset V^*$ and $0 < M < \infty$, we obtain

$$\sup_{\vartheta \in V_\varepsilon(\vartheta^*)} n^{-1}(\ell_n(\vartheta) - \ell_n(\vartheta_0))$$

$$\le n^{-1} \sum_{i=1}^{n} \sup_{\vartheta \in V_\varepsilon(\vartheta^*)} \log f(y_i | \theta_{x_i}(\beta), \phi) - n^{-1} \sum_{i=1}^{n} \log f(y_i | \theta_{x_i}(\beta_0), \phi_0)$$

$$\le n^{-1} \sum_{i=1}^{n} \sup_{\vartheta \in V_\varepsilon(\vartheta^*)} \max\{\log f(y_i | \theta_{x_i}(\beta), \phi), -M\} - n^{-1} \sum_{i=1}^{n} \log f(y_i | \theta_{x_i}(\beta_0), \phi_0).$$

Applying a series of convergence theorems will establish that this last expression is less than zero. By assumption (i) the expectation of the following positive part is finite:

$$\mathbb{E}\left(\left(\sup_{\vartheta \in V_\varepsilon(\vartheta^*)} \max\{\log f(Y | \theta_X(\beta), \phi), -M\}\right)^+\right) < \infty.$$

Furthermore, we have

$$\sup_{\vartheta \in V_\varepsilon(\vartheta^*)} \log f(y_i | \theta_{x_i}(\beta), \phi) \le \sup_{\vartheta \in V_\varepsilon(\vartheta^*)} \max\{\log f(y_i | \theta_{x_i}(\beta), \phi), -M\}$$

$$\le \left(\sup_{\vartheta \in V_\varepsilon(\vartheta^*)} \max\{\log f(y_i | \theta_{x_i}(\beta), \phi), -M\}\right)^+.$$

First, we apply the SLLN and obtain that

$$\limsup_{n \to \infty} \sup_{\vartheta \in V_\varepsilon(\vartheta^*)} n^{-1}(\ell_n(\vartheta) - \ell_n(\vartheta_0))$$

is less or equal to

$$\mathbb{E}\left(\sup_{\vartheta \in V_\varepsilon(\vartheta^*)} \max\{\log f(y_i | \theta_{x_i}(\beta), \phi), -M\}\right) - L(\vartheta_0, \vartheta_0).$$

By Lebegue's dominated convergence theorem this converges for $\varepsilon \to 0$ to

$$\mathbb{E}\left(\max\{\log f(y_i | \theta_{x_i}(\beta^*), \phi^*), -M\}\right) - L(\vartheta_0, \vartheta_0).$$

Finally, applying Loève (1977, Fatou-Lebesgue-Theorem, page 126), this converges for $M \to \infty$ to

$$L_H(\vartheta_0, \vartheta^*) - L_H(\vartheta_0, \vartheta_0) < 0.$$

The last inequality is a direct consequence of Lemma 5.51. Since U is compact there exist ε_i and ϑ_i^* such that $U \subset \bigcup_{i=1}^{m} V_{\varepsilon_i}(\vartheta_i^*)$. This completes the proof. $\square$

Note, the next corollary uses the same assumptions as Theorem 5.52 but assumption (ii) replaces the compactness of Ξ.

Corollary 5.53 *Assume that*

(i) for all $\vartheta^* \in \varXi$ exists an open neighborhood $V^* = V(\vartheta^*)$ of ϑ^* such that

$$\mathbb{E}\left(\sup_{\vartheta \in V^*} \log f(Y|\theta_X(\beta), \phi) \right) < \infty,$$

(ii) there exists a compact set C such that ϑ_0 is an interior point of C and

$$\mathbb{E}\left(\sup_{\vartheta \in \varXi \setminus C} \log f(Y|\theta_X(\beta), \phi) - \log f(Y|\theta_X(\beta_0), \phi_0) \right) < 0.$$

Under the assumption of Lemma 5.51 it holds that $\hat{\vartheta}_n \to \vartheta_0$ almost surely, where $\hat{\vartheta}_n$ is the maximum of $\ell_n(\cdot)$.

Proof Denote by V an arbitrary open neighborhood of ϑ_0. Following the proof of Theorem 5.52 it is sufficient to show

$$\mathbb{P}(\limsup_{n \to \infty} \sup_{\vartheta \in \varXi \setminus V} \ell_n(\vartheta) - \ell_n(\vartheta_0) < 0) = 1.$$

Since C is compact, using $U = C \setminus V$, we directly obtain from the proof of Theorem 5.52, that

$$\mathbb{P}(\limsup_{n \to \infty} \sup_{\vartheta \in U} \ell_n(\vartheta) - \ell_n(\vartheta_0) < 0) = 1.$$

Similar as in the proof of Theorem 5.52, but now using (ii), we conclude

$$\sup_{\vartheta \in \varXi \setminus C} n^{-1}(\ell_n(\vartheta) - \ell_n(\vartheta_0))$$

$$< n^{-1} \sum_{i=1}^{n} \sup_{\vartheta \in \varXi \setminus C} [\log f(y_i|\theta_{x_i}(\beta), \phi) - \log f(y_i|\theta_{x_i}(\beta_0), \phi_0)]$$

$$\to \mathbb{E}\left(\sup_{\vartheta \in \varXi \setminus C} \log f(Y|\theta_X(\beta), \phi) - \log f(Y|\theta_X(\beta_0), \phi_0) \right) < 0.$$

Therefore, we obtain

$$\mathbb{P}(\limsup_{n \to \infty} \sup_{\vartheta \in \varXi \setminus C} \ell_n(\vartheta) - \ell_n(\vartheta_0) < 0) = 1.$$

Without loss of generality we can assume that $V \subset C$. Hence, $\varXi \setminus V = \varXi \setminus C \cup U$, which finally leads to

$$\mathbb{P}(\limsup_{n\to\infty} \sup_{\vartheta\in\Xi\backslash V} \ell_n(\vartheta) - \ell_n(\vartheta_0) < 0)$$

$$= \mathbb{P}\left(\{\limsup_{n\to\infty} \sup_{\vartheta\in\Xi\backslash C} \ell_n(\vartheta) - \ell_n(\vartheta_0) < 0\} \cup \{\limsup_{n\to\infty} \sup_{\vartheta\in U} \ell_n(\vartheta) - \ell_n(\vartheta_0) < 0\}\right)$$

$$= 1.$$

This concludes the proof. □

The following lemma supports the upcoming proof of the asymptotic normality of the maximum likelihood estimator.

Lemma 5.54 *Let $(\Omega_n, \mathscr{A}_n, \mathbb{P}_n)$ be a sequence of probability spaces. Let X_n (defined on Ω_n) be a random p-vector converging in distribution to X and let A_n (defined on Ω_n) be a random matrix converging in probability to a constant invertible matrix A. If $X_n = A_n Y_n$ for all n for some random p-vector Y_n (defined on Ω_n), then $Y_n = A^{-1} X_n + o_{\mathbb{P}_n}(1)$.*

Proof Let $B_n = \{\det(A_n) \neq 0\}$. Since $\det(A) \neq 0$ and $A_n \to A$ in probability, we have $\mathbb{P}_n(B_n) \to 1$ and $\mathrm{I}_{\{B_n\}} A_n^{-1} X_n = \mathrm{I}_{\{B_n\}} Y_n = Y_n - \mathrm{I}_{\{B_n^c\}} Y_n$. Obviously, $\mathrm{I}_{\{B_n\}} A_n^{-1} = A^{-1} + o_{\mathbb{P}_n}(1)$ and for all $\varepsilon < 1$

$$\mathbb{P}_n(|\mathrm{I}_{\{B_n^c\}} Y_n| > \varepsilon) \leq \mathbb{P}_n(\mathrm{I}_{\{B_n^c\}} > \varepsilon) = 1 - \mathbb{P}_n(B_n) = o(1).$$

Furthermore, since X_n converges in distribution to X for all $\varepsilon > 0$ there exists a $K > 0$ such that $\mathbb{P}_n(\|X_n\|_\infty > K) < \varepsilon$, where $\|\cdot\|_\infty$ denotes the maximum norm on $\mathbb{R}^p$, which implies that $\|(A^{-1} - \mathrm{I}_{\{B_n\}} A_n^{-1}) X_n\|_\infty = o_{\mathbb{P}_n}(1)$. Altogether, we have

$$Y_n = \mathrm{I}_{\{B_n\}} A_n^{-1} X_n + o_{\mathbb{P}_n}(1) = A^{-1} X_n + o_{\mathbb{P}_n}(1).$$

This concludes the proof. □

For sake of compactness, for a map m depending on ϑ or only β or ϕ, denote by $D_r(m)$ and $D_{r,s}(m)$ the first partial derivative of m with respect to the r-th component and the second partial derivative of m with respect to the r-th and s-th component, respectively. Furthermore, if m is a map from $\mathbb{R}^p$ to $\mathbb{R}$, then $D(m)$ denotes the gradient of m and if m is a map from $\mathbb{R}^p$ to $\mathbb{R}^k$, then $D(m)$ denotes the Jacobi-matrix of m. For instance, $f(y|\theta_x(\beta), \phi)$ is a function of ϑ, therefore $D(f(y|\theta_x(\beta), \phi))$ denotes the gradient with respect to ϑ, whereas $\theta_x(\beta)$ is a function of β only and therefore $D(\theta_x(\beta))$ denotes the gradient with respect to β. Note also that $D_{p+1}(f(y|\theta_x(\beta), \phi))$ is the partial derivative of $f(y|\theta_x(\beta), \phi)$ with respect to the last component of ϑ which is ϕ. For a function like $c(y, \phi)$ that only depends on ϕ, we have $D(c(y, \phi)) = D_1(c(y, \phi))$.

Theorem 5.55 *If*

(i) $\log f(y|\theta_x(\beta), \phi)$ has continuous second derivatives with respect to ϑ and there exits an open neighborhood $V \subset \Xi$ of ϑ_0 such that for all $1 \leq r, s \leq p+1$

$$\mathbb{E}\left(\sup_{\vartheta \in V}\left|D_{r,s}(\log f(Y|\theta_X(\beta), \phi))\right|\right) < \infty,$$

(ii)

$$\int D_{p+1}(f(y|\theta_x(\beta_0), \phi_0))\nu(\mathrm{d}y)H(\mathrm{d}x) = 0,$$

(iii) *for all* $1 \le r, s \le p+1$

$$\int D_{r,s}(f(y|\theta_x(\beta_0), \phi_0))\nu(\mathrm{d}y)H(\mathrm{d}x) = 0,$$

(iv)

$$A := \phi_0^{-1}\mathbb{E}\left(\zeta''(\theta_X(\beta_0))D(\theta_X(\beta_0))(D(\theta_X(\beta_0)))^{\top}\right)$$

exist and is positive definite,

(v)

$$0 < B := \mathbb{E}\left(\left(D(\log(h(Y, \phi_0))) - \frac{\theta_X(\beta_0)Y - \zeta(\theta_X(\beta_0))}{\phi_0^2}\right)^2\right) < \infty,$$

(vi) $\hat{\vartheta}_n$ *converges in probability to* ϑ_0

holds, then $n^{1/2}(\hat{\vartheta}_n - \vartheta_0) \to Z$, *where* Z *is multivariate normally distributed with zero mean and covariance matrix*

$$\Sigma^{-1} = \begin{pmatrix} A & 0 \\ 0 & B \end{pmatrix}^{-1}.$$

Proof Define $s_n(\vartheta) := D(\ell_n(\vartheta))$ and note that

$$s_n(\hat{\vartheta}_n) - s_n(\vartheta_0) = \left(\int_0^1 Ds_n(\vartheta_0 + t(\hat{\vartheta}_n - \vartheta_0))\,\mathrm{d}t\right)(\hat{\vartheta}_n - \vartheta_0).$$

Note that the right-hand side is a matrix-vector product. First, we substitute the integral by $Ds_n(\vartheta_0)$. Define

$$\Delta_n := \int_0^1 Ds_n(\vartheta_0 + t(\hat{\vartheta}_n - \vartheta_0))\mathrm{d}t - Ds_n(\vartheta_0)$$

and $B_\varepsilon := \{\vartheta : \|\vartheta - \vartheta_0\| \le \varepsilon\}$. W.l.o.g. we assume that $B_\varepsilon \subset V$. We have by Markov's inequality for the r-th and s-th component of Δ_n, denoted by $\Delta_n^{(r,s)}$, that

$$\mathbb{P}(|\Delta_n^{(r,s)}/n| > \tilde{\varepsilon}) \leq \mathbb{P}(\hat{\vartheta}_n \notin B_\varepsilon) + \tilde{\varepsilon}^{-1} \mathbb{E}\left(\sup_{\vartheta \in B_\varepsilon} |D_{r,s}\ell_1(\vartheta) - D_{r,s}\ell_1(\vartheta_0)| \right).$$

$$(5.22)$$

Since $\hat{\vartheta}_n$ converges in probability to ϑ_0, the first term on the right-hand side converges to zero. By the continuity assumption of (i)

$$\lim_{\varepsilon \to 0} \sup_{\vartheta \in B_\varepsilon} |D_{r,s}\ell_1(\vartheta) - D_{r,s}\ell_1(\vartheta_0)| = 0.$$

Therefore, by assumption (i) and Lebesgue's dominated convergence theorem the second term on the right-hand side of (5.22) can be made arbitrarily small. Altogether, we obtain $n^{-1}\Delta_n = o_\mathbb{P}(1)$ and since $s_n(\hat{\vartheta}_n) = 0$ the initial equality becomes

$$-n^{-1/2}s_n(\vartheta_0) = (n^{-1}Ds_n(\vartheta_0) + o_\mathbb{P}(1)) \, n^{1/2}(\hat{\vartheta}_n - \vartheta_0). \qquad (5.23)$$

The final step is to apply the CTL to $s_n(\vartheta_0)$ and afterward Lemma 5.54. The function s_n consists of two parts, i.e.,

$$D_q \ell_n(\vartheta_0) = \frac{1}{\phi_0} \sum_{i=1}^n (y_i - \zeta'(\theta_{x_i}(\beta_0))) D_q(\theta_{x_i}(\beta_0))$$

for $1 \leq q \leq p$ and

$$D_{p+1}\ell_n(\vartheta_0) = \sum_{i=1}^n D(c(y_i, \phi_0)) - \frac{\theta_{x_i}(\beta_0)y_i - \zeta(\theta_{x_i}(\beta_0))}{\phi_0^2},$$

where $c(y, \phi) = \log h(y, \phi)$. Since $(Y_i, X_i)_{i=1,\dots,n}$ is an i.i.d. sequence, we consider in the following calculations of the first two moments only the i−th summand. Obviously, the first components, $1 \leq q \leq p$, of $s_n(\vartheta_0)$ are centered:

$$\mathbb{E}\left((Y_i - \zeta'(\theta_{X_i}(\beta_0)))D_q\theta_{X_i}(\beta_0)\right) = \mathbb{E}\left((\mathbb{E}(Y_i|X_i) - \zeta'(\theta_{X_i}(\beta_0)))D_q\theta_{X_i}(\beta_0)\right)$$

$$(5.24)$$

$$= 0,$$

since $\mathbb{E}(Y_i|X_i) = \zeta'(\theta_{X_i}(\beta_0))$. By assumption (ii) also the last component of $s_n(\vartheta_0)$ is centered:

$$\mathbb{E}\left(D(c(Y_i, \phi_0)) - \frac{\theta_{X_i}(\beta_0)Y_i - \zeta(\theta_{X_i}(\beta_0))}{\phi_0^2}\right) = \mathbb{E}\left(D_{p+1}(\ell_1(\vartheta_0))\right)$$

$$= \int D(f(y|\theta_x(\beta_0), \phi_0))\nu(\mathrm{d}y)H(\mathrm{d}x)$$

$$= 0.$$

For the second moments, we start with the covariance of the q-th component and the last component of $s_n(\vartheta_0)$. In order to simplify the notation, we write f for the density of Y. In general, for all $1 \le r, s \le p+1$, we have

$$D_{r,s}(\log f) = \frac{1}{f}\left(D_{r,s}f - \frac{1}{f}(D_r f)(D_s f)\right) = \frac{1}{f}\left(D_{r,s}f - f D_r(\log f) D_s(\log f)\right).$$

Therefore, considering the partial derivatives at ϑ_0, by assumption (iii), we obtain

$$\mathbb{E}\left(D_{r,s}(\log f)\right) = \int D_{r,s}(f)\nu(dy)H(dx) - \mathbb{E}\left(D_r(\log f)D_s(\log f)\right)$$
$$= 0 - \mathrm{COV}\left(D_r(\log f), D_s(\log f)\right). \tag{5.25}$$

In particular for $r = p+1$, we additional have for the second derivatives at ϑ_0 that

$$\mathbb{E}\left(\frac{\partial^2 \log f}{\partial\phi\partial\beta}\right) = -\phi_0^{-2}\mathbb{E}\left(\frac{\partial \log f}{\partial\beta}\right) = 0$$

by Eq. (5.24), where $\partial \log f/\partial\beta$ is the gradient of $\log f$ with respect to the vector β. This shows that the covariance of the q-th component ($1 \le q \le p$) and the last component of s_n equals zero. This is not surprising, since the likelihood equation of β is independent of ϕ. Therefore, the covariance matrix of s_n consists of two blocks. According to the equations for the conditional expectation and variance for Y, see (5.19), the first block is

$$\mathrm{COV}\left(\phi_0^{-1}(Y - \zeta'(\theta_X(\beta_0)))D(\theta_X(\beta_0))\right) = \phi_0^{-2}\mathbb{E}\left((Y - \zeta'(\theta_X(\beta_0)))^2 S(X)\right)$$
$$= \phi_0^{-2}\mathbb{E}\left(\mathbb{E}[(Y - E(Y|X))^2|X]S(X)\right)$$
$$= \phi_0^{-1}\mathbb{E}(\zeta''(\theta_X(\beta_0))S(X)),$$

where

$$S(X) = D(\theta_X(\beta_0))\left(D(\theta_X(\beta_0))\right)^\top.$$

Note that ϕ_0^{-1} in the last line is correct since $\mathrm{VAR}(Y|X) = \phi_0\zeta''(\theta_X(\beta_0))$. The second block is

$$\mathbb{E}\left(\left(D(c(Y,\phi_0)) - \frac{\theta_X(\beta_0)Y - \zeta(\theta_X(\beta_0))}{\phi_0^2}\right)^2\right).$$

Thus, $n^{-1/2}s_n(\beta_0)$ converges in distribution to a multivariate normally distributed random variable with zero mean and covariance matrix Σ that consists of those two blocks. Finally, $n^{-1}Ds_n(\vartheta_0)$ converges by the SLLN and (5.25) almost surely to $-\Sigma$. Representation (5.23) and Lemma 5.54 complete the proof. $\square$

The following corollary will be used later when we investigate goodness-of-fit-tests.

Corollary 5.56 *Under the assumptions of Theorem 5.55 it holds for*

$$L(X_i, Y_i, \vartheta_0) = \Sigma^{-1} D(\log(f(Y_i|\theta_{X_i}(\beta_0), \phi_0)))$$

that

1. $n^{1/2}(\hat{\vartheta}_n - \vartheta_0) = n^{-1/2} \sum_{i=1}^{n} L(X_i, Y_i, \beta_0, \phi_0) + o_{\mathbb{P}}(1)$,
2. $\mathbb{E}(L(X_i, Y_i, \beta_0, \phi_0)) = 0$,
3. $\mathbb{E}\left(L(X_i, Y_i, \beta_0, \phi_0)L^{\top}(X_i, Y_i, \beta_0, \phi_0)\right)$ *exists and is positive definite.*

Proof All calculations were already made in the proof of Theorem 5.55. Setting

$$L(X_i, Y_i, \beta_0, \phi_0) = \Sigma^{-1} D(\log(f(Y_i|\theta_{X_i}(\beta_0), \phi_0)))$$

yield again the representation (5.23) for $n^{1/2}(\hat{\vartheta}_n - \vartheta_0)$, where due to the SLLN $n^{-1}Ds_n(\vartheta_0)$ was substituted by $-\Sigma$. Since Σ is a constant matrix the calculations of the first and second moment for the components of $s_n(\vartheta_0)$ in the proof of Theorem 5.55 directly yield the assertions 2 and 3 of the corollary. This concludes the proof. □

5.3.2 Mathematical Framework of Bootstrap MLE

Since a GLM makes an explicit assumption about the density of the Y, it is possible to bootstrap the data in a parametric manner. After estimating the parameters on the original dataset, for instance in a Poisson regression, we can create/bootstrap a new dataset according to the fitted model. This is the backbone of RSS 5.42. In the following we investigate the behavior of the MLE estimator in such a bootstrap world. This will lead to the same consistency results we already obtained in the non-bootstrapped MLE in Sect. 5.3.1. Furthermore, the results of this chapter are used to construct goodness-of-fit-tests for GLMs.

Remark 5.57 Bootstrapping in according to Resampling Scheme 5.42 means that $X_{k;i}^*$ are constants in the bootstrap world. Therefore, in the bootstrap world the covariates have not a common distribution $\mathbb{P}_X$.

For ease of notation we suppress k in the following and due to Step (B) of the resampling scheme we obtain $X_i^* = X_i$. Similar as before we obtain that the log likelihood is

$$\ell_n^*(\vartheta) = \sum_{i=1}^{n} \frac{\theta_{x_i}(\beta)y_{in}^* - \zeta(\theta_{x_i}(\beta))}{\phi} + \log(h(y_{in}^*, \phi))$$

with the corresponding derivatives (components of the score function s_n^*)

$$D_q \ell_n^*(\vartheta) = \frac{1}{\phi} \sum_{i=1}^n (y_{in}^* - \zeta'(\theta_{x_i}(\beta))D_q(\theta_{x_i}(\beta))$$

for $1 \leq q \leq p$ and

$$D_{p+1}\ell_n^*(\vartheta) = \sum_{i=1}^n D(c(y_{in}^*, \phi)) - \frac{\theta_{x_i}(\beta)y_{in}^* - \zeta(\theta_{x_i}(\beta))}{\phi^2},$$

where $c(y, \phi) = \log h(y, \phi)$.

Lemma 5.58 *Assume $\hat{\vartheta}_n \to \vartheta_0$ w.p.1 and the density f is continuous in ϑ at ϑ_0. If there are open neighborhoods V_1 and V_2 of ϑ_0 such that*

$$\int \int \sup_{\vartheta_1 \in V_1} |A(y, x, \vartheta_1)| \sup_{\vartheta_2 \in V_2} f(y|\theta_x(\beta_2), \phi_2)\nu(\mathrm{d}y)H(\mathrm{d}x) < \infty,$$

then under Resampling Scheme 5.42, as $n \to \infty$,

$$n^{-1}\sum_{i=1}^n \mathbb{E}_n^*(A(Y_{in}^*, X_i, \hat{\vartheta}_n)) \longrightarrow \int \int A(y, x, \vartheta_0)f(y|\theta_x(\beta_0), \phi_0)\nu(\mathrm{d}y)H(\mathrm{d}x)$$

w.p.1 if A is continuous in ϑ at ϑ_0.

Proof Obviously by our assumption it also holds true that

$$\int \int \sup_{\vartheta_1 \in V} |A(y, x, \vartheta_1)| \sup_{\vartheta_2 \in V} |f(y|\theta_x(\beta_2), \phi_2) - f(y|\theta_x(\beta_0), \phi_0)| \, \nu(\mathrm{d}y)H(\mathrm{d}x) < \infty.$$

We have w.p.1

$$\left| n^{-1}\sum_{i=1}^n \mathbb{E}_n^*(A(Y_{in}^*, X_i, \hat{\vartheta}_n)) - n^{-1}\sum_{i=1}^n \int A(y, X_i, \hat{\vartheta}_n)f(y|\theta_{X_i}(\beta_0), \phi_0)\nu(\mathrm{d}y) \right|$$

$$\leq n^{-1}\sum_{i=1}^n \int \left| A(y, X_i, \hat{\vartheta}_n) \right| \left| f(y|\theta_{X_i}(\hat{\beta}_n), \hat{\phi}_n) - f(y|\theta_{X_i}(\beta_0), \phi_0) \right| \nu(\mathrm{d}y)$$

$$\leq n^{-1}\sum_{i=1}^n \int \sup_{\vartheta_1 \in V_1} |A(y, X_i, \vartheta_1)| \sup_{\vartheta_2 \in V_2} \left| f(y|\theta_{X_i}(\beta_2), \phi_2) - f(y|\theta_{X_i}(\beta_0), \phi_0) \right| \nu(\mathrm{d}y)$$

$$\to \int \int \sup_{\vartheta_1 \in V_1} |A(y, x, \vartheta_1)| \sup_{\vartheta_2 \in V_2} |f(y|\theta_x(\beta_2), \phi_2) - f(y|\theta_x(\beta_0), \phi_0)| \, \nu(\mathrm{d}y)H(\mathrm{d}x),$$

as $n \to \infty$, where the second inequality follows from the fact that $\hat{\vartheta}_n$ converges to ϑ_0 w.p.1 and the last step follows from the SLLN. By continuity of the density function with respect to ϑ and Lebegue's dominated convergence theorem the last expression converges to zero by shrinking V_2 toward the point set $\{\vartheta_0\}$. In the same manner we obtain, as $n \to \infty$,

$$\left| n^{-1} \sum_{i=1}^{n} \int (A(y, X_i, \hat{\vartheta}_n) - A(y, X_i, \vartheta_0)) f(y|\theta_{X_i}(\beta_0), \phi_0) v(\mathrm{d}y) \right|$$

$$\leq n^{-1} \sum_{i=1}^{n} \int \sup_{\vartheta_1 \in V_1} |A(y, X_i, \vartheta_1) - A(y, X_i, \vartheta_0)| f(y|\theta_{X_i}(\beta_0), \phi_0) v(\mathrm{d}y)$$

$$\to \int \int \sup_{\vartheta_1 \in V_1} |A(y, x, \vartheta_1) - A(y, x, \vartheta_0)| f(y|\theta_x(\beta_0), \phi_0) v(\mathrm{d}y) H(\mathrm{d}x),$$

which also converges to zero by the continuity of A at ϑ_0 and Lebegue's dominated convergence theorem if we shrink V_1 toward the point set $\{\vartheta_0\}$. Finally, one only needs to observe that

$$n^{-1} \sum_{i=1}^{n} \int A(y, X_i, \vartheta_0) f(y|\theta_{X_i}(\beta_0), \phi_0) v(\mathrm{d}y)$$

converges by the SLLN to

$$\int \int A(y, x, \vartheta_0) f(y|\theta_x(\beta_0), \phi_0) v(\mathrm{d}y) H(\mathrm{d}x),$$

which concludes the proof. $\qquad \square$

Theorem 5.59 *If Ξ is compact, the density f is continuous in ϑ at ϑ_0 and*

(i) *there exists an open neighborhood $V_0 = V(\vartheta_0)$ of ϑ_0 such that for all $\vartheta^* \in \Xi$ exists an open neighborhood $V^* = V(\vartheta^*)$ of ϑ^* with*

$$\int \int \left(\left| \sup_{\tilde{\vartheta} \in V^*} \log \left(\frac{f(y|\theta_x(\tilde{\beta}), \tilde{\phi})}{f(y|\theta_x(\beta_0), \phi_0)} \right) \right| \right) \sup_{\vartheta \in V_0} f(y|\theta_x(\beta), \phi) v(\mathrm{d}y) H(\mathrm{d}x) < \infty,$$

and

$$\int \int \left(\left| \sup_{\tilde{\vartheta} \in V^*} \log \left(\frac{f(y|\theta_x(\tilde{\beta}), \tilde{\phi})}{f(y|\theta_x(\beta_0), \phi_0)} \right) \right|^2 \right) \sup_{\vartheta \in V_0} f(y|\theta_x(\beta), \phi) v(\mathrm{d}y) H(\mathrm{d}x) < \infty,$$

then under the assumptions of Lemma 5.51 it holds w.p.1, as $n \to \infty$, that $\hat{\vartheta}_n^* \to \vartheta_0$ in probability with respect to $\mathbb{P}_n^*$, where $\hat{\vartheta}_n^*$ is the maximizer of $\ell_n^*(\cdot)$.

Proof Note that we might encounter measurability issues as in Theorem 5.52 for the MLE. Again, if this happens we consider the inner probability measure. The continuity of the density functions and the compactness of Ξ assure the existence of $\hat{\vartheta}_n^* \in \Xi$. Denote by $V(\subset V_0)$ an arbitrary open neighborhood of ϑ_0. Since

$\hat{\vartheta}_n \to \vartheta_0$ w.p.1, we can assume that $\hat{\vartheta}_n \in V$ for all $n \in \mathbb{N}$. Let $U = \Xi \backslash V$. Clearly, $\sup_{\vartheta \in U} \ell_n^*(\vartheta) < \ell_n^*(\vartheta_0)$ imply $\hat{\vartheta}_n^* \in V$. Therefore, it is sufficient to proof that w.p.1

$$\mathbb{P}_n^* \left(\sup_{\vartheta \in U} \ell_n^*(\vartheta) - \ell_n^*(\vartheta_0) < 0 \right) \longrightarrow 1, \quad \text{as } n \to \infty. \tag{5.26}$$

We will now find a finite cover $B_1, \ldots, B_m$ for U, where every B_k will have the property (5.26), i.e.,

$$\mathbb{P}_n^* \left(\sup_{\vartheta \in B_k} \ell_n^*(\vartheta) - \ell_n^*(\vartheta_0) \geq 0 \right) = o_{\mathbb{P}_n^*}(1), \quad \text{as } n \to \infty, \tag{5.27}$$

w.p.1, for $k = 1, \ldots, m$. For $\vartheta^* \in U$ choose V^* according to the assumption (i). In order to have a more compact notation we set

$$W_{in} = \sup_{\tilde{\vartheta} \in V^*} \log \left(\frac{f(Y_{in}^* | \theta_{X_i}(\tilde{\beta}), \tilde{\phi})}{f(Y_{in}^* | \theta_{X_i}(\beta_0), \phi_0)} \right).$$

We obtain

$$
\begin{aligned}
\sup_{\tilde{\vartheta} \in V^*} \ell_n^*(\tilde{\vartheta}) - \ell_n^*(\vartheta_0) &= n^{-1} \sup_{\tilde{\vartheta} \in V^*} \sum_{i=1}^n \log \left(\frac{f(Y_{in}^* | \theta_{X_i}(\tilde{\beta}), \tilde{\phi})}{f(Y_{in}^* | \theta_{X_i}(\beta_0), \phi_0)} \right) \\
&\leq n^{-1} \sum_{i=1}^n \sup_{\tilde{\vartheta} \in V^*} \log \left(\frac{f(Y_{in}^* | \theta_{X_i}(\tilde{\beta}), \tilde{\phi})}{f(Y_{in}^* | \theta_{X_i}(\beta_0), \phi_0)} \right) \\
&= n^{-1} \sum_{i=1}^n W_{in}.
\end{aligned}
$$

Equation (5.27) holds if we establish

$$\mathbb{P}_n^* \left(n^{-1} \sum_{i=1}^n W_{in} \geq 0 \right) = \mathbb{P}_n^* \left(n^{-1} \sum_{i=1}^n W_{in} - \mathbb{E}_n^*(W_{in}) \geq -n^{-1} \sum_{i=1}^n \mathbb{E}_n^*(W_{in}) \right) = o_{\mathbb{P}_n^*}(1).$$

For $\varepsilon > 0$ we get by Chebyshev's inequality

$$\mathbb{P}_n^* \left(n^{-1} \sum_{i=1}^n W_{in} - \mathbb{E}_n^*(W_{in}) \geq \varepsilon \right)$$

$$\leq (n\varepsilon)^{-2} \sum_{i=1}^n \mathbb{E}_n^*(W_{in}^2)$$

$$\leq (n\varepsilon)^{-2} \sum_{i=1}^{n} \int \left| \sup_{\tilde{\vartheta} \in V^*} \log \left(\frac{f(y|\theta_{X_i}(\tilde{\beta}), \tilde{\phi})}{f(y|\theta_{X_i}(\beta_0), \phi_0)} \right) \right|^2 \sup_{\vartheta \in V_0} f(y|\theta_{X_i}(\beta), \phi) \nu(\mathrm{d}y),$$

which converges w.p.1 to zero by assumption (i) and the SLLN, as $n \to \infty$. It remains to show that $n^{-1} \sum_{i=1}^{n} \mathbb{E}_n^*(W_{in})$ converges w.p.1 to a negative constant. Assumption (i) and Lemma 5.58 yield w.p.1, as $n \to \infty$,

$$n^{-1} \sum_{i=1}^{n} \mathbb{E}_n^*(W_{in}) \to \int \int \sup_{\tilde{\vartheta} \in V^*} \log \left(\frac{f(y|\theta_x(\tilde{\beta}), \tilde{\phi})}{f(y|\theta_x(\beta_0), \phi_0)} \right) f(y|\theta_x(\beta_0), \phi_0) \nu(\mathrm{d}y) H(\mathrm{d}x).$$

$$(5.28)$$

By assumption (i) and Lebegue's dominated convergence theorem the right-hand side of (5.28) converges to $L_H(\vartheta_0, \vartheta^*) - L_H(\vartheta_0, \vartheta_0)$ by shrinking V^* toward $\{\vartheta^*\}$. Finally, Lemma 5.51 implies $L_H(\vartheta_0, \vartheta^*) - L_H(\vartheta_0, \vartheta_0) < 0$.

In sum, w.p.1, for every $\varepsilon > 0$ we can choose for all ϑ^* an open neighborhood V^* of ϑ^* and an N such that

$$\mathbb{P}_n^*(\sup_{\vartheta \in V^*} \ell_n^*(\vartheta) - \ell_n^*(\vartheta_0) \geq 0) \leq \varepsilon$$

for $n \geq N$, where N maybe subject to ω. Since Ξ is compact, we can select from this cover of U a finite cover $B_1, \ldots, B_m$ which provides (5.26). Since V was chosen arbitrary, this concludes the proof. $\qquad\square$

Theorem 5.60 *If the density f is continuous in ϑ at ϑ_0 and*

(i) $\log f(y|\theta_x(\beta), \phi)$ has continuous second derivatives with respect to ϑ and there exist open neighborhoods $V_1, V_2 \subset \Xi$ of ϑ_0 such that for all $1 \leq r, s \leq p+1$

$$\int \int \sup_{\vartheta_1 \in V_1} |D_r(\log f(y|\theta_x(\beta_1), \phi_1))|^2 \sup_{\vartheta_2 \in V_2} f(y|\theta_x(\beta_2), \phi_2) \nu(\mathrm{d}y) H(\mathrm{d}x) < \infty$$

and

$$\int \int \sup_{\vartheta_1 \in V_1} |D_{r,s}(\log f(y|\theta_x(\beta_1), \phi_1))| \sup_{\vartheta_2 \in V_2} f(y|\theta_x(\beta_2), \phi_2) \nu(\mathrm{d}y) H(\mathrm{d}x) < \infty,$$

(ii) for all $\vartheta \in V_2$ it holds that

$$\int D_{p+1}(f(y|\theta_x(\beta), \phi)) \nu(\mathrm{d}y) H(\mathrm{d}x) = 0,$$

(iii) for all $1 \leq r, s \leq p+1$ and all $\vartheta \in V_2$ it holds that

$$\int D_{r,s}(f(y|\theta_x(\beta), \phi)) \nu(\mathrm{d}y) H(\mathrm{d}x) = 0,$$

(iv) for every $x \in \mathbb{R}^p$ the function

$$R_1(x, \beta) = \zeta''(\theta_x(\beta)) D(\theta_x(\beta))(D(\theta_x(\beta)))^\top$$

is continuous in β at β_0 and

$$\int \sup_{\vartheta_1 \in V_1} |R_1(x, \beta_1)| H(\mathrm{d}x) < \infty$$

and

$$A = \phi_0^{-1} \mathbb{E}\left(R_1(X, \beta_0)\right)$$

   exists and is positive definite,
(v) for every $x \in \mathbb{R}^p$ and $y \in \mathbb{R}$ the function

$$R_2(y, x, \vartheta) = D(\log(h(y, \phi))) - \frac{\theta_x(\beta)y - \zeta(\theta_x(\beta))}{\phi^2}$$

is continuous in ϑ at ϑ_0 and

$$\int\int \sup_{\vartheta_1 \in V_1} R_2^2(y, x, \vartheta_1) \sup_{\vartheta_2 \in V_2} f(y|\theta_x(\beta_2), \phi_2) \nu(\mathrm{d}y) H(\mathrm{d}x) < \infty,$$

and

$$0 < B = \mathbb{E}\left(R_2^2(Y, X, \vartheta_0)\right) < \infty,$$

(vi) $\hat{\vartheta}_n^* - \hat{\vartheta}_n = o_{\mathbb{P}_n^*}(1)$ w.p.1,
(vii) $\hat{\vartheta}_n$ converges w.p.1 to ϑ_0

holds, then $n^{1/2}(\hat{\vartheta}_n^* - \hat{\vartheta}_n) \to Z$, where Z is multivariate normally distributed with zero mean and covariance matrix

$$\Sigma^{-1} = \begin{pmatrix} A & 0 \\ 0 & B \end{pmatrix}^{-1}.$$

Remark 5.61 Note that the covariance matrix Σ of Theorem 5.60 equals the covariance matrix of Theorem 5.55, which is the CLT for the original MLE.

   Proof (of Theorem 5.60) Note, this proof is closely in line with the proof of Theorem 5.55 and we partially reuse calculations from that previous proof. In order to have more compact notation during the proof, define $\ell(y, x, \vartheta) = \log(f(y|\theta_x(\beta), \phi))$ and denote by s_n^* the gradient of ℓ_n^* and let Ds_n^* be the Jacobian matrix of the score function s_n^*. As before we also use D to denote by $D_r g$ and $D_{r,s} g$ the first partial derivative of g with respect to the r-th component of ϑ and the second partial derivative of g with respect to the r-th and s-th component of ϑ, respectively.

Note that

$$s_n^*(\hat{\vartheta}_n^*) - s_n^*(\hat{\vartheta}_n) = \left(\int_0^1 Ds_n^*(\hat{\vartheta}_n + t(\hat{\vartheta}_n^* - \hat{\vartheta}_n))dt \right) (\hat{\vartheta}_n^* - \hat{\vartheta}_n),$$

where the right-hand side is a matrix-vector product. First, we substitute the integral by $Ds_n^*(\hat{\vartheta}_n)$. Define

$$\Delta_n = \int_0^1 Ds_n^*(\hat{\vartheta}_n + t(\hat{\vartheta}_n^* - \hat{\vartheta}_n))dt - Ds_n^*(\hat{\vartheta}_n)$$

and $B_\varepsilon = \{\vartheta : \|\vartheta - \vartheta_0\| \leq \varepsilon\}$. W.l.o.g. we assume that $B_\varepsilon \subset V_2$. We have by Markov's inequality for the r−th and s−th component of Δ_n, denoted by $\Delta_n^{(r,s)}$, that

$$\mathbb{P}_n^*(|\Delta_n^{(r,s)}/n| > \tilde{\varepsilon}) \leq \mathbb{P}_n^*(\hat{\vartheta}_n^* \notin B_\varepsilon) + \tilde{\varepsilon}^{-1}\mathbb{E}_n^* \left(\mathbb{I}_{\{\hat{\vartheta}_n^* \in B_\varepsilon\}} |\Delta_n^{(r,s)}/n| \right). \qquad (5.29)$$

Since $\hat{\vartheta}_n^* - \hat{\vartheta}_n = o_{\mathbb{P}_n^*}(1)$ w.p.1 and $\hat{\vartheta}_n$ converges w.p.1 to ϑ_0, the first term on the right-hand side converges to zero w.p.1. The second term on the right-hand side converges also to zero as follows. For the sake of simplicity, we ignore the leading $\tilde{\varepsilon}$ since it is simply a constant. Due to the almost sure convergence of $\hat{\vartheta}_n$ to ϑ_0 we can assume that $\hat{\vartheta}_n \in B_\varepsilon$ almost surely. Therefore, we have

$$\mathbb{E}_n^* \left(\mathbb{I}_{\{\hat{\vartheta}_n^* \in B_\varepsilon\}} |\Delta_n^{(r,s)}/n| \right)$$
$$\leq \mathbb{E}_n^* \left(\sup_{\vartheta \in B_\varepsilon} \left| n^{-1} \sum_{i=1}^n D_{r,s}\ell(Y_{in}^*, X_i, \vartheta) - D_{r,s}\ell(Y_{in}^*, X_i, \hat{\vartheta}_n) \right| \right)$$
$$\leq n^{-1} \sum_{i=1}^n \mathbb{E}_n^* \left(\sup_{\vartheta, \tilde{\vartheta} \in B_\varepsilon} \left| D_{r,s}\ell(Y_{in}^*, X_i, \vartheta) - D_{r,s}\ell(Y_{in}^*, X_i, \tilde{\vartheta}) \right| \right).$$

By the assumptions on the second derivatives in (i) and Lemma 5.58, the last expression converges w.p.1 to

$$\int \int \sup_{\vartheta, \tilde{\vartheta} \in B_\varepsilon} \left| D_{r,s}\ell(y, x, \vartheta) - D_{r,s}\ell(y, x, \tilde{\vartheta}) \right| f(y|\theta_x(\beta_0), \phi_0) v(dy) H(dx),$$

which converges to zero if ε tends to zero due to the continuity of the second derivatives of $\log f$, see assumption (i), and Lebegue's dominated convergence theorem. Altogether, we obtain $n^{-1}\Delta_n = o_{\mathbb{P}_n^*}(1)$ and since $s_n^*(\hat{\vartheta}_n^*) = 0$ the initial equality becomes

$$-n^{-1/2}s_n^*(\hat{\vartheta}_n) = \left(n^{-1}Ds_n^*(\hat{\vartheta}_n) + o_{\mathbb{P}_n^*}(1) \right) \left(n^{1/2}(\hat{\vartheta}_n^* - \hat{\vartheta}_n) \right). \qquad (5.30)$$

We now prepare the application of the CLT by investigating the limit of the variance of $n^{-1/2}s_n^*(\hat{\vartheta}_n)$. The function s_n^* consists of two parts, i.e.,

$$D_q\ell_n^*(\hat{\vartheta}_n) = \sum_{i=1}^{n} D_q\ell(Y_{in}^*, X_i, \hat{\vartheta}_n) = \frac{1}{\hat{\phi}_n}\sum_{i=1}^{n}(Y_{in}^* - \zeta'(\theta_{X_i}(\hat{\beta}_n)))D_q(\theta_{X_i}(\hat{\beta}_n))$$

for $1 \le q \le p$ and

$$D_{p+1}\ell_n^*(\hat{\vartheta}_n) = \sum_{i=1}^{n} D_{p+1}\ell(Y_{in}^*, X_i, \hat{\vartheta}_n) = \sum_{i=1}^{n} D(c(Y_{in}^*, \hat{\phi}_n)) - \frac{\theta_{X_i}(\hat{\beta}_n)Y_{in}^* - \zeta(\theta_{X_i}(\hat{\beta}_n))}{\hat{\phi}_n^2},$$

where $c(y, \phi) = \log h(y, \phi)$. Following the proof of Theorem 5.55 we easily conclude (under assumption (ii)) that every summand of $s_n^*(\hat{\vartheta}_n)$ is centered. Another relation that can be directly reused (under assumption (iii)) from the proof of Theorem 5.55 is that

$$\mathbb{E}_n^* \left(D_{r,s}(\log f_{in})\right) = -\text{COV}_n^* \left(D_r(\log f_{in}), D_s(\log f_{in})\right) \qquad (5.31)$$

for all $1 \le r, s \le p + 1$, where f_{in} is the density of Y_{in}^*. In particular,

$$\text{COV}_n^* \left(D_{p+1}(\log f_{in}), D_q(\log f_{in})\right)$$

equals

$$-\mathbb{E}_n^* \left(\frac{\partial^2 \log f_{in}}{\partial \phi \partial \beta_q}\right) = \hat{\phi}_n^{-2}\mathbb{E}_n^* \left(\frac{\partial \log f_{in}}{\partial \beta_q}\right) = 0$$

for all $1 \le q \le p$, which is quite expectable because the likelihood equation of β is independent of ϕ. By construction, $Y_{1n}^*, \dots, Y_{nn}^*$ is an independent sequence and therefore, the covariance matrix of $n^{-1/2}s_n^*(\hat{\vartheta}_n)$ consists of two blocks, and following the proof of Theorem 5.55 we obtain

$$\text{COV}_n^* \left((n^{1/2}\hat{\phi}_n)^{-1}\sum_{i=1}^{n}(Y_{in}^* - \zeta'(\theta_{X_i}(\hat{\beta}_n)))D(\theta_{X_i}(\hat{\beta}_n))\right) = (n\hat{\phi}_n)^{-1}\sum_{i=1}^{n}\mathbb{E}_n^*(R_1(X_i, \hat{\beta}_n)).$$

The right-hand side converges by assumption (iv) and Lemma 5.58 w.p.1 to

$$A = \phi_0^{-1}\mathbb{E}(R_1(X, \beta_0)). \qquad (5.32)$$

Due to independence, the second block of $n^{-1/2}s_n^*(\hat{\vartheta}_n)$ equals

$$\mathbb{E}_n^* \left(\left(n^{-1/2}\sum_{i=1}^{n} R_2(Y_{in}^*, X_i, \hat{\vartheta}_n)\right)^2\right) = n^{-1}\sum_{i=1}^{n}\mathbb{E}_n^* \left(R_2^2(Y_{in}^*, X_i, \hat{\vartheta}_n)\right).$$

By assumption (v) and again Lemma 5.58, we conclude that the second block of $\text{COV}_n^*(n^{-1/2}s_n^*(\hat{\vartheta}_n))$ converges w.p.1 to

$$B = \mathbb{E}\left(R_2^2(Y, X, \vartheta_0)\right). \tag{5.33}$$

Note that due to equation (5.31) $-n^{-1}Ds_n^*(\hat{\vartheta}_n)$ converges also to the asymptotic covariance matrix of $n^{-1/2}s_n^*(\hat{\vartheta}_n)$.

The final step is to apply the CLT to $s_n^*(\hat{\vartheta}_n)$ and afterward Lemma 5.54. According to the Cramér-Wold device, we have to investigate $n^{-1/2}a^\top s_n^*(\hat{\vartheta}_n)$ for $a \in \mathbb{R}^{p+1}\backslash\{0\}$ arbitrary. Obviously, every summand of the linear combination is centered because every component of $s_n^*(\hat{\vartheta}_n)$ is centered. Hence, it remains to proof that the Lindeberg condition holds. But since the variance of $n^{-1/2}a^\top s_n^*(\hat{\vartheta}_n)$ converges w.p.1, the Lindeberg condition simplifies to

$$\sum_{i=1}^n \int_{\{|n^{-1/2}\sum_{q=1}^{p+1} a_q D_q \ell(y, X_i, \hat{\vartheta}_n)| \geq \delta\}} \left(n^{-1/2}\sum_{q=1}^{p+1} a_q D_q \ell(y, X_i, \hat{\vartheta}_n)\right)^2 d\mathbb{P}_n^* \longrightarrow 0, \quad \text{as } n \to \infty,$$

w.p.1, where $\delta > 0$. The left-hand side is eventually bounded by

$$n^{-1}\sum_{i=1}^n \mathbb{E}_n^*\left(\sup_{\vartheta \in B_\varepsilon} I_{\{|\sum_{q=1}^{p+1} a_q D_q \ell(y, X_i, \vartheta)| \geq \delta K^{1/2}\}} \left(\sum_{q=1}^{p+1} a_q D_q \ell(y, X_i, \vartheta)\right)^2\right)$$

for all $K \in \mathbb{N}$ which converges w.p.1, as $n \to \infty$, to

$$\mathbb{E}\left(\sup_{\vartheta \in B_\varepsilon} I_{\{|\sum_{q=1}^{p+1} a_q D_q \ell(Y, X, \vartheta)| \geq \delta K^{1/2}\}} \left(\sum_{q=1}^{p+1} a_q D_q \ell(Y, X, \vartheta)\right)^2\right).$$

This expression tends to zero by the assumption on the first derivative in (i) for $K \to \infty$, which proofs that the Lindeberg condition holds.

To sum up, the left-hand side of equation (5.30) is asymptotically normal distributed with an asymptotic variance consisting of the two blocks (5.32) and (5.33), i.e., Σ. Furthermore, we know that $n^{-1}Ds_n^*(\vartheta_0)$ converges to $-\Sigma$, as $n \to \infty$. Applying Lemma 5.54 yields the result and concludes the proof. $\qquad\square$

Corollary 5.62 *Under the assumptions of Theorem 5.60 it holds for*

$$L(X_i, Y_{in}^*, \hat{\beta}_n, \hat{\phi}_n) = \Sigma^{-1}D(\log(f(Y_{in}^*|\theta_{X_i}(\hat{\beta}_n), \hat{\phi}_n)))$$

that

1. $n^{1/2}(\hat{\vartheta}_n^* - \hat{\vartheta}_n) = n^{-1/2}\sum_{i=1}^n L(X_i, Y_{in}^*, \hat{\beta}_n, \hat{\phi}_n) + o_{\mathbb{P}^*}(1)$, *as $n \to \infty$, w.p.1,*
2. $\mathbb{E}^*(L(X_i, Y_{in}^*, \hat{\beta}_n, \hat{\phi}_n)) = 0$ *for all $n \in \mathbb{N}$,*

3. $n^{-1} \sum_{i=1}^{n} \mathbb{E}^* \left(L(X_i, Y_{in}^*, \hat{\beta}_n, \hat{\phi}_n) L^\top (X_i, Y_{in}^*, \hat{\beta}_n, \hat{\phi}_n) \right)$ *converges w.p.1 to* Σ^{-1}.

Proof All calculations were already made in the proof of Theorem 5.60. According to the representation (5.30) and Lemma 5.54 we can set

$$L(X_i, Y_{in}^*, \hat{\beta}_n, \hat{\phi}_n) = \Sigma^{-1} D(\log(f(Y_{in}^* | \theta_{X_i}(\hat{\beta}_n), \hat{\phi}_n)))$$

to obtain assertion 1, since $n^{-1} Ds_n^*(\hat{\vartheta}_n)$ converges to $-\Sigma$. Note, these are the summands of $s_n^*(\hat{\vartheta}_n)$ from the proof of Theorem 5.60 multiplied by Σ^{-1}. In the proof it was shown that the summands of $s_n^*(\hat{\vartheta}_n)$ are centered and the arithmetic mean of the covariance of the summands converges w.p.1 to Σ. Since Σ is a constant matrix the proof of Theorem 5.60 directly yield the assertions 2 and 3 of the corollary.   □

5.4   Semi-parametric Model

Recall the situation of the classical linear model, where $Y = \beta^\top X + \varepsilon$. This was extended to the parametric generalized linear model assuming that Y given X has a distribution belonging to the exponential family and additionally that there exists a link function g such that $g(\mathbb{E}(Y|X = x)) = m(x, \beta) = \beta^\top x$. Another way to extend the classical linear model is to consider $Y = m(\beta^\top X) + \varepsilon$ and leave the distribution of ε unspecified. Hence, we have the parametric component β and the non-parametric component ε. In summary, we get

Definition 5.63 Let $(Y, X) \in \mathbb{R}^{1+p}$ and let $g : \mathbb{R} \to \mathbb{R}$ be an invertible link function. If there exists $\beta_0 \in \mathbb{R}^p$ such that for $\mathbb{E}(Y \mid X = x)$, the conditional distribution of Y given $X = x$,

$$\mathbb{E}(Y \mid X = x) = g^{-1}(\beta_0^\top x) \equiv m(\beta_0^\top x), \quad \text{for all } x \in \mathbb{R}^p,$$

applies, then (Y, X) follows a *semi-parametric generalized linear model* with link function g.

Note that we also write m instead of g^{-1} to uniform the presentation.

Most of the time in this section we will only assume

$$Y = m(X, \vartheta) + \varepsilon,$$

i.e., we are not restricted to $\beta^\top X$. One of the model definitions, see Definition 5.68, is $\mathbb{E}(\varepsilon|X) = 0$, and therefore yields $\mathbb{E}(Y|X) = m(X, \vartheta)$.

The parametric bootstrap is not applicable anymore here because no parametric form of ε is assumed. In this section, we will focus on the wild bootstrap, where the resampling scheme is very similar to the resampling scheme we used for linear models, see RSS 5.23. The only difference is how the estimators for the model parameter and residuals are determined.

Resampling Scheme 5.64

(A) *Based on the i.i.d. observations* $(Y_i, X_i)_{1 \le i \le n} \subset \mathbb{R}^{1+p}$ *calculate the* $\hat{\vartheta}_n$.
(B) *Determine the estimated residuals* $\hat{\varepsilon}_{i,n} = Y_i - m(X_i, \hat{\vartheta}_n)$.
(C) *Define the wild bootstrap residuals by* $\varepsilon^*_{i,n} = \hat{\varepsilon}_{i,n} \cdot \tau_i^*$, *where* $\tau_1^*, \ldots, \tau_n^*$ *is an i.i.d. sequence of Rademacher rvs. which is independent of* $(X_1, \varepsilon_1), \ldots, (X_n, \varepsilon_n)$.
(D) *Set* $X_i^* = X_i$, $Y_{i,n}^* = m(X_i, \hat{\vartheta}_n) + \varepsilon^*_{i,n}$.
(E) *Determine* $\hat{\vartheta}_n^*$ *based on* $(Y_{i,n}^*, X_i^*)$.

R-Example 5.65 The dataset in this example follows

$$m(X, \vartheta) + \varepsilon = \vartheta_a \exp(X/\vartheta_b) + \vartheta_c \exp(X/\vartheta_d) + \varepsilon$$

with $\vartheta_0 = (4, -2, -3, -10)$, $\varepsilon \sim N(0, 0.25^2)$ and X uniformly distributed on $[1, 30]$. The following R-code generates 400 samples and fits a model.

```
set.seed(123,kind ="Mersenne-Twister",normal.kind ="Inversion")
semiparametric_data <-
  data.frame(X = runif(400, min = 1, max = 30)) %>%
  dplyr::mutate(
    mu = 4 * exp(-X/2) - 3 * exp(-X/10),
    epsilon = rnorm(400, sd = 0.25),
    Y = mu + epsilon)

fit_sp <- minpack.lm::nlsLM(
  formula = Y ~ a * exp(X/b) + c * exp(X/d),
  data = semiparametric_data,
  start = c(a = 4, b = -2, c = -3, d = -10),
  control = nls.control(maxiter = 1000))
fit_sp


  ## Nonlinear regression model
  ##    model: Y ~ a * exp(X/b) + c * exp(X/d)
  ##     data: semiparametric_data
  ##       a       b       c       d
  ##   3.707  -2.105  -3.025  -9.797
  ##   residual sum-of-squares: 23.76
  ##
  ## Number of iterations to convergence: 3
  ## Achieved convergence tolerance: 1.49e-08

confint(fit_sp)

## Waiting for profiling to be done...

  ##            2.5%       97.5%
  ## a      3.174945   4.269019
```

```
## b  -2.824567 -1.609529
## c  -3.844516 -2.601336
## d -10.959331 -8.551295
```

These large number of samples are necessary because otherwise estimating the confidence intervals via *confint* is problematic and quickly results in an error. This is also the reason why we started the optimization in ϑ_0 which is unknown in practice. Now, we implement the wild bootstrap and apply it to the fitted model.

```
rrademacher <- function(n) {
  2 * rbinom(n = n, size = 1, prob = 1/2) - 1
}

bootstrap_sp <- function(data, fit_obj) {
  # Step B
  epsilon_hat <- residuals(fit_obj)
  # Step C
  boot_epsilon <- rrademacher(length(epsilon_hat)) * epsilon_hat
  # Step D
  boot_X <- data$X
  boot_Y <- predict(fit_obj) + boot_epsilon
  # Step E
  minpack.lm::nlsLM(
    formula = boot_Y ~ a * exp( boot_X/b) + c * exp(boot_X/d),
    start = coef(fit_obj),
    control = nls.control(warnOnly = T, maxiter = 1000))
}
fit_wb <- lapply(
  1:200,
  function(dummy) bootstrap_sp(semiparametric_data, fit_sp))

coef_wb <- sapply(fit_wb, coef) %>%
  t() %>%
  as.data.frame()
tail(coef_wb)
```

```
##             a         b         c          d
## 195 3.988986 -2.127204 -3.145468  -9.381500
## 196 3.925056 -2.417854 -3.346528  -9.234672
## 197 3.892880 -1.869759 -2.908396  -9.994309
## 198 3.573355 -2.123758 -3.050824  -9.367015
## 199 3.997472 -1.589187 -2.686212 -10.280919
## 200 3.552934 -1.917992 -2.792621 -10.195711
```

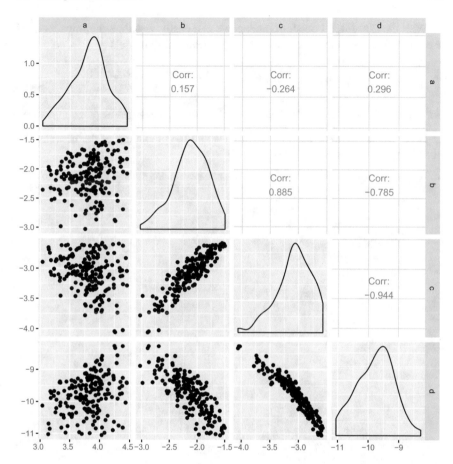

Fig. 5.11 Simulated non-linear model. Matrix of plots showing the distribution of the bootstrapped parameters

This allows us to obtain 95% confidence intervals using quantiles

```
apply(coef_wb, 2, quantile, prob = c(0.025, 0.975))
```

```
##            a         b         c          d
## 2.5%   3.180270 -2.802138 -3.727098 -10.975106
## 97.5%  4.386482 -1.556582 -2.613631  -8.652354
```

However, there is strong correlation between the four components, see Fig. 5.11.

```
coef_wb %>%
  GGally::ggpairs()
```

With the 200 fitted bootstrap models we can easily visualize the impact on the estimated function. First, we gather the predictions of all models

```
pred_wb <- sapply(fit_wb, predict) %>%
  as.data.frame() %>%
  dplyr::mutate(X = semiparametric_data$X) %>%
  tidyr::gather(boot_model, y_pred_wb, -X)
```

Here, we see an excerpt of the covariates and the prediction of the first and last bootstrapped models:

```
head(pred_wb)
```

```
##              X boot_model   y_pred_wb
## 1   9.339748          V1  -1.1281292
## 2  23.860849          V1  -0.2593153
## 3  12.860331          V1  -0.8058073
## 4  26.607505          V1  -0.1948618
## 5  28.273551          V1  -0.1638439
## 6   2.321138          V1  -1.1879945
```

```
tail(pred_wb)
```

```
##               X boot_model   y_pred_wb
## 79995  4.057115        V200  -1.4473640
## 79996  7.948244        V200  -1.2243636
## 79997  8.845801        V200  -1.1374968
## 79998  3.930696        V200  -1.4415745
## 79999  4.419501        V200  -1.4556303
## 80000 29.745860        V200  -0.1509946
```

Next, we plot the original observations with the corresponding model fit as well as all 200 bootstrapped models, see Fig. 5.12.

```
semiparametric_data %>%
  dplyr::mutate(y_pred = predict(fit_sp))  %>%
  ggplot(aes(x = X, y = Y)) +
  geom_point() +
  geom_line(data = pred_wb,
            aes(x = X, y = y_pred_wb, group = boot_model),
            alpha = 0.1) +
  geom_line(aes(y = y_pred), color = "red") +
  theme_minimal()
```

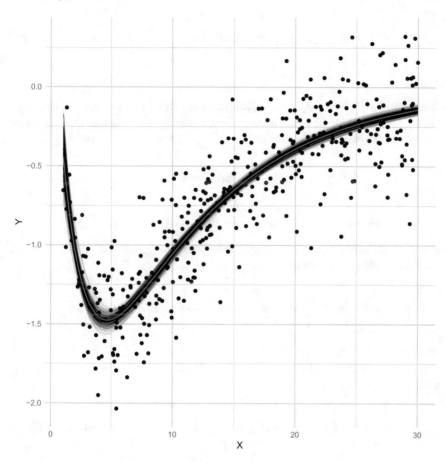

Fig. 5.12 Simulated non-linear model. Fitted model as solid red line and 200 bootstrapped models as solid black lines

5.4.1 Mathematical Framework of LSE

The proofs rely heavily on Jennrich (1969). Especially, Theorem 2 of Jennrich (1969) will be used multiple times. Therefore, we explicitly state the theorem next.

Theorem 5.66 (Theorem 2, Jennrich 1969) *Let m be a function on $\mathscr{X} \times \Theta$ where $\mathscr{X}$ is a Euclidean space and Θ is a compact subset of a Euclidean space. Let $m(x, \vartheta)$ be a continuous function of ϑ for each x and a measurable function of x for each ϑ. Assume also that $|m(x, \vartheta)| \leq M(x)$ for all x and ϑ, where M is integrable with respect to a probability distribution function F on $\mathscr{X}$. If $X_1, X_2, \ldots, X_n$ is an i.i.d. sample with distribution function F, then*

$$\left\| n^{-1} \sum_{i=1}^{n} m(X_i, \vartheta) - \int m(x, \vartheta) F(\mathrm{d}x) \right\|_{\vartheta \in \Theta} \longrightarrow 0, \quad as \ n \to \infty,$$

w.p.1.

Corollary 5.67 *Let $\vartheta_1, \vartheta_2, \ldots, \vartheta_n$ be a sequence of random variables with codomain Θ. Under the assumptions of Theorem 5.66, but only assuming that there exists an open neighborhood V of ϑ_0 such that $|m(x, \vartheta)| \leq M(x)$ for all x and $\vartheta \in V$, then*

$$n^{-1} \sum_{i=1}^{n} m(X_i, \vartheta_n) \longrightarrow \mathbb{E}(m(X, \vartheta_0)), \quad as \ n \to \infty,$$

w.p.1 (in probability), if ϑ_n converges w.p.1 (in probability) to $\vartheta_0 \in \Theta$.

Proof First assume that ϑ_n converges almost surely to ϑ_0. Let $\tilde{V} \subset V$ be a compact subset such that ϑ_0 is an inner point of $\tilde{V}$. Obviously,

$$\left| n^{-1} \sum_{i=1}^{n} m(X_i, \vartheta_n) \mathrm{I}_{\{\vartheta_n \notin \tilde{V}\}} \right| \longrightarrow 0, \quad as \ n \to \infty,$$

w.p.1 because ϑ_n converges to ϑ_0 w.p.1.
The corresponding counterpart $|n^{-1} \sum_{i=1}^{n} m(X_i, \vartheta_n) \mathrm{I}_{\{\vartheta_n \in \tilde{V}\}} - \mathbb{E}(m(X, \vartheta_0))|$ is bounded by

$$\left\| n^{-1} \sum_{i=1}^{n} m(X_i, \vartheta) - \mathbb{E}(m(X, \vartheta)) \right\|_{\vartheta \in \tilde{V}} + |\mathbb{E}(m(X, \vartheta_n) \mathrm{I}_{\{\vartheta_n \in \tilde{V}\}} - m(X, \vartheta_0))|.$$

The first term converges to zero by Theorem 5.66 w.p.1 because $\tilde{V}$ is compact. By the assumption, the difference $|m(x, \vartheta_n) \mathrm{I}_{\{\vartheta_n \in \tilde{V}\}} - m(x, \vartheta_0)|$ is dominated by $2M(x)$ and converges w.p.1 to zero since ϑ_n converges to ϑ_0 w.p.1. Applying Lebegue's dominated convergence theorem to $\mathbb{E}(|m(X, \vartheta_n) \mathrm{I}_{\{\vartheta_n \in \tilde{V}\}} - m(X, \vartheta_0)|)$ yields the first part of the corollary.

Now assume that ϑ_n converges in probability to ϑ_0. Then for every sub-sequence n_k exists a further sub-sequence $n_{k'}$ such that $\vartheta_{n_{k'}}$ converges to ϑ_0 w.p.1. Applying the first part of this corollary, we obtain

$$n_{k'}^{-1} \sum_{i=1}^{n_{k'}} m(X_i, \vartheta_{n_{k'}}) \longrightarrow \mathbb{E}(m(X, \vartheta_0)), \quad as \ k' \to \infty,$$

w.p.1. This implies the convergence in probability for the original sequence and completes the proof. $\square$

We now list some general assumptions (GA) which will be used frequently in this section.

General Assumptions 5.68

(i) Θ compact.

(ii) $X, X_1, ..., X_n$ is an i.i.d. sample with codomain $\mathscr{X}$.

(iii) $\varepsilon, \varepsilon_1, ..., \varepsilon_n$ is an i.i.d. sample, $\mathbb{E}(\varepsilon|X) = 0$ w.p.1, $\mathbb{E}(\varepsilon^2) = \sigma^2$.

(iv) $Y_i = m(X_i, \vartheta_0) + \varepsilon_i, \vartheta_0 \in \Theta$.

(v) $Q(\vartheta) = \mathbb{E}((m(X, \vartheta_0) - m(X, \vartheta))^2)$ has a unique minimum at $\vartheta = \vartheta_0$.

(vi) $m(x, \vartheta)$ continuous in ϑ for all $x \in \mathscr{X}$ and measurable in x for all $\vartheta \in \Theta$.

(vii) there exists a measurable function $M(x)$ with $m^2(x, \vartheta) \leq M(x)$ for all $x \in \mathscr{X}$ and $\vartheta \in \Theta$; $\mathbb{E}(M(X)) < \infty$.

(viii) $\mathbb{E}(M(X)|\varepsilon|) < \infty$.

Lemma 5.69 *Under the GA 5.68,*

$$\left\| n^{-1} \sum_{i=1}^{n} m(X_i, \vartheta)\varepsilon_i \right\|_{\vartheta \in \Theta} \longrightarrow 0, \quad as \ n \to \infty,$$

w.p.1.

Proof By the assumption of continuity and domination, i.e., assumption (vi)–(viii), we directly obtain from Theorem 5.66 that $n^{-1} \sum_{i=1}^{n} m(X_i, \vartheta)\varepsilon_i$ converges w.p.1 uniformly in ϑ to $\mathbb{E}(m(X, \vartheta)\varepsilon) = \mathbb{E}(m(X, \vartheta)\mathbb{E}(\varepsilon|X))$ which equals zero by assumption (iii). $\square$

Lemma 5.70 *Under the GA 5.68,*

$$\left\| n^{-1} \sum_{i=1}^{n} (Y_i - m(X_i, \vartheta))^2 - Q(\vartheta) - \sigma^2 \right\|_{\vartheta \in \Theta} \longrightarrow 0, \quad as \ n \to \infty,$$

w.p.1.

Proof Setting $D(x, \vartheta) := m(x, \vartheta_0) - m(x, \vartheta)$, we obtain

$$n^{-1} \sum_{i=1}^{n} (Y_i - m(X_i, \vartheta))^2 = n^{-1} \sum_{i=1}^{n} (m(X_i, \vartheta_0) + \varepsilon_i - m(X_i, \vartheta))^2$$

$$= n^{-1} \sum_{i=1}^{n} D^2(X_i, \vartheta) + 2n^{-1} \sum_{i=1}^{n} D(X_i, \vartheta)\varepsilon_i + n^{-1} \sum_{i=1}^{n} \varepsilon_i^2.$$

Since m^2 is dominated, i.e., assumption (vii), Theorem 5.66 implies that the first term converges uniformly in ϑ to $Q(\vartheta)$ w.p.1. The second term converges uniformly in ϑ to zero w.p.1 by Lemma 5.69. Finally, the last term, which is independent of ϑ, converges by the SLLN to σ^2 w.p.1. This concludes the proof. $\square$

Theorem 5.71 *Under the GA 5.68, $\hat{\vartheta}_n$ converges to ϑ_0, as $n \to \infty$, w.p.1.*

Proof Let $Q_n(\vartheta) = n^{-1} \sum_{i=1}^{n} (Y_i - m(X_i, \vartheta))^2$. Since Θ is compact and f is continuous in ϑ, there exists a $\hat{\vartheta}_n$ that minimizes Q_n. By virtue of Lemma 5.70, Q_n converges uniformly and almost surely to $Q + \sigma^2$. Therefore, it exists a set $\Omega_0 \subset \Omega$ with $\mathbb{P}(\Omega_0) = 1$ such that Q_n converges uniformly and the sequence $\hat{\vartheta}_n$ minimizes Q_n for all $\omega \in \Omega_0$. The following arguments are restricted to a fixed $\omega \in \Omega_0$. Since Θ is compact, $\hat{\vartheta}_n$ has a limit point $\tilde{\vartheta}$. We can assume that $\hat{\vartheta}_n$ converges to $\tilde{\vartheta}$. By Corollary 5.67 we have $Q_n(\hat{\vartheta}_n) \to Q(\tilde{\vartheta}) + \sigma^2$ and $Q_n(\vartheta_0) \to \sigma^2$ because $Q(\vartheta_0) = 0$. Since $\hat{\vartheta}_n$ minimizes Q_n, it also holds for all $n \in \mathbb{N}$ that $Q_n(\hat{\vartheta}_n) \leq Q_n(\vartheta_0)$. Therefore, $Q(\tilde{\vartheta}) + \sigma^2 \leq \sigma^2$, which implies $Q(\tilde{\vartheta}) = 0$. The uniqueness assumption (v) yields that $\tilde{\vartheta} = \vartheta_0$. Since $\mathbb{P}(\Omega_0) = 1$, this concludes the proof. $\qquad\square$

Corollary 5.72 *Under the GA 5.68, $n^{-1} \sum_{i=1}^{n} (Y_i - m(X_i, \hat{\vartheta}_n))^2$ converges to σ^2, as $n \to \infty$, w.p.1.*

Proof Obviously,

$$n^{-1} \sum_{i=1}^{n} (Y_i - m(X_i, \hat{\vartheta}_n))^2 = n^{-1} \sum_{i=1}^{n} (m(X_i, \vartheta_0) + \varepsilon_i - m(X_i, \hat{\vartheta}_n))^2$$

$$\xrightarrow[n \to \infty]{} \mathbb{E}\left((m(X, \vartheta_0) + \varepsilon - m(X, \vartheta_0))^2 \right)$$

$$= \sigma^2,$$

w.p.1, where the convergence is due to the consistency of the estimator $\hat{\vartheta}_n$ and Corollary 5.67. $\qquad\square$

Theorem 5.73 *In addition to the GA 5.68, assume*

(i) *the first and second partial derivatives of f with respect to ϑ are continuous in ϑ for all $x \in \mathscr{X}$ and measurable in x for all $\vartheta \in \Theta$*

(ii)

$$A = \left(\mathbb{E}\left(\frac{\partial m(X, \vartheta_0)}{\partial \vartheta_s} \frac{\partial m(X, \vartheta_0)}{\partial \vartheta_t} \right) \right)_{1 \leq s,t \leq p}$$

is positive definite

(iii)

$$A_\sigma = \left(\mathbb{E}\left(\varepsilon^2 \frac{\partial m(X, \vartheta_0)}{\partial \vartheta_s} \frac{\partial m(X, \vartheta_0)}{\partial \vartheta_t} \right) \right)_{1 \leq s,t \leq p}$$

is positive definite

(iv) *there exists $\delta > 0$ and $M_2(x)$ such that*

$$\left| \frac{\partial^2 m(x, \vartheta)}{\partial \vartheta_s \partial \vartheta_t} \right| \leq M_2(x)$$

for all x and ϑ in a closed ball $B_\delta(\vartheta_0)$ with $\mathbb{E}(M_2(X)|\varepsilon|) < \infty$

(v) there exists $\delta > 0$ and $M_3(x)$ such that

$$\left| \frac{\partial m(x, \vartheta)}{\partial \vartheta_s} \frac{\partial m(x, \vartheta)}{\partial \vartheta_t} \right| \leq M_3(x)$$

for all x and ϑ in a closed ball $B_\delta(\vartheta_0)$ with $\mathbb{E}(M_3(X)) < \infty$

(vi) there exists $\delta > 0$ and $M_4(x)$ such that

$$\left| m(x, \tilde{\vartheta}) \frac{\partial^2 m(x, \vartheta)}{\partial \vartheta_s \partial \vartheta_t} \right| \leq M_4(x)$$

for all x and $\tilde{\vartheta}$ and ϑ in a closed ball $B_\delta(\vartheta_0)$ with $\mathbb{E}(M_4(X)) < \infty$

(vii) $\hat{\vartheta}_n$ minimizes $\sum_{i=1}^n (m(X_i, \vartheta) - Y_i)^2$

(viii) $\hat{\vartheta}_n$ converges almost surely to ϑ_0 and ϑ_0 is an inner point of Θ,

then

$$n^{1/2}(\hat{\vartheta}_n - \vartheta_0) \to Z, \quad \text{as } n \to \infty,$$

in distribution, where Z is normally distributed with mean zero and variance $A^{-1} A_\sigma A^{-\top}$.

Proof Set $Q_n(\vartheta) := (2n)^{-1} \sum_{i=1}^n (m(X_i, \vartheta) - Y_i)^2$. Since $\hat{\vartheta}_n \to \vartheta_0$ and ϑ_0 is an inner point of Θ, we can assume that $\hat{\vartheta}_n$ is also an inner point of Θ for $n > N$. We have

$$0 = \frac{\partial Q_n(\hat{\vartheta}_n)}{\partial \vartheta} = \frac{\partial Q_n(\vartheta_0)}{\partial \vartheta} + \left(\frac{\partial^2 Q_n(\tilde{\vartheta}_n)}{\partial \vartheta \partial \vartheta^\top} \right) (\hat{\vartheta}_n - \vartheta_0)$$

with $\|\tilde{\vartheta}_n - \vartheta_0\| \leq \|\hat{\vartheta}_n - \vartheta_0\|$. Consider the first term on the right-hand side,

$$n^{1/2} \frac{\partial Q_n(\vartheta_0)}{\partial \vartheta} = n^{-1/2} \sum_{i=1}^n (m(X_i, \vartheta_0) - Y_i) \frac{\partial m(X_i, \vartheta_0)}{\partial \vartheta} = -n^{-1/2} \sum_{i=1}^n \varepsilon_i \frac{\partial m(X_i, \vartheta_0)}{\partial \vartheta}.$$

According to the CLT this converges in distribution to a centered normal random variable with covariance matrix A_σ.

We now focus on the components of the second partial derivatives of Q_n at $\tilde{\vartheta}_n$, i.e.,

$$\frac{\partial^2 Q_n(\tilde{\vartheta}_n)}{\partial \vartheta \partial \vartheta^\top} = n^{-1} \sum_{i=1}^n \frac{\partial m(X_i, \tilde{\vartheta}_n)}{\partial \vartheta} \frac{\partial m(X_i, \tilde{\vartheta}_n)}{\partial \vartheta^\top} + n^{-1} \sum_{i=1}^n (m(X_i, \tilde{\vartheta}_n) - Y_i) \frac{\partial^2 m(X_i, \tilde{\vartheta}_n)}{\partial \vartheta \partial \vartheta^\top}$$

$$= n^{-1} \sum_{i=1}^n \frac{\partial m(X_i, \tilde{\vartheta}_n)}{\partial \vartheta} \frac{\partial m(X_i, \tilde{\vartheta}_n)}{\partial \vartheta^\top} - n^{-1} \sum_{i=1}^n \varepsilon_i \frac{\partial^2 m(X_i, \tilde{\vartheta}_n)}{\partial \vartheta \partial \vartheta^\top}$$

$$+ n^{-1} \sum_{i=1}^n \left(m(X_i, \tilde{\vartheta}_n) - m(X_i, \vartheta_0) \right) \frac{\partial^2 m(X_i, \tilde{\vartheta}_n)}{\partial \vartheta \partial \vartheta^\top}.$$

Since $\hat{\vartheta}_n$ converges to ϑ_0 w.p.1 and $\|\tilde{\vartheta}_n - \vartheta_0\| \le \|\hat{\vartheta}_n - \vartheta_0\|$, we can assume that $\tilde{\vartheta}_n \in B_\delta(\vartheta_0)$ for all $n > N$. By the continuity assumptions and assumption (vi), Corollary 5.67 implies that the third term converges to

$$\mathbb{E}\left((m(X, \vartheta_0) - m(X, \vartheta_0)) \frac{\partial^2 m(X, \vartheta_0)}{\partial\vartheta\,\partial\vartheta^\top} \right) = 0.$$

Similar, by the continuity assumptions and assumption (iv), Corollary 5.67 implies that the second term converges to

$$\mathbb{E}\left(\frac{\partial^2 m(X, \vartheta_0)}{\partial\vartheta\,\partial\vartheta^\top}\varepsilon \right) = \mathbb{E}\left(\frac{\partial^2 m(X, \vartheta_0)}{\partial\vartheta\,\partial\vartheta^\top}\mathbb{E}(\varepsilon|X) \right),$$

which is also zero because $\mathbb{E}(\varepsilon|X) = 0$. Again, by the continuity assumptions and assumption (v), Corollary 5.67 implies that the first term converges to

$$\mathbb{E}\left(\frac{\partial m(X, \vartheta_0)}{\partial\vartheta} \frac{\partial m(X, \vartheta_0)}{\partial\vartheta^\top} \right) = A.$$

At the beginning we stated that

$$-n^{1/2}\frac{\partial Q_n(\vartheta_0)}{\partial\vartheta} = \left(\frac{\partial^2 Q_n(\tilde{\vartheta}_n)}{\partial\vartheta\,\partial\vartheta^\top} \right)\left(n^{1/2}(\hat{\vartheta}_n - \vartheta_0) \right). \tag{5.34}$$

The left-hand side converges in distribution to a centered normal distributed random variable with covariance matrix A_σ. Furthermore, the partial derivatives on the right-hand side converge to A w.p.1. Since A is positive definite, Lemma 5.54 concludes the proof. □

The last theorem gives the following asymptotic representation of the estimator.

Corollary 5.74 *Under the assumptions of Theorem 5.73 it holds for*

$$L(x, y, \vartheta_0) = A^{-1}(y - m(x, \vartheta_0))\frac{\partial m(x, \vartheta_0)}{\partial\vartheta}$$

that

1. $n^{1/2}(\hat{\vartheta}_n - \vartheta_0) = n^{-1/2}\sum_{i=1}^n L(X_i, Y_i, \vartheta_0) + o_{\mathbb{P}}(1)$, *as* $n \to \infty$,
2. $\mathbb{E}(L(X, Y, \vartheta_0)) = 0$,
3. $\mathbb{E}\left(L(X, Y, \vartheta_0)L^\top(X, Y, \vartheta_0) \right)$ *exists and is positive definite.*

Proof As shown in the proof of Theorem 5.73, we have that

$$\frac{\partial^2 Q_n(\tilde{\vartheta}_n)}{\partial\vartheta\,\partial\vartheta^\top} \longrightarrow A, \quad \text{as } n \to \infty,$$

w.p.1. Hence, according to Equation (5.34) we obtain the first result, i.e.,

$$n^{1/2}(\hat{\vartheta}_n - \vartheta_0) = o_{\mathbb{P}}(1) + n^{-1/2} \sum_{i=1}^{n} A^{-1}(Y_i - m(X_i, \vartheta_0)) \frac{\partial m(X_i, \vartheta_0)}{\partial \vartheta},$$

as $n \to \infty$. Due to the assumption that $\mathbb{E}(\varepsilon | X) = 0$ we obtain the second result. Finally, $\mathbb{E}\left(L(X, Y, \vartheta_0)L^{\top}(X, Y, \vartheta_0)\right) = A^{-1}A_\sigma A^{-\top}$ is positive definite since A and A_σ are positive definite. □

5.4.2 Mathematical Framework of Wild Bootstrap LSE

In the wild bootstrap setup, as we have already stated in Sect. 5.2.2, we use $\mathbb{P}^*$ instead of $\mathbb{P}_n^*$ for the underlying probability measure of the bootstrap.

Lemma 5.75 Let $Z_1, Z_2, \ldots, Z_n$ be an i.i.d. sequence of random variables and assume that $\mathbb{E}\left(|Z_1|^{2+\delta}\right) < \infty$ for some $\delta > 0$. Then

$$\sum_{i \geq 1}(Z_i/i)^2 < \infty$$

w.p.1.

Proof Let $\kappa = 1/(1 + \delta/2)$. We have the following bound

$$\sum_{i \geq 1} \frac{Z_i^2}{i^2} = \sum_{i \geq 1} \frac{Z_i^2}{i^\kappa} \frac{1}{i^{2-\kappa}} \leq \sum_{i \geq 1} \frac{Z_i^2}{i^\kappa} \frac{1}{i^{2-\kappa}} I_{\{Z_i^2 > i^\kappa\}} + \sum_{i \geq 1} \frac{1}{i^{2-\kappa}}.$$

The second sum on the right-hand side converges because $\kappa < 1$. The first sum on the right-hand side is finite because $\limsup_{i \to \infty} Z_i^2/i^\kappa \leq 1$ w.p.1. This is due to the Borel-Cantelli lemma and the following inequality,

$$\sum_{i \geq 1} \mathbb{P}\left(\frac{Z_i^2}{i^\kappa} > 1\right) \leq \sum_{i \geq 1} \mathbb{P}\left(\frac{|Z_i|^{2/\kappa}}{i} > 1\right)$$

$$= \sum_{i \geq 1} \int_{[i-1,i)} \mathbb{P}\left(|Z_1|^{2+\delta} > i\right) \mathrm{d}z$$

$$\leq \sum_{i \geq 1} \int_{[i-1,i)} \mathbb{P}\left(|Z_1|^{2+\delta} > z\right) \mathrm{d}z$$

$$= \int_0^\infty \mathbb{P}\left(|Z_1|^{2+\delta} > z\right) \mathrm{d}z$$

$$= \mathbb{E}(|Z_1|^{2+\delta})$$

$$< \infty.$$

This concludes the proof. □

Lemma 5.76 *Under the GA 5.68, Resampling Scheme 5.64 and the assumptions*

(i) *there exists a $\delta > 0$ such that for all $\vartheta \in \Theta$ the expectation $\mathbb{E}(|m(X, \vartheta)\varepsilon|^{2+\delta})$ is finite,*

(ii) *$\mathbb{E}(M(X)\varepsilon^2) < \infty$, compare GA 5.68 (vii) and (viii),*

(iii) *for all $\delta > 0$ exists a $\tilde{\delta} > 0$ such that $|m(x, \vartheta_1) - m(x, \vartheta_2)| < \delta$ for all $x \in \mathcal{X}$ and $\|\vartheta_1 - \vartheta_2\| < \tilde{\delta}$,*

then

$$\left\| n^{-1} \sum_{1 \leq i \leq n} m(X_i^*, \vartheta)\varepsilon_i \tau_i^* \right\|_{\vartheta \in \Theta} = o_{\mathbb{P}^*}(1)$$

w.p.1.

Proof Define $c_{i,\omega}(\vartheta) = m(X_i(\omega), \vartheta)\varepsilon_i(\omega)$. Due to Definition 5.68 and assumption (ii), Theorem 5.66 guarantees that $n^{-1} \sum_{i=1}^n c_{i,\omega}^2(\vartheta)$ converges uniformly in ϑ w.p.1. Hence, there exist an Ω_0, independent of ϑ, with $\mathbb{P}(\Omega_0) = 1$ such that $n^{-1} \sum_{i=1}^n c_{i,\omega}^2(\vartheta)$ converge for all $\vartheta \in \Theta$ and $\omega \in \Omega_0$. By definition of the Rademacher rvs. $\text{VAR}^*(\tau_i^*) = 1$ and therefore we have by Lemma 5.75 that

$$\sum_{i \geq 1} \frac{\text{VAR}^*(c_{i,\omega}(\vartheta)\tau_i^*)}{i^2} = \sum_{i \geq 1} \frac{c_{i,\omega}^2(\vartheta)}{i^2} < \infty$$

for all $\omega \in \Omega_0$ and $\vartheta \in \Theta$. This allows to apply Shorack (2000, Theorem 10.4.4) which implies

$$n^{-1} \sum_{i=1}^n m(X_i(\omega), \vartheta)\varepsilon_i(\omega)\tau_i^*(\omega^*) \longrightarrow 0, \quad \text{as } n \to \infty, \qquad (5.35)$$

almost surely with respect to $\mathbb{P}^*$, for all $\omega \in \Omega_0$ and all $\vartheta \in \Theta$. The final step is to extend this result to uniform convergence in ϑ. Denote the sum on the left-hand side of (5.35) by $Z_{n,\omega}(\omega^*, \vartheta)$. In order to achieve uniform convergence, we have to show that $\{Z_{n,\omega}(\omega^*, \vartheta), \omega^* \in \Omega^*, n \geq 1\}$ is equicontinuous. By the equicontinuity of m there exists for all $\delta > 0$ a $\tilde{\delta}$ such that $|m(x, \vartheta_1) - m(x, \vartheta_2)| \leq \delta$ for all $x \in \mathcal{X}$ and $\|\vartheta_1 - \vartheta_2\| \leq \tilde{\delta}$. Since $|\tau_i^*| = 1$, we obtain

$$|Z_{n,\omega}(\omega^*, \vartheta_1) - Z_{n,\omega}(\omega^*, \vartheta_2)|$$

$$\leq n^{-1} \sum_{i=1}^n |m(X_i(\omega), \vartheta_1) - m(X_i(\omega), \vartheta_2)| \, |\varepsilon_i(\omega)| \, |\tau_i^*(\omega^*)|$$

$$\leq \delta 2\mathbb{E}(|\varepsilon|),$$

where the last inequality holds for $n > N(\omega)$ and $\|\vartheta_1 - \vartheta_2\| \leq \tilde{\delta}$. Since Θ is compact, for all $\omega \in \Omega_0$, Yuan (1997, Lemma) yields that $\|Z_{n,\omega}(\omega^*, \vartheta)\|_{\vartheta \in \Theta}$ converges to zero almost surely with respect to $\mathbb{P}^*$, which also implies convergence in probability with respect to $\mathbb{P}^*$. Since $\mathbb{P}(\Omega_0) = 1$, this concludes the proof. $\square$

Lemma 5.77 *Under the assumptions of Lemma 5.76,*

$$\left\| n^{-1} \sum_{i=1}^n m(X_i^*, \vartheta) \varepsilon_{i,n}^* \right\|_{\vartheta \in \Theta} = o_{\mathbb{P}^*}(1), \quad as\ n \to \infty,$$

w.p.1.

Proof By definition $\varepsilon_{i,n}^* = \tau_i^* \hat{\varepsilon}_{i,n} = \tau_i^*(Y_i - m(X_i, \hat{\vartheta}_n)) = \tau_i^*(m(X_i, \vartheta_0) + \varepsilon_i - m(X_i, \hat{\vartheta}_n))$. Hence, for $\delta > 0$,

$$\mathbb{P}^* \left(\left\| n^{-1} \sum_{i=1}^n m(X_i, \vartheta) \varepsilon_{i,n}^* \right\|_{\vartheta \in \Theta} > \delta \right)$$

$$= \mathbb{P}^* \left(\left\| n^{-1} \sum_{i=1}^n m(X_i, \vartheta) \tau_i^*(Y_i - m(X_i, \hat{\vartheta}_n)) \right\|_{\vartheta \in \Theta} > \delta \right)$$

$$\leq \mathbb{P}^* \left(\left\| n^{-1} \sum_{i=1}^n m(X_i, \vartheta) \tau_i^* \varepsilon_i \right\|_{\vartheta \in \Theta} > \delta/2 \right)$$

$$+ \mathbb{P}^* \left(\left\| n^{-1} \sum_{i=1}^n m(X_i, \vartheta) \tau_i^*(m(X_i, \vartheta_0) - m(X_i, \hat{\vartheta}_n)) \right\|_{\vartheta \in \Theta} > \delta/2 \right)$$

$$= o_{\mathbb{P}^*}(1) + \mathbb{P}^* \left(\left\| n^{-1} \sum_{i=1}^n m(X_i, \vartheta) \tau_i^*(m(X_i, \vartheta_0) - m(X_i, \hat{\vartheta}_n)) \right\|_{\vartheta \in \Theta} > \delta/2 \right),$$

where the last equality is due to Lemma 5.76. It remains to investigate the second term. Let $\tilde{\delta} > 0$ and $B_{\tilde{\delta}}(\vartheta_0)$ be a ball around ϑ_0. Since $\hat{\vartheta}_n$ converges to ϑ_0 w.p.1 and $|\tau_i^*| = 1$, the corresponding norm is bound by

$$n^{-1} \sum_{i=1}^n \left\| m(X_i, \vartheta) \tau_i^*(m(X_i, \vartheta_0) - m(X_i, \hat{\vartheta}_n)) \right\|_{\vartheta \in \Theta}$$

$$\leq n^{-1} \sum_{i=1}^n \|m(X_i, \vartheta)\|_{\vartheta \in \Theta} |\tau_i^*| |m(X_i, \vartheta_0) - m(X_i, \hat{\vartheta}_n)|$$

$$\leq n^{-1} \sum_{i=1}^n \|m(X_i, \vartheta)\|_{\vartheta \in \Theta} \|m(X_i, \vartheta_0) - m(X_i, \tilde{\vartheta})\|_{\tilde{\vartheta} \in B_{\tilde{\delta}}(\vartheta_0)}$$

$$\xrightarrow[n \to \infty]{} \mathbb{E} \left(\|m(X, \vartheta)\|_{\vartheta \in \Theta} \|m(X, \vartheta_0) - m(X, \tilde{\vartheta})\|_{\tilde{\vartheta} \in B_{\tilde{\delta}}(\vartheta_0)} \right)$$

$$\xrightarrow[\tilde{\delta} \to 0]{} 0,$$

where the last convergence is due to Lebegue's dominated convergence theorem because $\|m(X, \vartheta)\|_{\vartheta \in \Theta} \|m(X, \vartheta_0) - m(X, \tilde{\vartheta})\|_{\tilde{\vartheta} \in B_{\tilde{\delta}}(\vartheta_0)}$ converges to zero if $\tilde{\delta}$ converges to zero and is dominated by $2M(X)$ according to the GA 5.68. Since $\tilde{\delta}$ was arbitrary chosen, this concludes the proof.   □

Lemma 5.78 *Under the assumptions of Lemma 5.76,*

$$\left\| n^{-1} \sum_{i=1}^{n} (Y_{i,n}^* - m(X_i^*, \vartheta))^2 - Q(\vartheta) - \sigma^2 \right\|_{\vartheta \in \Theta} = o_{\mathbb{P}^*}(1), \quad as \ n \to \infty,$$

w.p.1.

Proof Define $\Delta(x, \vartheta_1, \vartheta_2) = m(x, \vartheta_1) - m(x, \vartheta_2)$, then

$$n^{-1} \sum_{i=1}^{n} (Y_{i,n}^* - m(X_i^*, \vartheta))^2 = n^{-1} \sum_{i=1}^{n} (m(X_i, \hat{\vartheta}_n) + \varepsilon_{i,n}^* - m(X_i, \vartheta))^2$$

$$= n^{-1} \sum_{i=1}^{n} \Delta^2(X_i, \hat{\vartheta}_n, \vartheta) + 2n^{-1} \sum_{i=1}^{n} \Delta(X_i, \hat{\vartheta}_n, \vartheta)\varepsilon_{i,n}^*$$

$$+ n^{-1} \sum_{i=1}^{n} \varepsilon_{i,n}^{*2}.$$

Due to Lemma 5.77 we have

$$\mathbb{P}^* \left(\left\| n^{-1} \sum_{i=1}^{n} (Y_{i,n}^* - m(X_i^*, \vartheta))^2 - Q(\vartheta) - \sigma^2 \right\|_{\vartheta \in \Theta} > \delta \right)$$

$$\leq \mathbb{P}^* \left(\left\| n^{-1} \sum_{i=1}^{n} \Delta^2(X_i, \hat{\vartheta}_n, \vartheta) - Q(\vartheta) \right\|_{\vartheta \in \Theta} > \delta/3 \right) + o_{\mathbb{P}^*}(1)$$

$$+ \mathbb{P}^* \left(\left\| n^{-1} \sum_{i=1}^{n} \varepsilon_{i,n}^{*2} - \sigma^2 \right\|_{\vartheta \in \Theta} > \delta/3 \right).$$

By definition $\tau_{i,n}^{*2} = 1$, therefore the third term becomes

$$\mathbb{I}_{\{|n^{-1} \sum_{i=1}^{n} \hat{\varepsilon}_{i,n}^2 - \sigma^2| > \delta/3\}},$$

which converges to zero by the strong consistency of the estimated residuals, see Corollary 5.72. It remains to investigate

$$\left\| n^{-1} \sum_{i=1}^{n} \Delta^2(X_i, \hat{\vartheta}_n, \vartheta) - Q(\vartheta) \right\|_{\vartheta \in \Theta},$$

which is bounded by

$$
\left\| n^{-1} \sum_{i=1}^{n} \Delta^2(X_i, \vartheta_1, \vartheta_2) - \tilde{Q}(\vartheta_1, \vartheta_2) \right\|_{(\vartheta_1, \vartheta_2) \in \Theta^2} + \left\| \tilde{Q}(\hat{\vartheta}_n, \vartheta) - \tilde{Q}(\vartheta_0, \vartheta) \right\|_{\vartheta \in \Theta},
$$

where $\tilde{Q}(\vartheta_1, \vartheta_2) = \mathbb{E}\left((m(X, \vartheta_1) - m(X, \vartheta_2))^2 \right)$. Note, $Q(\vartheta) = \tilde{Q}(\vartheta_0, \vartheta)$. Since $\Delta^2(X, \hat{\vartheta}_n, \vartheta)$ is dominated by $4M(X)$ and Θ^2 is compact, we can apply Theorem 5.66 and obtain

$$
n^{-1} \sum_{i=1}^{n} \Delta^2(X_i, \vartheta_1, \vartheta_2) \longrightarrow \tilde{Q}(\vartheta_1, \vartheta_2), \quad \text{as } n \to \infty,
$$

uniformly in $(\vartheta_1, \vartheta_2) \in \Theta^2$ w.p.1. Note that $\tilde{Q}$ is a continuous function in $(\vartheta_1, \vartheta_2)$ because m^2 is dominated by M which guarantees the continuity by Lebegue's dominated convergence theorem. Due to the compactness of Θ^2 it is also uniform continuous. Therefore, $\left\| \tilde{Q}(\hat{\vartheta}_n, \vartheta) - \tilde{Q}(\vartheta_0, \vartheta) \right\|_{\vartheta \in \Theta}$ converges to zero because $\hat{\vartheta}_n$ converges to ϑ_0 w.p.1. This concludes the proof. $\qquad \square$

Theorem 5.79 *Under Resampling Scheme 5.64 and the assumptions of Lemma 5.76,*

$$
\|\hat{\vartheta}_n^* - \vartheta_0\| = o_{\mathbb{P}^*}(1), \quad \text{as } n \to \infty,
$$

w.p.1.

Proof First observe that for all $\delta > 0$ there exists an $\varepsilon > 0$ such that $|\vartheta - \vartheta_0| > \delta$ implies $|Q(\vartheta) - Q(\vartheta_0)| > \varepsilon$. This can be seen by contradiction. Assume that there exists a $\delta > 0$ such that for all $n \in \mathbb{N}$ we find a ϑ_n with $|\vartheta_n - \vartheta_0| > \delta$ and $|Q(\vartheta_n) - Q(\vartheta_0)| \leq n^{-1}$. Since Θ is compact we can assume that ϑ_n converges to $\tilde{\vartheta}$. By the continuity of Q we also have $Q(\tilde{\vartheta}) = Q(\vartheta_0) = 0$. By the uniqueness assumption for ϑ_0, we obtain $\tilde{\vartheta} = \vartheta_0$. But this contradicts our assumption that $|\vartheta_n - \vartheta_0| > \delta$ for all n. This yields the bound $\mathbb{P}^*(|\hat{\vartheta}_n^* - \vartheta_0| > \delta) \leq \mathbb{P}^*(|Q(\hat{\vartheta}_n^*) - Q(\vartheta_0)| > \varepsilon)$. Let $Q_n^*(\vartheta) = n^{-1} \sum_{i=1}^{n} (Y_{i,n}^* - m(X_i^*, \vartheta))^2$. We have w.p.1 that

$$
\begin{aligned}
Q(\hat{\vartheta}_n^*) + \sigma^2 &= o_{\mathbb{P}^*}(1) + Q_n^*(\hat{\vartheta}_n^*) \\
&= o_{\mathbb{P}^*}(1) + \inf_{\vartheta \in \Theta} Q_n^*(\vartheta) \\
&= o_{\mathbb{P}^*}(1) + \inf_{\vartheta \in \Theta} (o_{\mathbb{P}^*}(1) + Q(\vartheta) + \sigma^2) \\
&= o_{\mathbb{P}^*}(1) + \inf_{\vartheta \in \Theta} Q(\vartheta) + \sigma^2 \\
&= o_{\mathbb{P}^*}(1) + Q(\vartheta_0) + \sigma^2,
\end{aligned}
$$

where the first, third and fourth equality are due to the uniform convergence of Q_n^*, see Lemma 5.78, and the second and last equality are simply the definition of $\hat{\vartheta}_n^*$ and

ϑ_0. Therefore, $\mathbb{P}^*(|Q(\hat{\vartheta}_n^*) - Q(\vartheta_0)| > \varepsilon)$ converges to zero with probability one for all $\varepsilon > 0$. This concludes the proof. $\square$

Theorem 5.80 *Under Resampling scheme 5.64, assuming the GA 5.68 and in addition*

(i) *the first and second partial derivatives of m with respect to ϑ are continuous in ϑ for all $x \in \mathscr{X}$ and measurable in x for all $\vartheta \in \Theta$,*

(ii)

$$A = \left(\mathbb{E} \left(\frac{\partial m(X, \vartheta_0)}{\partial \vartheta_s} \frac{\partial m(X, \vartheta_0)}{\partial \vartheta_t} \right) \right)_{1 \le s, t \le p}$$

is positive definite,

(iii)

$$A_\sigma = \left(\mathbb{E} \left(\varepsilon^2 \frac{\partial m(X, \vartheta_0)}{\partial \vartheta_s} \frac{\partial m(X, \vartheta_0)}{\partial \vartheta_t} \right) \right)_{1 \le s, t \le p}$$

is positive definite,

(iv) *there exists $\delta > 0$ and $M_0(x)$, $M_1(x)$ and $M_2(x)$ such that for $k = 0, 1, 2$ and $s = 1, \ldots, p$,*

$$\left| m^k(x, \tilde{\vartheta}_1) \right| \left| \frac{\partial m(x, \tilde{\vartheta}_2)}{\partial \vartheta_s} \right|^2 \le M_k(x)$$

for all $x \in \mathscr{X}$ and $\tilde{\vartheta}_1$ and $\tilde{\vartheta}_2$ in a closed ball $B_\delta(\vartheta_0)$ with $\mathbb{E}(M_k(X)|\varepsilon|^{2-k}) < \infty$ for $k = 0, 1, 2$ and $\mathbb{E}(M_0(X)) < \infty$,

(v) *there exists $\delta > 0$ and $\tilde{M}_0(x)$, $\tilde{M}_1(x)$ and $\tilde{M}_2(x)$ such that for $k = 0, 1, 2$, $s = 1, \ldots, p$ and $t = 1, \ldots, p$,*

$$\left| m^k(x, \tilde{\vartheta}_1) \right| \left| \frac{\partial^2 m(x, \tilde{\vartheta}_2)}{\partial \vartheta_s \partial \vartheta_t} \right|^2 \le \tilde{M}_k(x)$$

for all $x \in \mathscr{X}$ and $\tilde{\vartheta}_1$ and $\tilde{\vartheta}_2$ in a closed ball $B_\delta(\vartheta_0)$ with $\mathbb{E}(\tilde{M}_k(X)|\varepsilon|^{2-k}) < \infty$ for $k = 0, 1, 2$,

(vi) *$\hat{\vartheta}_n$ converges to ϑ_0 w.p.1 and ϑ_0 is an inner point of Θ,*

(vii) *$\|\hat{\vartheta}_n^* - \vartheta_0\| = o_{\mathbb{P}^*}(1)$, as $n \to \infty$, w.p.1.*

Then w.p.1

$$n^{1/2}(\hat{\vartheta}_n^* - \hat{\vartheta}_n) \to Z, \quad as \ n \to \infty,$$

in distribution with respect to $\mathbb{P}^*$, where Z is normally distributed with mean zero and variance $A^{-1} A_\sigma A^{-\top}$.

Proof Set $Q_n^*(\vartheta) = (2n)^{-1} \sum_{i=1}^n (m(X_i^*, \vartheta) - Y_{i,n}^*)^2$ and let $V \subset \Theta$ be an open neighborhood of ϑ_0. Since all points in V are inner points of Θ, we have

$$0 = \frac{\partial Q_n^*(\hat{\vartheta}_n^*)}{\partial \vartheta} \mathrm{I}_{\{\hat{\vartheta}_n^* \in V\}} = \frac{\partial Q_n^*(\hat{\vartheta}_n)}{\partial \vartheta} \mathrm{I}_{\{\hat{\vartheta}_n^* \in V\}} + \left(\frac{\partial^2 Q_n^*(\tilde{\vartheta}_n)}{\partial \vartheta \, \partial \vartheta^\top} \mathrm{I}_{\{\hat{\vartheta}_n^* \in V\}} \right) \left(\hat{\vartheta}_n^* - \hat{\vartheta}_n \right)$$

$$(5.36)$$

with $\|\tilde{\vartheta}_n - \hat{\vartheta}_n\| \le \|\hat{\vartheta}_n^* - \hat{\vartheta}_n\|$. Note, $\|\hat{\vartheta}_n^* - \hat{\vartheta}_n\| = o_{\mathbb{P}^*}(1)$ due to the convergence of $\hat{\vartheta}_n^*$ as well as $\hat{\vartheta}_n$ to ϑ_0. Consider the first term on the right-hand side of (5.36). Since $Y_{i,n}^* = m(X_i, \hat{\vartheta}_n) + \tau_i^* \hat{\varepsilon}_{i,n}$,

$$n^{1/2} \frac{\partial Q_n^*(\hat{\vartheta}_n)}{\partial \vartheta} = -n^{-1/2} \sum_{i=1}^n \tau_i^* \hat{\varepsilon}_{i,n} \frac{\partial m(X_i, \hat{\vartheta}_n)}{\partial \vartheta}. \tag{5.37}$$

We now apply the Cramér-Wold device and verify the Lindeberg condition to show that the right-hand side converges to a multivariate normal distribution. Let $a \in \mathbb{R}^p$ be arbitrary but fixed and define $Z_{i,n}^* = n^{-1/2} \tau_i^* \hat{\varepsilon}_{i,n} \partial m(X_i, \hat{\vartheta}_n)/\partial \vartheta$. Obviously, $\mathbb{E}^*(a^\top Z_{i,n}^*) = 0$ and $\mathrm{VAR}^*(a^\top Z_{i,n}^*) = n^{-1} \hat{\varepsilon}_{i,n}^2 (a^\top \partial m(X_i, \hat{\vartheta}_n)/\partial \vartheta)^2$. The sum of these variances, denoted by s_n^2, appear in the Lindeberg condition. Therefore, we investigate its behavior. We have

$$s_n^2 = \sum_{i=1}^n \mathrm{VAR}^*(a^\top Z_{i,n}^*)$$

$$= n^{-1} \sum_{i=1}^n \hat{\varepsilon}_{i,n}^2 \left(a^\top \frac{\partial m(X_i, \hat{\vartheta}_n)}{\partial \vartheta} \right)^2$$

$$= n^{-1} \sum_{i=1}^n (m(X_i, \vartheta_0) - m(X_i, \hat{\vartheta}_n))^2 \left(a^\top \frac{\partial m(X_i, \hat{\vartheta}_n)}{\partial \vartheta} \right)^2$$

$$+ 2n^{-1} \sum_{i=1}^n (m(X_i, \vartheta_0) - m(X_i, \hat{\vartheta}_n)) \varepsilon_i \left(a^\top \frac{\partial m(X_i, \hat{\vartheta}_n)}{\partial \vartheta} \right)^2$$

$$+ n^{-1} \sum_{i=1}^n \varepsilon_i^2 \left(a^\top \frac{\partial m(X_i, \hat{\vartheta}_n)}{\partial \vartheta} \right)^2$$

$$\longrightarrow \mathbb{E} \left(\left(\varepsilon a^\top \frac{\partial m(X, \vartheta_0)}{\partial \vartheta} \right)^2 \right), \quad \text{as } n \to \infty, \tag{5.38}$$

w.p.1, where the convergence is due to assumption (iv) and Corollary 5.67 applied to each individual sum.

Now, we check the validity of the Lindeberg condition. For $\tilde{\varepsilon} > 0$,

$$\sum_{i=1}^n \frac{1}{s_n^2} \int_{|a^\top Z_{i,n}^*| > \tilde{\varepsilon} s_n} (a^\top Z_{i,n}^*)^2 \mathrm{d}\mathbb{P}^*$$

becomes

$$\frac{1}{ns_n^2} \sum_{i=1}^{n} \hat{\varepsilon}_{i,n}^2 \left(a^\top \frac{\partial m(X_i, \hat{\vartheta}_n)}{\partial \vartheta} \right)^2 \mathrm{I}_{\{|\hat{\varepsilon}_{i,n} a^\top \partial m(X_i, \hat{\vartheta}_n)/\partial \vartheta| > n^{1/2} \tilde{\varepsilon} s_n\}}$$

because $|\tau_i^*| = 1$. We now introduce a function J that bounds the indicator in a continuous way. Let

$$J(t) = \begin{cases} 1 & \text{if } 1 \le |t|, \\ 2|t| - 1 & \text{if } 1/2 < |t| < 1, \\ 0 & \text{if } |t| \le 1/2. \end{cases}$$

Due to this definition we have that $\mathrm{I}_{\{|y| > x\}} \le J(y/x)$ for $x > 0$. According to (5.38), it is therefore sufficient to show that

$$\frac{1}{ns_0^2/2} \sum_{i=1}^{n} \hat{\varepsilon}_{i,n}^2 \left(a^\top \frac{\partial m(X_i, \hat{\vartheta}_n)}{\partial \vartheta} \right)^2 J \left(\frac{\hat{\varepsilon}_{i,n} a^\top \partial m(X_i, \hat{\vartheta}_n)/\partial \vartheta}{n^{1/2} \tilde{\varepsilon} s_0/2} \right)$$

converges to zero, where s_0^2 denotes the limit of s_n^2. For fixed $K > 0$, this is eventually bounded by

$$\frac{1}{ns_0^2/2} \sum_{i=1}^{n} \hat{\varepsilon}_{i,n}^2 \left(a^\top \frac{\partial m(X_i, \hat{\vartheta}_n)}{\partial \vartheta} \right)^2 J \left(\frac{\hat{\varepsilon}_{i,n} a^\top \partial m(X_i, \hat{\vartheta}_n)/\partial \vartheta}{K} \right),$$

which converges w.p.1, as $n \to \infty$, by Corollary 5.67, see the argumentation for $\sum_{i=1}^{n} \mathrm{VAR}^*(a^\top Z_{i,n}^*)$, to

$$2 s_0^{-2} \mathbb{E} \left(\left(\varepsilon a^\top \frac{\partial m(X, \vartheta_0)}{\partial \vartheta} \right)^2 J \left(\frac{\varepsilon a^\top \partial m(X, \vartheta_0)/\partial \vartheta}{K} \right) \right) \xrightarrow[K \to \infty]{} 0.$$

The last convergence to zero is guaranteed by the definition of $J(t)$ and assumption (iv). This verifies the Lindeberg condition. According to the definition of A_σ in assumption (iii), $s_0^2 = a^\top A_\sigma A_\sigma^\top a$ which yields w.p.1

$$n^{1/2} \frac{\partial Q_n^*(\hat{\vartheta}_n)}{\partial \vartheta} \longrightarrow Z, \quad \text{as } n \to \infty,$$

in distribution with respect to $\mathbb{P}^*$, where Z is a centered multivariate normally distributed random variable with covariance matrix A_σ. Note that with assumption (vii) this also implies

$$n^{1/2} \frac{\partial Q_n^*(\hat{\vartheta}_n)}{\partial \vartheta} \mathrm{I}_{\{\hat{\vartheta}_n^* \notin V\}} = o_{\mathbb{P}^*}(1).$$

We now focus on the components of the second partial derivatives of Q_n at $\tilde{\vartheta}_n$, i.e., second term on the right-hand side of (5.36),

$$
\begin{aligned}
\frac{\partial^2 Q_n^*(\tilde{\vartheta}_n)}{\partial\vartheta\,\partial\vartheta^\top} &= n^{-1}\sum_{i=1}^n \frac{\partial m(X_i,\tilde{\vartheta}_n)}{\partial\vartheta}\frac{\partial m(X_i,\tilde{\vartheta}_n)}{\partial\vartheta^\top} + n^{-1}\sum_{i=1}^n (m(X_i,\tilde{\vartheta}_n)-Y_{i,n}^*)\frac{\partial^2 m(X_i,\tilde{\vartheta}_n)}{\partial\vartheta\,\partial\vartheta^\top} \\
&= n^{-1}\sum_{i=1}^n \frac{\partial m(X_i,\tilde{\vartheta}_n)}{\partial\vartheta}\frac{\partial m(X_i,\tilde{\vartheta}_n)}{\partial\vartheta^\top} - n^{-1}\sum_{i=1}^n \tau_i^*\hat{\varepsilon}_{i,n}\frac{\partial^2 m(X_i,\tilde{\vartheta}_n)}{\partial\vartheta\,\partial\vartheta^\top} \\
&\quad + n^{-1}\sum_{i=1}^n \big(m(X_i,\tilde{\vartheta}_n)-m(X_i,\hat{\vartheta}_n)\big)\frac{\partial^2 m(X_i,\tilde{\vartheta}_n)}{\partial\vartheta\,\partial\vartheta^\top}.
\end{aligned}
\tag{5.39}
$$

Since $\hat{\vartheta}_n$ and $\tilde{\vartheta}_n$ converges in probability (with respect to $\mathbb{P}^*$) to ϑ_0, the continuity assumptions, assumption (v) and Corollary 5.67 imply that the third term on the right-hand side of (5.39) converges w.p.1 to

$$
\mathbb{E}\left((m(X,\vartheta_0)-m(X,\vartheta_0))\frac{\partial^2 m(X,\vartheta_0)}{\partial\vartheta\,\partial\vartheta^\top}\right) = 0, \quad \text{as } n\to\infty,
$$

in probability with respect to $\mathbb{P}^*$. In a similar way as we handled $\sum_{i=1}^n \mathrm{VAR}^*(a^\top Z_{i,n}^*)$, assumption (v) and Corollary 5.67 provide w.p.1 that

$$
n^{-1}\sum_{i=1}^n\left(\hat{\varepsilon}_{i,n}\frac{\partial^2 m(X_i,\tilde{\vartheta}_n)}{\partial\vartheta\,\partial\vartheta^\top}\right)^2 \longrightarrow \mathbb{E}\left(\left(\varepsilon\frac{\partial^2 m(X,\vartheta_0)}{\partial\vartheta\,\partial\vartheta^\top}\right)^2\right), \quad \text{as } n\to\infty,
$$

in probability with respect to $\mathbb{P}^*$. Therefore, by Chebyshev's inequality, w.p.1 the second term on the right-hand side of (5.39), i.e.,

$$
n^{-1}\sum_{i=1}^n \tau_i^*\hat{\varepsilon}_{i,n}\frac{\partial^2 m(X_i,\tilde{\vartheta}_n)}{\partial\vartheta\,\partial\vartheta^\top}
$$

converges in probability (with respect to $\mathbb{P}^*$) to zero. Finally, by assumption (iv) and again Corollary 5.67 w.p.1 the first term converges in probability (with respect to $\mathbb{P}^*$) to A. In sum, with assumption (vii), we have w.p.1

$$
\frac{\partial^2 Q_n^*(\tilde{\vartheta}_n)}{\partial\vartheta\,\partial\vartheta^\top}\mathrm{I}_{\{\hat{\vartheta}_n^*\in V\}} = A + o_{\mathbb{P}^*}(1)
\tag{5.40}
$$

and as mentioned before

$$
n^{1/2}\frac{\partial Q_n^*(\hat{\vartheta}_n)}{\partial\vartheta}\mathrm{I}_{\{\hat{\vartheta}_n^*\notin V\}} = o_{\mathbb{P}^*}(1).
$$

Altogether, we obtain w.p.1 from (5.36)

$$-n^{1/2}\frac{\partial Q_n^*(\hat{\vartheta}_n)}{\partial \vartheta} + o_{\mathbb{P}^*}(1) = \left(A + o_{\mathbb{P}^*}(1)\right)\left(n^{1/2}(\hat{\vartheta}_n^* - \hat{\vartheta}_n)\right). \tag{5.41}$$

Since A has an inverse we apply Lemma 5.54 to obtain w.p.1 that $n^{1/2}(\hat{\vartheta}_n^* - \hat{\vartheta}_n)$ converges in distribution to a centered multivariate normally distributed random variable with covariance matrix $A^{-1}A_\sigma A^{-\top}$. This concludes the proof. □

The last theorem shows that the asymptotic covariance of the bootstrapped estimator is the same as the covariance of Theorem 5.73 and gives the following asymptotic representation of the estimator.

Corollary 5.81 *Under the assumptions of Theorem 5.80 it holds for*

$$L(x, y, \tau, \vartheta) = A^{-1}\tau(y - m(x, \vartheta))\frac{\partial m(x, \vartheta)}{\partial \vartheta}$$

that

1. $n^{1/2}(\hat{\vartheta}_n^* - \hat{\vartheta}_n) = n^{-1/2}\sum_{i=1}^n L(X_i, Y_{i,n}^*, \tau_i^*, \hat{\vartheta}_n) + o_{\mathbb{P}^*}(1)$, *as* $n \to \infty$, *w.p.1,*
2. $\mathbb{E}^*(L(X_i, Y_{i,n}^*, \tau_i^*, \hat{\vartheta}_n)) = 0$ *for all* n,
3. $n^{-1}\sum_{i=1}^n \mathbb{E}^*\left(L(X_i, Y_{i,n}^*, \tau_i^*, \hat{\vartheta}_n)L^\top(X_i, Y_{i,n}^*, \tau_i^*, \hat{\vartheta}_n)\right) \longrightarrow A^{-1}A_\sigma A^{-\top}$,
   as $n \to \infty$, *w.p.1.*

Proof According to Eq. 5.37 and 5.41 we obtain the first assertion from the proof of Theorem 5.80. The second result follows directly from $\mathbb{E}^*(\tau_i^*) = 0$. Finally, due to $\mathbb{E}^*(\tau_i^{*2}) = 1$ we obtain

$$\mathbb{E}^*\left(L(X_i, Y_{i,n}^*, \tau_i^*, \hat{\vartheta}_n)L^\top(X_i, Y_{i,n}^*, \tau_i^*, \hat{\vartheta}_n)\right) = A^{-1}\hat{\varepsilon}_{i,n}^2 \frac{\partial m(X_i, \hat{\vartheta}_n)}{\partial \vartheta}\left(\frac{\partial m(X_i, \hat{\vartheta}_n)}{\partial \vartheta}\right)^\top A^{-\top}.$$

Using a similar argumentation as for Equation (5.38) in proof of Theorem 5.80, we obtain with Corollary 5.67 and assumption (v) of Theorem 5.80 that

$$n^{-1}\sum_{i=1}^n \hat{\varepsilon}_{i,n}^2 \frac{\partial m(X_i, \hat{\vartheta}_n)}{\partial \vartheta}\left(\frac{\partial m(X_i, \hat{\vartheta}_n)}{\partial \vartheta}\right)^\top \longrightarrow A_\sigma, \quad \text{as } n \to \infty,$$

w.p.1. Since A is a constant matrix, we directly obtain assertion 3, which completes the proof. □

5.5 Exercises

Exercise 5.82 Simulate observations $(Y_i, x_i)_{1 \le i \le n}$, with $n = 50$, according to the model

$$Y_i = x_i \beta + \varepsilon_i, \qquad x_i = i/n,$$

where $\beta = 0.5$, $\sigma^2 = 4$, and $\varepsilon_1, \ldots, \varepsilon_n \sim \mathcal{N}(0, \sigma^2)$ are i.i.d.

 (i) Use Theorem 5.10 to construct an approximative confidence interval for β to the confidence level 0.9.
 (ii) Use Theorem 5.17 with 1000 bootstrap replications to construct an approximative confidence interval to the level 0.9.
 (iii) Repeat the steps (i) and (ii) 100 times. Determine the mean interval widths for the 100 intervals based on normal approximation and for the 100 intervals based on bootstrap approximation. Furthermore, obtain the coverage levels corresponding to the two approximations.

Exercise 5.83 Take the model given under Exercise 5.82.

 (i) Use Theorem 5.17 to construct a bootstrap-based test for

$$H_0 : \beta = 0.4 \quad \text{against} \quad H_1 : \beta > 0.4$$

and determine the approximative p−value based on 1000 bootstrap replications.
 (ii) Repeat the generation of the observations according to the model 100 times and use the bootstrap test developed under (i) for each dataset to calculate the corresponding p−values. Visualize the edf. of the 100 p−values and interpret the result.

Exercise 5.84 Use the model

$$Y_i = x_i \beta + \varepsilon_i, \qquad x_i = i/n,$$

where $\varepsilon_1 = x_1 \delta_1, \ldots, \varepsilon_n = x_n \delta_n$ and $\delta_1, \ldots, \delta_n \sim \mathcal{N}(0, \sigma^2)$ are i.i.d., $\beta = 0.5$, and $\sigma^2 = 4$. Note, in this case the error terms in the model, i.e., ε_i, are not homoscedastic anymore! Repeat the simulation studies of Exercises 5.82 and 5.83 with this model.

Exercise 5.85 Let the true model be $Y = 10 + 5x + \varepsilon$, where $\varepsilon \sim \mathcal{N}(0, 1)$ and x ranges from 1 to 20. Fit a linear model using only the x variable but no intercept. (Using an R-formula, this can be achieved by Y ~ x - 1). Why would the classical bootstrap scheme 5.31 and the wild bootstrap scheme 5.23 return very different bootstrap distributions for $\hat{\beta}$?

Exercise 5.86 Try to reproduce the estimation from Example 5.2 using Equation (5.2). Note, the diabetes status has to be recoded into 0 and 1.

Exercise 5.87 Try to reproduce the estimation from Example 5.2 using Remark 5.1 via the R-functions "stats::optim" or "stats:nlm". Note, the diabetes status has to be recoded into 0 and 1.

Exercise 5.88 Proof that RSS 5.7 works.

Exercise 5.89 Prove Lemma 5.37.

Exercise 5.90 Prove Lemma 5.38.

References

Billingsley P (1968) Convergence of probability measures. Wiley, New York
Dua D, Graff C (2017) UCI machine learning repository. URL http://archive.ics.uci.edu/ml.
    Accessed on 23 Dec 2019
Fanaee TH, Gama J (2013) Event labeling combining ensemble detectors and background knowl-
    edge. Prog Artif Intell 2:113–127
Jennrich RI (1969) Asymptotic properties of non-linear least squares estimators. Ann Math Stat
    40(2):633–643
Liu RY (1988) Bootstrap procedures under some non-i.i.d. models. Ann Stat 16(4):1696–1708
Loève M (1977) Probability theory. I, 4th edn. Springer, New York
Perlman MD (1972) On the strong consistency of approximate maximum likelihood estimates. In
    Proceedings of sixth Berk symposium math statistics and probability. University of California
    Press, Berkeley, CA, pp 263–281
Shorack GR (2000) Probability for statisticians. Springer texts in statistics. Springer, New York
Stute W (1990) Bootstrap of the linear correlation model. Statistics 21(3):433–436
Wu CFJ (1986) Jackknife, bootstrap and other resampling methods in regression analysis. Ann Stat
    14(4):1261–1350
Yuan KH (1997) A theorem on uniform convergence of stochastic functions with applications. J
    Multivar Anal 62(1):100–109

Chapter 6
Goodness-of-Fit Test for Generalized Linear Models

Goodness-of-fit (GOF) tests in regression analysis are mainly based on the observed residuals. In a series of articles, starting with Stute (1997), Stute established a general approach for GOF tests which is based on a marked empirical process (MEP), a standardized cumulative sum process obtained from the observed residuals. Resting upon the asymptotic limiting process of the MEP under the null hypothesis, Kolmogorov-Smirnov or Cramér-von Mises type tests can be stated as GOF tests. Their asymptotic distributions are derived through an application of the continuous mapping theorem. Since, in most cases, the asymptotic distributions depend on the model and, therefore, are not distribution free, further concepts are necessary to obtain the critical values for these tests.

In the literature, two approaches are discussed to handle the complicated structure of the limiting process of the MEP under the null hypothesis. In the first approach, the MEP is transformed in such a way that the resulting limiting process is a time-transformed Brownian motion with an assessable time transformation, compare Nikabadze and Stute (1997) and (Stute and Zhu, 2002). Originally, this technique was introduced by Khmaladze (1982) in the context of GOF tests based on estimated empirical processes. The second concept is based on the bootstrap, where the resampling scheme mimics the model under the null hypothesis. Resting upon the bootstrap data, the (bootstrap) MEP is derived. If one can show that this MEP tends to the same asymptotic process as the MEP of the original data does under the null hypothesis, the bootstrap MEP can be used to determine the critical value for the GOF statistic. Among others, this approach was used in Stute et al (1998) for parametric regression, in Dikta et al (2006) for binary regression, and in van Heel et al (2019) for multivariate binary regression models.

According to the general idea of bootstrap-based tests outlined in the introduction of Chap. 4, the bootstrap data has to be generated under the null hypothesis or close to it. If the asymptotic distribution of the bootstrapped statistic is the same as the corresponding one of the original data under the null hypothesis, critical values obtained from the bootstrap statistic can be used since they are derived under the null

© Springer Nature Switzerland AG 2021
G. Dikta and M. Scheer, *Bootstrap Methods*,
https://doi.org/10.1007/978-3-030-73480-0_6

hypothesis (the bootstrap data are generated under the null hypothesis) regardless whether the original data are following the null hypothesis or the alternative.

Denote, as usual, by $\mathbb{E}(Y \mid X = x)$ the regression function of Y at x (the conditional expectation of Y given $X = x$), and let

$$\mathcal{M} = \left\{ m(\beta^{\top} \cdot, \theta) \; : \; (\beta, \theta) \in \mathbb{R}^p \times \Theta \subset \mathbb{R}^{p+q} \right\}$$

define a parametric class based on a known function m. The general test problem for the GOF test is now

$$\mathbb{E}(Y \mid X = \cdot) \in \mathcal{M} \quad \text{versus} \quad \mathbb{E}(Y \mid X = \cdot) \notin \mathcal{M}.$$

Within the context of GLM with link function g, whether parametric or semi-parametric, there exists a $\beta_0 \in \mathbb{R}^p$ such that

$$\mathbb{E}(Y \mid X = x) = g^{-1}(\beta_0^{\top} x), \quad \text{for all } x \in \mathbb{R}^p.$$

Therefore, the MEP

$$\bar{R}_n^1 : \quad [-\infty, \infty] \ni u \longrightarrow \bar{R}_n^1(u) = n^{-1/2} \sum_{i=1}^{n} \left(Y_i - g^{-1}(\beta_n^{\top} X_i) \right) \mathrm{I}_{\{\beta_n^{\top} X_i \leq u\}} \quad (6.1)$$

can be used for the original data and

$$R_n^{1*} : \quad [-\infty, \infty] \ni u \longrightarrow R_n^{1*}(u) = n^{-1/2} \sum_{i=1}^{n} \left(Y_i^* - g^{-1}(\beta_n^{*\top} X_i) \right) \mathrm{I}_{\{\beta_n^{\top} X_i \leq u\}}$$

$$(6.2)$$

as bootstrap-based MEP, where the exact definition is given in Definitions 6.17 and 6.23, respectively.

In a parametric regression setup, where MEP-based statistics will be used for GOF tests, the following details will guarantee the validity of the bootstrap-based test:

1. Estimate the model parameter and build the MEP $\bar{R}_n^1$.
2. Determine the limit process of the MEP under the null hypothesis.
3. Generate bootstrap data according to the model, where the estimated parameters are used.
4. Repeat step (1) based on the bootstrap data and use R_n^{1*} as bootstrap-based MEP.
5. Verify that the bootstrap-based MEP tends to the limit process which is derived under (2).

The parameter estimation under (1) depends on the type of regression model. If we consider a semi-parametric GLM setup, LSE will be used to estimate the parameter since no further information about the distribution type of the error term is available. In this case, the wild bootstrap will be used. Otherwise, in the parametric GLM case, MLE will be applied and the bootstrap will be implemented parametrically.

Note that the indicator function in R_n^{1*} is based on β_n and not on β_n^*, as one would expect. This is mainly for performance reasons, see Remark 6.24. As shown in Sects. 6.4 and 6.5, both processes converge in distribution to the same centered Gaussian process $\bar{R}_\infty^1$ under the null hypothesis in the parametric and in the semi-parametric setup, if the appropriate assumptions can be guaranteed. Furthermore, the paths of $\bar{R}_\infty^1$ can be assumed to be continuous functions. Based on this result, Kolmogorov-Smirnov (D_n) and Cramér-von Mises (W_n^2) statistic are defined analogously to (4.7) and (4.8), respectively, by

$$D_n = \sup_{-\infty \le t \le \infty} \left| \bar{R}_n^1(t) \right|, \quad W_n^2 = n^{-1} \sum_{i=1}^{n} \left(\bar{R}_n^1(\beta_n^\top X_i) \right)^2.$$

Both statistics can be used to reveal discrepancies between the assumed model and the observations. By replacing $\bar{R}_n^1$ with R_n^{1*}, we get

$$D_n^* = \sup_{-\infty \le t \le \infty} \left| R_n^{1*}(t) \right|, \quad W_n^{*2} = n^{-1} \sum_{i=1}^{n} \left(R_n^{1*}(\beta_n^\top X_i) \right)^2,$$

the corresponding bootstrap statistics. Since both processes $\bar{R}_n^1$ and R_n^{1*} converge against the same Gaussian process under the null hypothesis, it follows, applying the continuous mapping theorem, that D_n and D_n^* as well as W_n^2 and W_n^{*2} also converge against the same limit distribution. But since the bootstrap data are always generated under the null hypothesis, we can now approximate the p-values of D_n and W_n^2 as usual by Monte Carlo application.

Our R-package `bootGOF` contains methods for performing the bootstrap tests we describe in this chapter. It is available on https://github.com/MarselScheer/bootGOF and CRAN. A brief introduction to the package can be found in the appendix. However, we deliberately do not use the `bootGOF`- package here because we want to illustrate how such complex resampling schemes can be implemented from scratch using simple (understandable) R-commands.

6.1 MEP in the Parametric Modeling Context

Usually modeling data is an iterative process where by fitting a model and investigating diagnostic aspects, like plots and test for assumptions, give ideas about potential improvements or serious misspecification. The GOF test based on the MEP is an additional tool that helps to detect if a fitted model contradicts the data one tries to model.

In this section, we apply the GOF test, based on the marked empirical process, to a real dataset in order to choose between a Poisson-, normal-, or negative-binomial model. Afterward, the GOF test is applied to artificial datasets in order to get a feeling for the test in situation where the truth is known.

Assume a parametric GLM with link function g. Under the notation stated in Definition 5.45, the following resampling scheme will be used for the GOF test.

Resampling Scheme 6.1

(A) Calculate the MLE $\hat{\beta}_n$ and $\hat{\phi}_n$ for $(Y_1, X_1), \ldots, (Y_n, X_n)$.

(B) Obtain the MEP (6.1) and calculate D_n and/or W_n^2 accordingly.

(C) Set $X_{\ell;i}^* = X_i$ for all $i = 1, \ldots, n$ and all $\ell = 1, \ldots, m$.

(D) Generate $Y_{\ell;i}^*$ according to the density $f(\cdot, \hat{\beta}_n, \hat{\phi}_n, X_i)$ for all $i = 1, \ldots, n$ and all $\ell = 1, \ldots, m$.

(E) Calculate the MLE $\hat{\beta}_{\ell;n}^*$ and $\hat{\phi}_{\ell;n}^*$ based on $(Y_{\ell;1}^*, X_{\ell;1}^*), \ldots, (Y_{\ell;n}^*, X_{\ell;n}^*)$, the MEP $R_{\ell;n}^{*1}$ according to (6.2), $D_{\ell;n}^*$ and/or $W_{\ell;n}^{*2}$, for $\ell = 1, \ldots, m$.

(F) Determine the p$-$value of D_n within the simulated $D_{\ell;n}^*$, $1 \leq \ell \leq m$ and/or W_n^2 the p-value of W_n^2 within the simulated $W_{\ell;n}^{*2}$, $1 \leq \ell \leq m$, respectively.

6.1.1 Implementation

First, we need the test statistic that will be resampled. The Cramér-von Mises test can be implemented as follows:

```
Rn1 <- function(mod, est_b_time_x) {

  # mod            - a model fit,
  # est_b_time_x - scalar product of the covariates and
  #                 estimator of beta

  o_idx <- order(est_b_time_x)
  ordered_res <- residuals(mod, type = "response")[o_idx]
  dplyr::tibble(est_b_time_x = est_b_time_x[o_idx],
             res = ordered_res,
             Rn1_x = cumsum(ordered_res) / sqrt(length(o_idx)),
             ordering = o_idx)
}


CvM <- function(mod, est_b_time_x) {

  # mod            - a model fit,
  # est_b_time_x - scalar product of the covariates and
  #                 estimator of beta

  Wn2 <- mean(Rn1(mod, est_b_time_x)$Rn1_x^2)
  Wn2
}
```

Note that this function itself uses the generic functions *predict* and *residuals* with a specific *type*-parameter. A fit created with "stats::glm" can be safely passed to the function because the corresponding functions "predict.glm" and "residuals.glm" respect the defined *type*-parameter. However, other packages can be used to fit a generalize linear model. Such packages usually provide their own set of *predict*- and *residuals*-function. In that case, the *type*-parameter of the corresponding package-specific function might have a different meaning or ignore the parameter completely, which then could lead to the wrong test statistic or an error message. Although "stats::glm" can fit various distributions, it does not offer the possibility to fit a negative-binomial model. One option, which works properly with our function for the test statistic, is "MASS::glm.nb".

Next, we implement the Resampling Scheme 6.1. Fortunately, R provides a lot of infrastructure that allows an easy implementation.

```
gof_model_boot <- function(model, data, B = 1000) {

  # mod   - a model fit,
  #   + residuals(mod, type = "response") must return
  #       Y - m_est(X), where is the estimator of the
  #       regression function m
  #   + predict(model, type = "link") must return
  #       the scalar product of the covariates and
  #       estimator of beta
  #   + simulate(model) must generate generate
  #       target/dependent variables according to
  #       the fitted model
  # data - observed data
  # B    - number of bootstrapped MEPs

  # progress bar that appears if calculations will take more
  # than 1 second
  pb <- dplyr::progress_estimated(B, min_time = 1)

  est_b_time_x <- predict(model, type = "link")
  # Calculate the statistic for the original MEP
  Wn2 <- CvM(model, est_b_time_x = est_b_time_x)

  # copy to build up the bootstrap data set
  data_boot <- data

  # name of the target/dependent variable
  y_name <- all.vars(formula(model), max.names = 1)

  # bootstrap the statistic
  Wn2_boot <- sapply(seq_len(B), function(i) {

    pb$tick()$print() # print progress

    # due to Step C only the target/dependent variable
    # needs to be updated.
    data_boot[[y_name]] <- simulate(model)[,1]
```

```r
    # refit the model using the bootstrapped data set
    m_boot <- update(model, formula. = formula(model),
                      data = data_boot)

    # Calculate the statistic for the bootstrapped MEP
    CvM(m_boot, est_b_time_x)
  })
  ret <- list(Wn2_boot = Wn2_boot,
              Wn2 = Wn2,
              pvalue_cvm = mean(Wn2_boot > Wn2))
  ret
}
```

The following is only a convenient function for displaying the estimated marked empirical process and model residuals while also showing bootstrapped versions.

```r
plot_Rn1_and_residuals <- function(model, data, B) {
  # mod  - a model fit,
  #    + residuals(mod, type = "response") must return
  #      Y - m_est(X), where is the estimator of the
  #      regression function m
  #    + predict(model, type = "link") must return
  #      the scalar product of the covariates and
  #      estimator of beta
  #    + simulate(model) must generate generate
  #      target/dependent variables according to
  #      the fitted model
  # data - observed data
  # B    - number of bootstrapped MEPs

  y_name <- all.vars(formula(model), max.names = 1)
  est_b_time_x <- predict(model, type = "link")
  # MEP of the original model
  org_model <- Rn1(model, est_b_time_x) %>% dplyr::as_tibble()

  # bootstrapped MEP
  boot_model <- purrr::map_dfr(seq_len(B), function(boot_idx){
    # due to Step C only the target/dependent variable
    # needs to be updated.
    data[[y_name]] <- simulate(model, data = data)[,1]

    # refit the model using the bootstrapped data set
    # and calculate the MEP
    update(model, formula. = formula(model), data = data) %>%
      Rn1(est_b_time_x = est_b_time_x) %>%
      dplyr::as_tibble() %>%
      dplyr::mutate(original = FALSE, idx = boot_idx)
  })

  # statistics for the bootstrapped models
  Wn2_boot <- boot_model %>%
    dplyr::group_by(idx) %>%
```

```
    dplyr::summarise(CvM = mean(Rn1_x^2))

  pvalue_cvm <- mean(Wn2_boot$CvM > mean(org_model$Rn1_x^2))

  plot_Rn1 <- boot_model %>%
    ggplot(aes(x = est_b_time_x, y = Rn1_x)) +
    geom_line(aes(group = idx), alpha = 0.1) +
    geom_line(data = org_model, color = "red") +
    ggtitle(paste0("p-value (CvM) = ", pvalue_cvm))

  plot_res <- boot_model %>%
    ggplot(aes(x = est_b_time_x, y = res)) +
    geom_point(alpha = 0.1) +
    geom_point(data = org_model, color = "red")

  cowplot::plot_grid(plot_Rn1, plot_res, nrow = 2)
}
```

Similar as before, this function uses generic functions, namely, "simulate" and "update". A fit created with "stats::glm" or "MASS::glm.nb" can be safely passed to this function. If another package is used, one should check that "simulate" really simulates the dependent variable and "update" refits the model using the generated dataset.

6.1.2 Bike Sharing Data

In Sect. 5.3, we prepared and analyzed the ridership data, which resulted in four model candidates. The corresponding diagnostic plots were already presented and briefly discussed in that section. Here, we apply the bootstrap-based goodness-of-fit test to obtain another indicator for inappropriate models.

As a reminder, we briefly repeat the steps from Sect. 5.3, i.e., import and preprocess/wrangle the dataset and subset it to the dates before hurricane "Sandy":

```
ridership <- readr::read_csv("day.csv") %>%
  data_preprocess()

## Parsed with column specification:
## cols(
##   instant = col_double(),
##   dteday = col_date(format = ""),
##   season = col_double(),
##   yr = col_double(),
##   mnth = col_double(),
##   holiday = col_double(),
##   weekday = col_double(),
##   workingday = col_double(),
##   weathersit = col_double(),
##   temp = col_double(),
```

```
##    atemp = col_double(),
##    hum = col_double(),
##    windspeed = col_double(),
##    casual = col_double(),
##    registered = col_double(),
##    cnt = col_double()
## )

ridership <-
  ridership %>%
  dplyr::filter(dteday < lubridate::ymd("2012-10-29"))
```

In order to get an idea how the upcoming plots of the residuals and the estimated marked empirical process would look like if the model is correct, we take the ridership data and generate the target according to a fitted model and then apply the GOF test, see Fig. 6.1.

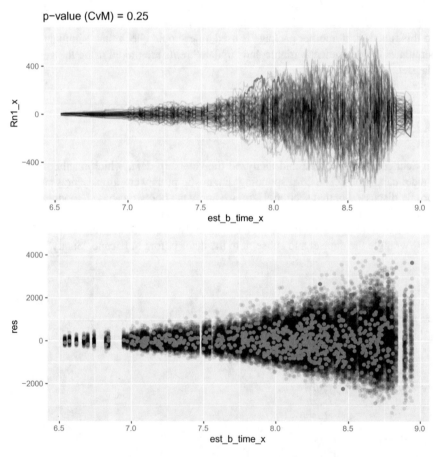

Fig. 6.1 Estimated marked empirical process and residuals in red and the corresponding boot-strapped versions in black if the ridership data would follow a negative-binomial model

```
frml <- y ~ temp + I(temp^2) + hum_imp + I(hum_imp^2) +
    windspeed + yr*season + workingday +
    weathersit + holiday + christmas
fit_nb <- MASS::glm.nb(frml, data = ridership)
ridership_generated <- ridership
# generate riderships that follow a negative-binomial
# distribution according to the fitted model
set.seed(123,kind ="Mersenne-Twister",normal.kind ="Inversion")
ridership_generated$y <- simulate(fit_nb, data = data)[,1]
fit_nb_generated <- MASS::glm.nb(frml, data = ridership_generated)
plot_Rn1_and_residuals(fit_nb_generated,
                       data = ridership_generated, B = 100)
```

Obviously, the estimated marked empirical process in Fig. 6.1 does not show more extreme behavior than the 100 bootstrapped versions and the residuals show a similar pattern as the residuals of the 100 bootstrapped model fits.

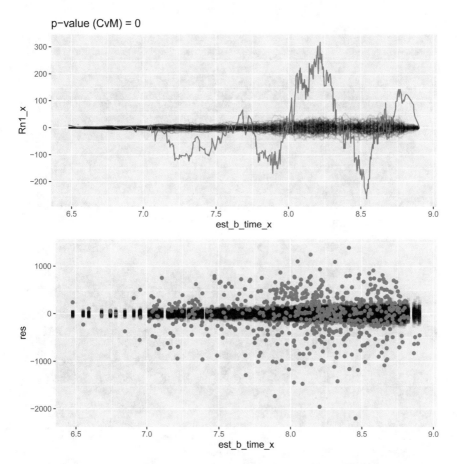

Fig. 6.2 Estimated marked empirical process and residuals in red and the corresponding bootstrapped versions in black for the Poisson model

Now, we apply the goodness-of-test to the four model candidates from the previous section. We start with the Poisson model, see Sect. 5.3 for the model output.

```
fit_poi <- glm(frml, data = ridership, family = poisson())
set.seed(123,kind ="Mersenne-Twister",normal.kind ="Inversion")
plot_Rn1_and_residuals(fit_poi, data = ridership, B = 100)
```

Figure 6.2 reveals that the estimated marked empirical process (as well as the residuals) in the observed data behave very differently than its bootstrapped version. This results in rejecting the corresponding null hypothesis of the GOF test for our fitted Poisson model. Fitting a quasi-Poisson model is possible but the parametric bootstrap is not possible because the distribution is not fully defined. Therefore, for the quasi-Poisson model one would have to use other diagnostic checks.

```
fit_qpoi <- glm(frml, data = ridership, family = quasipoisson())
```

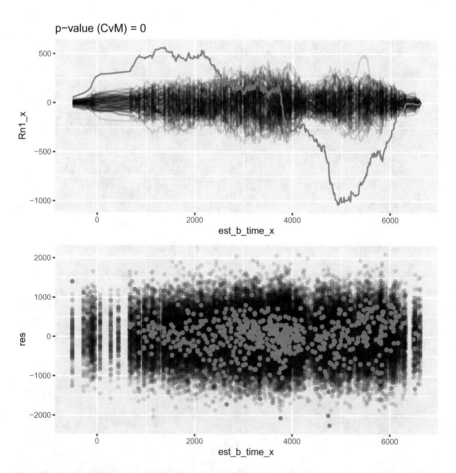

Fig. 6.3 Estimated marked empirical process and residuals in red and the corresponding boot-strapped versions in black for the Gaussian model

Trying the normal distributions without log-transformation also reveals that the estimated marked empirical process behaves very differently as its bootstrapped version, see Fig. 6.3.

```
fit_norm <- glm(frml, data = ridership, family = gaussian())
set.seed(123,kind ="Mersenne-Twister",normal.kind ="Inversion")
plot_Rn1_and_residuals(fit_norm, data = ridership, B = 100)
```

As in the last section, the normal distribution with log-transformations behaves surprisingly well, though the residuals seem to behave differently compared to the bootstrapped residuals, see Fig. 6.4.

```
fit_lognorm <-
  ridership %>%
  mutate(y = log(y)) %>%
  glm(frml, data = ., family = gaussian())
set.seed(123,kind ="Mersenne-Twister",normal.kind ="Inversion")
plot_Rn1_and_residuals(fit_lognorm, data = ridership, B = 100)
```

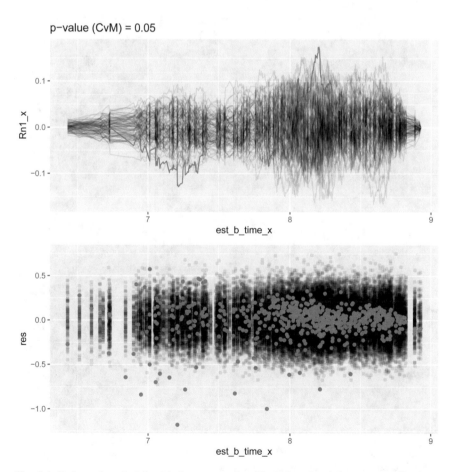

Fig. 6.4 Estimated marked empirical process and residuals in red and the corresponding bootstrapped versions in black for the Gaussian model with log-transformed target

Finally, using the negative-binomial distribution shows not too much deviations of the estimated marked empirical process from its bootstrapped versions, see Fig. 6.5. However, the residuals at the right end of the plot seem to indicate that the bootstrapped residuals have larger variance compared to the variance of the residuals based on the original data.

```
fit_nb <- MASS::glm.nb(frml, data = ridership)
set.seed(123,kind ="Mersenne-Twister",normal.kind ="Inversion")
plot_Rn1_and_residuals(fit_nb, data = ridership, B = 100)
```

Anyway, at this point, one would probably decide to go on with the negative-binomial model maybe also with the log-transformed Gaussian model (if the diagnostic checks for the quasi-Poisson model also indicate that it does not fit the data well) and start investigating the low residuals that seem to stand apart from the bootstrapped residuals as well as try to find the root cause for the smaller variance.

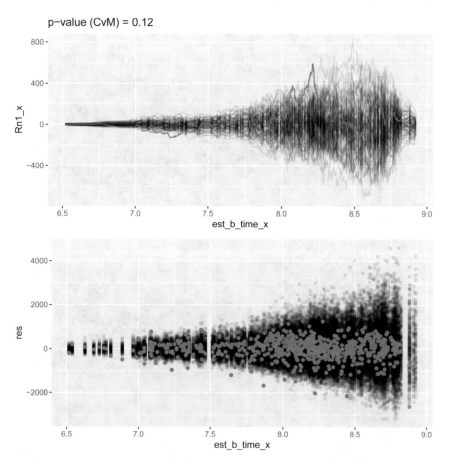

Fig. 6.5 Estimated marked empirical process and residuals in red and the corresponding bootstrapped versions in black for the negative-binomial model

6.1.3 Artificial Data

By generating the datasets we are able to judge if the result of the GOF test is correct. This provides at least some ideas about the limits of the GOF test. Of course, the simulations in this section are far from being exhaustive and, for instance, changing a β of the true model or the distribution of the covariates may lead to different results. Furthermore, a practitioner probably wants to investigate the GOF test himself in a specific situation when he has created reasonable model candidates. Consider the bike sharing example from the last section. It probably makes more sense in that particular case to take the negative-binomial model that passed the GOF test and artificially introduce additional covariates, for instance, a squared term, simulate the outcome variable and then check whether and when the GOF test is able to detect that a model without that new covariate is misspecified or just to get an idea of what we could expect if the model would be correct like Fig. 6.1.

We use a simple linear (Gaussian) model

$$Y = \beta_1 X_1^2 + \beta_2 X_2 + \beta_3 X_3 + \varepsilon,$$

where X_1 and X_2 are uniformly distributed, X_3 is Bernoulli distributed, see Fig. 6.6.

```r
genData <- function(N, coef_x1_square, coef_x2, coef_x3) {
    # N - sample size
    # data is generated according to
    # normal distribution with variance one
    # and mean
    # 10 + coef_x1_square * X1^2 + coef_x2 * X2 + coef_x3 * X3

    d <- data.frame(
        X1 = runif(N, 0, 3),
        X2 = runif(N, 1, 2),
        X3 = rbinom(N, size = 1, prob = 0.3),
        noise1 = runif(N),
        noise2 = runif(N)
    )
    lin_comb <- 10 + coef_x1_square * d$X1^2 +
        coef_x2 * d$X2 +
        coef_x3 * d$X3
    d$X3 <- as.factor(d$X3)
    d$Y <- rnorm(N, mean = lin_comb, sd = 1)
    return(d)
}
set.seed(123, kind ="Mersenne-Twister", normal.kind ="Inversion")
gaus_data <- genData(200, coef_x1_square = 1, coef_x2 = 2,
                     coef_x3 = 3)


GGally::ggpairs(gaus_data[, c("X1", "X2", "X3", "Y")])
```

One way to approach this dataset is to start with a backward selection.

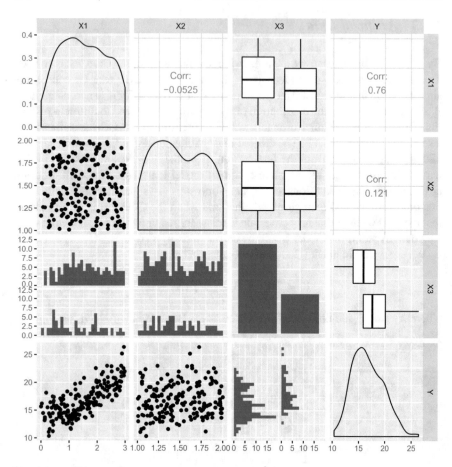

Fig. 6.6 Artificial dataset following the model $Y = \beta_1 X_1^2 + \beta_2 X_2 + \beta_3 X_3 + \varepsilon$

```
fit <- glm(formula = Y ~ X1 + X2 + X3 + noise1 + noise2,
    data = gaus_data, family = "gaussian")
(fit)


  ##
  ## Call: glm(formula = Y ~ X1 + X2 + X3 + noise1 + noise2,
  ## family = "gaussian",
  ##      data = gaus_data)
  ##
  ## Coefficients:
  ## (Intercept)              X1              X2             X31
  ##      8.3225          3.0601          1.9339          3.2109
  ##      noise1          noise2
```

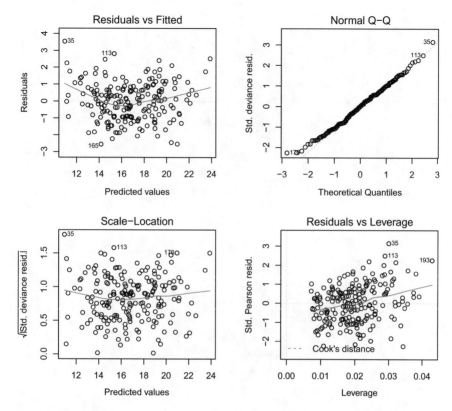

Fig. 6.7 Diagnostic plots for a linear model that only incorporate first-degree terms for X_1, X_2, and X_3

```
##        0.1959      -0.3021
##
## Degrees of Freedom: 199 Total (i.e. Null);   194 Residual
## Null Deviance:         1699
## Residual Deviance: 253.8      AIC: 629.3
```

This rules out the noise variables and the usual diagnostic plots already look quite promising, see Fig. 6.7.

```
fit <- glm(formula = Y ~ X1 + X2 + X3,
           data = gaus_data, family = "gaussian")
par(mfrow = c(2,2))
plot(fit)
```

However, the GOF test rejects the model, see Fig. 6.8. Though that figure does not indicate how to improve the model the residual plot in Fig. 6.7 indicates non-linearity.

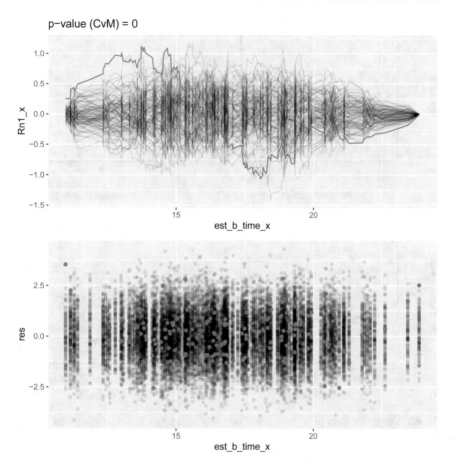

Fig. 6.8 Estimated marked empirical process and residuals in red and the corresponding boot-strapped versions in black for a linear model that only incorporates first-degree terms for X_1, X_2, and X_3

```
plot_Rn1_and_residuals(fit, gaus_data, B = 100)
```

Therefore, we try second-order terms

```
fit <- glm(formula = Y ~ X1 + X2 + X3 + I(X1^2) + I(X2^2) +
              X1:X2 + X1:X3 + X2:X3,
           data = gaus_data, family = "gaussian")
step(fit)
```

```
## Start:  AIC=576.44
## Y ~ X1 + X2 + X3 + I(X1^2) + I(X2^2) + X1:X2 + X1:X3 + X2:X3
##
```

```
##                Df Deviance    AIC
## - X1:X2     1    189.18 574.45
## - X2:X3     1    189.28 574.56
## - I(X2^2)   1    189.36 574.65
## - X1:X3     1    190.19 575.51
## <none>           189.17 576.44
## - I(X1^2)   1    254.21 633.54
##
## Step:  AIC=574.45
## Y ~ X1 + X2 + X3 + I(X1^2) + I(X2^2) + X1:X3 + X2:X3
##
##                Df Deviance    AIC
## - X2:X3     1    189.28 572.56
## - I(X2^2)   1    189.38 572.66
## - X1:X3     1    190.19 573.52
## <none>           189.18 574.45
## - I(X1^2)   1    254.30 631.61
##
## Step:  AIC=572.56
## Y ~ X1 + X2 + X3 + I(X1^2) + I(X2^2) + X1:X3
##
##                Df Deviance    AIC
## - I(X2^2)   1    189.50 570.79
## - X1:X3     1    190.31 571.64
## - X2        1    190.79 572.15
## <none>           189.28 572.56
## - I(X1^2)   1    254.72 629.95
##
## Step:  AIC=570.79
## Y ~ X1 + X2 + X3 + I(X1^2) + X1:X3
##
##                Df Deviance    AIC
## - X1:X3     1    190.50 569.84
## <none>           189.50 570.79
## - I(X1^2)   1    255.20 628.32
## - X2        1    268.75 638.67
##
## Step:  AIC=569.84
## Y ~ X1 + X2 + X3 + I(X1^2)
##
##                Df Deviance    AIC
## - X1        1    190.82 568.17
## <none>           190.50 569.84
## - I(X1^2)   1    255.89 626.86
```

```
## - X2          1     271.00 638.34
## - X3          1     582.17 791.27
##
## Step:   AIC=568.17
## Y ~ X2 + X3 + I(X1^2)
##
##                Df  Deviance     AIC
## <none>               190.82 568.17
## - X2          1     273.42 638.11
## - X3          1     584.96 790.22
## - I(X1^2)     1    1471.54 974.72
##
## Call: glm(formula = Y ~ X2 + X3 + I(X1^2), family =
## "gaussian", data = gaus_data)
##
## Coefficients:
## (Intercept)              X2          X31        I(X1^2)
##       9.6133          2.2093       3.0953         0.9832
##
## Degrees of Freedom: 199 Total (i.e. Null);   196 Residual
## Null Deviance:          1699
## Residual Deviance: 190.8      AIC: 568.2
```

The diagnostic plots for the resulting model show that the non-linearity was reduced, see Fig. 6.9 and also the GOF test does not reject the new model, see Fig. 6.10.

```
fit <- glm(formula = Y ~ I(X1^2) + X2 + X3,
           data = gaus_data, family = "gaussian")
par(mfrow = c(2,2))
plot(fit)


plot_Rn1_and_residuals(fit, gaus_data, B = 100)
```

In this particular situation, the GOF test clearly rejected our first model, while the diagnostic plots only slightly indicated that the model is not correct. One should be aware of the fact that this might be also the other way around. In order to illustrate this, we generate a dataset, where the Bernoulli-distributed variable has a larger impact. The diagnostic plots make it obvious that the model is misspecified, see Fig. 6.11, but the GOF test is not able to detect that because this drastically increases the variance of the bootstrapped MEP, see Fig. 6.12.

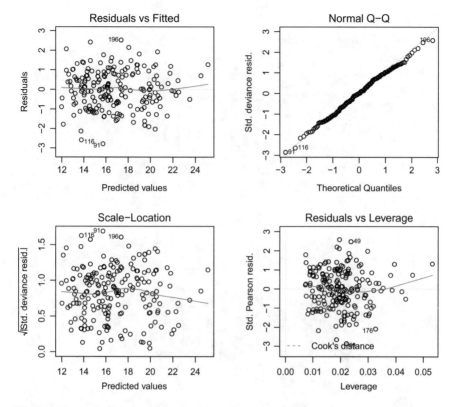

Fig. 6.9 Diagnostic plots for a linear model that incorporate all terms of the true model

```
set.seed(123,kind ="Mersenne-Twister",normal.kind ="Inversion")
gaus_data2 <- genData(200, coef_x1_square = 1, coef_x2 = 2,
                     coef_x3 = 6)
fit <- glm(formula = Y ~ I(X1^2) + X2, data = gaus_data2,
           family = "gaussian")


plot_Rn1_and_residuals(fit, gaus_data2, B = 100)
```

In this particular situation and this particular example, the GOF test rejected the model without X_1^2. In order to get a feeling for how reproducible this outcome would be, Fig. 6.13 shows the results of a small simulation study. Furthermore, in that simulation study, we add a model that misses term X_3 to see the performance of the GOF test with respect to this alternative.

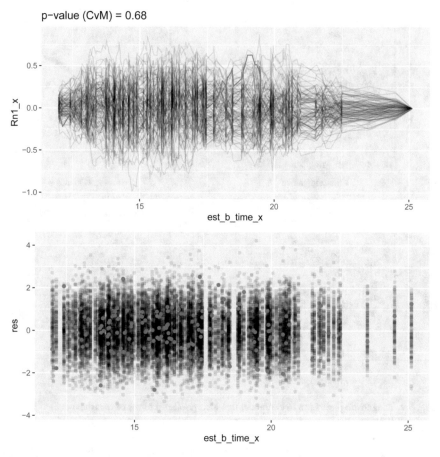

Fig. 6.10 Estimated marked empirical process and residuals in red and the corresponding boot-strapped versions in black for a linear model that incorporate all terms of the true model

```
gof_boot <- function(data, formula_str) {
  # fits a guassian model, performs
  # parametric GOF test and returns
  # the corresponding p-values

  # data - original data set
  # formula_str - a formula as a string

  frml <- as.formula(formula_str)
  m <- glm(frml, data = data, family = gaussian())

  gof <- gof_model_boot(m, data, B = 100)
  gof$pvalue_cvm
}
```

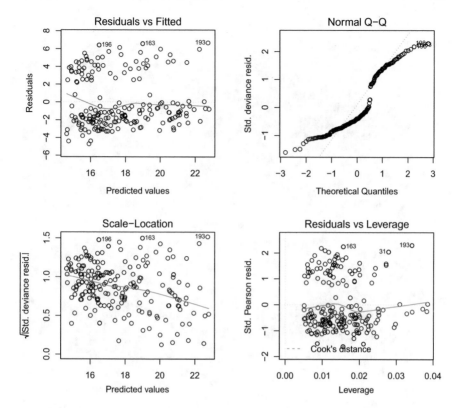

Fig. 6.11 Diagnostic plots for a linear model that incorporates all terms of the true model besides X_3

```
dg <- simTool::expand_tibble(
 proc = "genData",
 N = 200,
 coef_x1_square = 1,
 coef_x2 = 2,
 coef_x3 = 6)
pg <- simTool::expand_tibble(
 fun = c("gof_boot"),
 formula_str = c("Y ~ X1 + X2 + X3",
                 "Y ~ I(X1^2) + X2")
 )

eg <- simTool::eval_tibbles(
 data_grid = dg, proc_grid = pg,
 replications = 100, ncpus = 3,
 cluster_global_objects = ls())
```

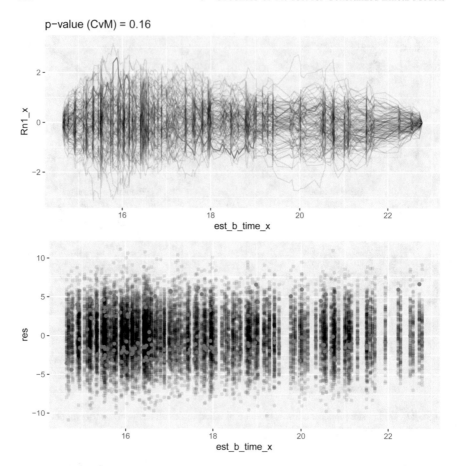

Fig. 6.12 Estimated marked empirical process and residuals in red and the corresponding boot-strapped versions in black for a linear model that incorporates all terms of the true model besides X_3

```
eg$simulation %>%
ggplot(aes(x = results, color = formula_str)) +
stat_ecdf() +
geom_abline(slope = 1, intercept = 0) +
#facet_grid(formula_str ~ N) +
theme(legend.position = "top")
```

As one can see from Fig. 6.13, the GOF test rejects the model with missing X_1^2 with high probability but has a hard time if X_3 is not part of the model. But excluding X_3 from the model if it has such a large impact and then applying the GOF test makes no sense. From that point of view, this aspect of the simulation makes no sense. However, X_3 might not have been recorded during the creation of the dataset. In such a case, it would not be possible to include X_3 in the model and the GOF test

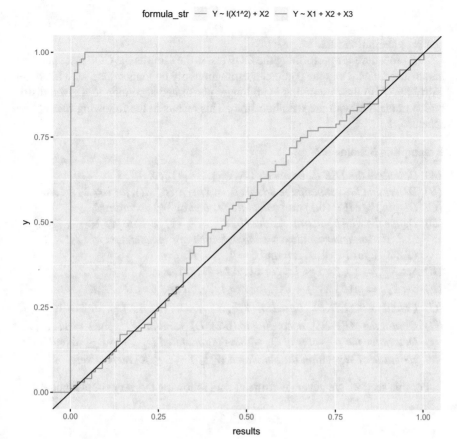

Fig. 6.13 Empirical cumulative distribution function of the p-values of the parametric GOF test

has only limited power to detect this. This shows that it makes it necessary to still consult other tests and plots to get an overall picture of misspecifications.

6.2 MEP in the Semi-parametric Modeling Context

In Sect. 5.4, it was assumed that

$$Y = m(X, \vartheta) + \varepsilon.$$

In the GLM context, this is specialized to

$$Y = m(\beta^\top X) + \varepsilon,$$

compare Definition 5.63.

The procedure for performing the GOF test is the same as the GOF test under the parametric GLM. Only the parameter estimations are no longer done with MLE but with LSE. Also the resampling is no longer performed according to a given distribution model but with the wild bootstrap. This results in the following resampling scheme.

Resampling Scheme 6.2

(A) *Calculate the LSE $\hat{\beta}_n$ based on $(Y_1, X_1), \ldots, (Y_n, X_n)$.*

(B) *Determine the estimated residuals $\hat{\varepsilon}_i = Y_i - m(\beta_n^\top X_i)$, for $i = 1, \ldots, n$.*

(C) *Obtain the MEP (6.1) and calculate D_n and/or W_n^2 accordingly.*

(D) *Define the wild bootstrap residual by $\varepsilon_{\ell,i}^* = \hat{\varepsilon}_i \cdot \tau_{\ell,i}^*$, where $(\tau_{\ell,i}^*)_{1 \le \ell \le K, 1 \le i \le n}$ are i.i.d. Rademacher random variables which are independent of $(Y_1, X_1), \ldots, (Y_n, X_n)$, for $i = 1, \ldots, n$ and $\ell = 1, \ldots, K$.*

(E) *Set $X_{\ell;i}^* = X_i$, for $i = 1, \ldots, n$ and $\ell = 1, \ldots, K$.*

(F) *Set $Y_{\ell;i}^* = m(\beta_n^\top X_{\ell;i}^*) + \varepsilon_{\ell;i}^*$, for $i = 1, \ldots, n$ and $\ell = 1, \ldots, K$.*

(G) *Calculate the LSE $\hat{\beta}_{\ell;n}^*$ based on $(Y_{\ell;1}^*, X_{\ell;1}^*), \ldots, (Y_{\ell;n}^*, X_{\ell;n}^*)$, for $\ell = 1, \ldots, K$.*

(H) *Obtain the MEP $R_{\ell;n}^{*1}$ according to (6.2), $D_{\ell;n}^*$ and/or $W_{\ell;n}^{*2}$, for $\ell = 1, \ldots, K$.*

(I) *Determine the p−value of D_n within the simulated $D_{\ell;n}^*$, $1 \le \ell \le K$ and/or the p−value of W_n^2 within the simulated $W_{\ell;n}^{*2}$, $1 \le \ell \le K$, respectively.*

For this section, we generate artificial data following the very simple model

$$Y = \sin(0.5X) + \varepsilon,$$

where X is uniformly distributed and ε is normally distributed.

```
set.seed(123,kind ="Mersenne-Twister",normal.kind ="Inversion")
gen_data <- function(N = 200, sd = 0.2)  {
  dplyr::mutate(
    data.frame(X = runif(N, min = 6, max = 14)),
    mu = sin(0.5 * X),
    epsilon = rnorm(N, sd = sd),
    Y = mu + epsilon)
}
nonlinear <- gen_data()
```

Assuming that we did not know the model, Fig. 6.14 clearly indicates a polynomial relation.

```
GGally::ggpairs(nonlinear[, c("X", "Y")])
```

One way to model such data (within a linear model) is to start with a simple model, in this case a polynomial of order two, and then gradually increase the complexity by increasing the degree of a polynomial. If there are some indications (maybe due

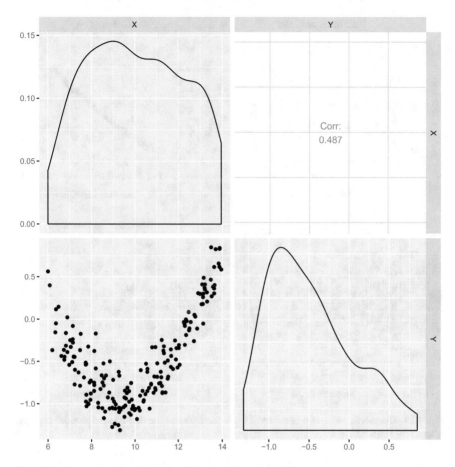

Fig. 6.14 Scatterplot of artificial data following $Y = \sin(0.5X) + \varepsilon$

to the theory of the problem at hand) that the pattern follows the sine function and one still wishes to model it with a linear model, it makes more sense to add the terms from the corresponding Taylor series, which in case of the sine function are only odd monomials. The common diagnostic plots for linear models do not indicate serious problems for a simple quadratic model, see Fig. 6.15

```
par(mfrow = c(2,2))
quadratic_fit <- glm(Y ~ X + I(X^2), data = nonlinear)
plot(quadratic_fit)
```

However, the wild bootstrap GOF test rejects the model (p-value = 0.024). The following two sections will implement the GOF test based on the wild bootstrap for the model specified in this section and apply it in a simulation study.

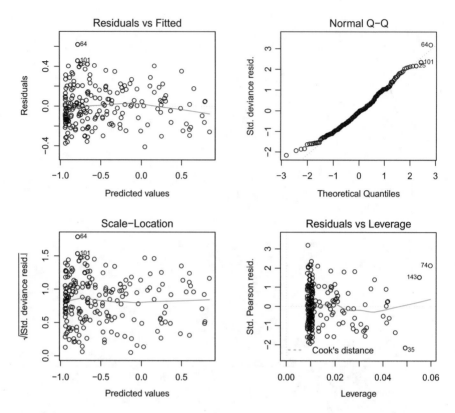

Fig. 6.15 Diagnostic plots of a linear model that incorporates the first two polynomial degrees, where $Y = \sin(0.5X) + \varepsilon$

6.2.1 Implementation

The implementation of the wild bootstrap is tailored to the model

$$Y = \sin(aX) + \varepsilon.$$

However, it is very similar to the implementation of GOF test using the parametric bootstrap. Basically, the difference is how the Y is generated and how the model is fitted. But the implementation is not so generic as for the parametric case. The calculation of $\beta_n^\top X$ is tailored to the situation that X is univariate. The main reason is that we will also use "minpack::nlsLM" for fitting a model and there seems to be no easy way to get this linear combination from the fit. Therefore, we prefer this simple implementation instead of a more generic but more complicated version.

```r
rrademacher <- function(n) {
  2 * rbinom(n = n, size = 1, prob = 1/2) - 1
}

gof_wb_boot <- function(model, data, B = 1000) {
  # mod   - a model fit (stats::glm or minpack.lm::nlsLM)
  #    + for models based on nlsLM it is assumed that
  #      the formula is of the type fun(para * X), where
  #      'para' is the parameter and 'X' is the covariate
  # data - observed data, column with name 'X'
  #        is the only covariate
  # B     - number of bootstrapped MEPs

  # progress bar that appears if calculations will take more
  # than 1 second
  pb <- dplyr::progress_estimated(B, min_time = 1)

  if (inherits(model, "nls")) {
    # only models of type fun(para * X) are supported
    est_b_time_x <- data$X * coef(model)
  } else {
    est_b_time_x <- predict(model, type = "response")
  }

  # statistics for the original model
  Wn2 <- CvM(model, est_b_time_x = est_b_time_x)
  epsilon_hat <- residuals(model)
  y_hat <- predict(model)

  # copy to build up the bootstrap data set
  data_boot <- data
  y_name <- all.vars(formula(model), max.names = 1)

  # statistics for the boostrap models
  Wn2_boot <- sapply(seq_len(B), function(i) {

    pb$tick()$print() # print progress

    # according to Step E only the target/dependent
    # variable needs to be updated
    tau <- rrademacher(length(epsilon_hat))
    data_boot[[y_name]] <- y_hat + tau * epsilon_hat

    # refit the model using the bootstrapped data set
    m_boot <- update(model, formula. = formula(model),
                     data = data_boot)
    # statistic for the boostrapped model fit
    CvM(m_boot, est_b_time_x)
  })
  ret <- list(Wn2_boot = Wn2_boot,
              Wn2 = Wn2,
              pvalue_cvm = mean(Wn2_boot > Wn2))
  ret
}
```

6.2.2 *Artificial Data*

We use linear models with different polynomial degrees in this simulation and the wild bootstrap GOF test to check them. Note, in Sect. 6.3, we will come back to a similar situation and compare the parametric and wild bootstrap version of the GOF test.

```r
gof_boot_nls <- function(data) {
  # performs a least square estimation
  # for sin(a * X) and a
  # semi-parametric GOF test
  # returns the corresponding p-values

  # data - original data set

  fit <- minpack.lm::nlsLM(Y ~ sin(a * X),
            data = data,
            start = c(a = 0.5),
            control = nls.control(maxiter = 500))
  gof <- gof_wb_boot(fit, data, B = 100)
  gof$pvalue_cvm
}

gof_boot_lm <- function(data, formula_str) {
  # fits a guassian model, performs
  # semi-parametric GOF test and returns
  # the corresponding p-values

  # data - original data set
  # formula_str - a formula as a string

  frml <- as.formula(formula_str)
  fit <- glm(frml, data = data, family = gaussian())
  gof <- gof_wb_boot(fit, data, B = 100)
  gof$pvalue_cvm
}
dg <- simTool::expand_tibble(proc = "gen_data", N = 100,
                             sd = 0.2)
pg <- dplyr::bind_rows(
  simTool::expand_tibble(fun = "gof_boot_nls"),
  simTool::expand_tibble(
    fun = "gof_boot_lm",
    formula_str = c("Y ~ X + I(X^2)",
                    "Y ~ X + I(X^2) + I(X^3)",
                    "Y ~ X + I(X^3) + I(X^5)"
                    ))
)
eg <- simTool::eval_tibbles(
  data_grid = dg, proc_grid = pg,
  replications = 100, ncpus = 3,
  cluster_global_objects = ls())
```

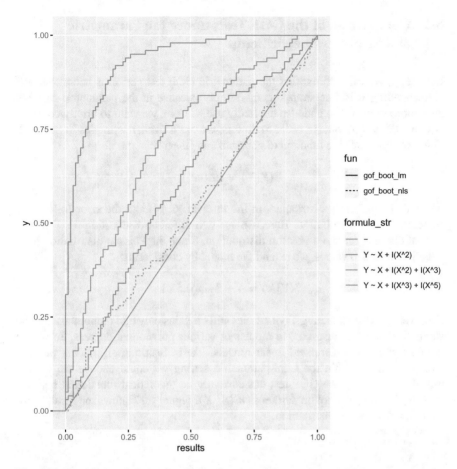

Fig. 6.16 Empirical cumulative distribution function of the p-values of GOF test based on the wild bootstrap for the semi-parametric model and of the parametric GOF test for the linear models, $Y = \sin(0.5X) + \varepsilon$ is conditionally normal distributed

Figure 6.16 shows the results of the simulation study. First note that the wild bootstrap shows a uniform distribution for the $p-$values, as expected since this is the correct model. Furthermore, the quadratic model as before shows a high chance to be rejected by the GOF test. Of course, increasing the complexity results in less rejections which is plausible because the sine function can be approximated this way. However, it is more effective to just use polynomials of an odd degree, which is also reflected by Fig. 6.16.

```
eg$simulation %>%
  dplyr::mutate(formula_str = ifelse(is.na(formula_str), "-",
                                      formula_str)) %>%
  ggplot(aes(x = results, linetype = fun, color = formula_str)) +
  stat_ecdf() +
  stat_function(fun = identity)
```

6.3 Comparison of the GOF Tests under the Parametric and Semi-parametric Setup

In general, we can assume that the parametric GOF test performs better than the corresponding wild bootstrap version, simply because in the parametric case we have more information and also explicitly use it. Here, we want to briefly compare both bootstrap versions. In order to do this, we use a similar setting as in Sect. 6.2. There we used the sine function to generate non-linear relation, i.e.,

$$\mathbb{E}(Y|X) = \sin(aX),$$

where X is uniformly distributed on the interval [6, 14] and the error followed a centered normal distribution. Here, we use two different distribution for Y, i.e., a normal distribution and a Poisson distribution. Since the Poisson distribution does not allow negative values, we extend the model by considering

$$\mathbb{E}(Y|X) = 4 + 2\sin(0.5X).$$

However, the corresponding Taylor series still contains only odd monomials and the simulations are also restricted to models of various polynomial degrees. So within the framework of generalized linear models, like in Sect. 5.3, all models we pick will be wrong. Within the semi-parametric setting we could choose the correct model but applying the GOF test has currently no theoretical foundation because $\beta_1 + \beta_2 \sin(\beta_3 X)$ cannot be written as $m(\beta^\top X)$. Figure 6.17 shows the results with conditionally normal distribution.

```
eg_para_vs_wb$simulation %>%
  ggplot(aes(x = results, linetype = fun, color = rhs)) +
  stat_ecdf() +
  facet_grid(N~., labeller = label_both) +
  stat_function(fun = identity, color = "black")
```

Since the least square estimator and maximum likelihood estimator are the same in this setting, any differences are only due to the generation of Y in the bootstrap world. At the first glance, it seems that wild bootstrap outperforms the parametric bootstrap for the small sample size $N = 10$. Although the theory is currently not rich enough, we applied also the semi-parametric GOF test, which shows that the GOF test is too liberate, i.e., the red dashed curve is above the diagonal. This, of course, is just an indicator of why the performance seems to be better. Furthermore, the models that are closer to the true model got rejected more often, which, of course, is a bit unusual. Another indicator that the performance advantage of the semi-parametric GOF test is probably spurious is that the same simulation based on sample size $N = 200$ shows that the performance of the semi-parametric GOF test degrades for the models with higher polynomials. For instance, according to ecdf of the p–values for the semi-parametric GOF test under the model $X + I(X^3) + I(X^5)$, around 25% of the p–values are below 0.05 for $N = 10$ and this decreases to around 5% for

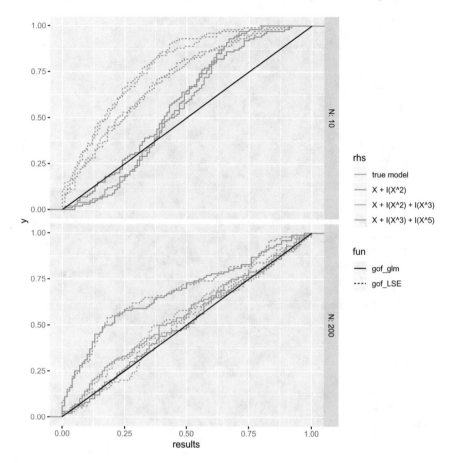

Fig. 6.17 Empirical cumulative distribution function of the p-values of GOF test based on the wild bootstrap (gof_LSE) for the semi-parametric model and of the parametric GOF test for the linear models (gof_glm), where $\mathbb{E}(Y|X) = 4 + 2\sin(0.5X)$ and Y is conditionally normal distributed. Sample size of the generated dataset is denoted by N. The right-hand side (rhs) describes which model was tested

$N = 200$. Note also that Fig. 6.17 shows that the p-values of the semi-parametric GOF test under the true model now seem to follow a uniform distribution. In this particular situation, both methods seem to have roughly equal performance, where for small sample size the semi-parametric GOF test may be too liberal. One reason why the semi-parametric GOF test is too liberal could be the Radermacher random variables, because this only changes the signs of the residuals and hence this only introduces little variation in the bootstrap datasets if the sample size is small.

Changing the conditional distribution to Poisson changes the results as expected, i.e., that the parametric GOF test results in more rejections if the sample size is

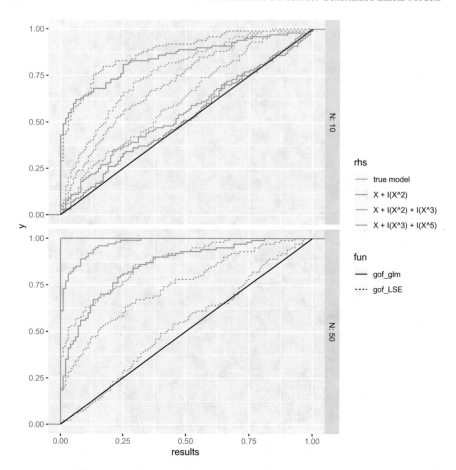

Fig. 6.18 Empirical cumulative distribution function of the p-values of GOF test based on the wild bootstrap (gof_LSE) for the semi-parametric model and of the parametric GOF test for the linear models (gof_glm), where $\mathbb{E}(Y|X) = 4 + 2\sin(0.5X)$ and Y is conditionally Poisson distributed. Sample size of the generated dataset is denoted by N. The right-hand side (rhs) describes which model was tested

sufficient. Furthermore, both GOF tests indicate that it is more efficient to use only odd polynomial degrees which corresponds also to our expectations, see Fig. 6.18.

```
eg_para_vs_wb2$simulation %>%
  ggplot(aes(x = results, linetype = fun, color = rhs)) +
  stat_ecdf() +
  facet_grid(N~., labeller = label_both) +
  stat_function(fun = identity, color = "black")
```

Again, for small sample size it seems that the performance gain of the semi-parametric GOF test is probably spurious for same reasons as before.

6.4 Mathematical Framework: Marked Empirical Processes

This excursion outlines some fundamental results of marked empirical processes (MEP) based on residuals given in Stute (1997) and Stute and Zhu (2002).

Since the following explanations are quite complex in their notation, we provide a short guideline in advance. In general, all analyzed MEPs are cumulative sum (cusum) error processes, which each propagate in a one-dimensional direction. The direction of the propagation is given within each indicator variable. If the indicator variable contains an estimated parameter, we speak here of an MEP that propagates in an estimated direction. We will consider three basic types of MEPs.

1. If the process is based on the true error and unfolds in a fixed, not estimated direction, then the process is called BMEP in the following and is always denoted with R_n.
2. If the MEP is based on estimated errors and unfolds in a fixed direction, then R_n^1 is chosen to denote the process. Processes of this kind are called EMEP in the following text.
3. Finally, there is a third type which will be called EMEPE. These processes are based on estimated errors and also on an estimated propagation direction. For these processes, we use the notation $\bar{R}_n^1$.

Furthermore, in our considerations, we make constant use of mathematical rules for conditional expectation without explicitly stating them in each case. A list of these rules can be found in Shorack (2000, Chapter 8.4 – 8.6). Only the concept of conditional variance is explained in more detail at this point. Let $Y \in L^2(\Omega, \mathscr{A}, \mathbb{P})$ and X be another random variable over $(\Omega, \mathscr{A}, \mathbb{P})$. Then we denote in the following with

$$\text{VAR}(Y|X) = \mathbb{E}\big((Y - \mathbb{E}(Y|X))^2 \big| X\big)$$

the conditional variance of Y given X.

The space $D[0, 1]$ provided with the Skorokhod topology is the metric space for investigating the convergence in distribution of the empirical process, see Billingsley (1968, Chapter 3). The processes to be examined in this section will usually be in $D[-\infty, \infty]$.

Definition 6.3 Define $D[-\infty, \infty]$ as the collection of all right continuous functions $f : \mathbb{R} \to \mathbb{R}$ whose left-sided limits exist and for which $\lim_{x \to \infty} f(x)$ and $\lim_{x \to -\infty} f(x)$ exist in $\mathbb{R}$ also applies.

Remark 6.4 Now consider a continuous, strictly increasing transformation

$$A : \quad [-\infty, \infty] \longrightarrow [0, 1].$$

For example, a continuous, strictly increasing distribution function for A can be used here. Then the transformation

$$T : D[0, 1] \ni f \longrightarrow T(f) = f \circ A \equiv f_A \in D[-\infty, \infty]$$

is a bijective transformation. Let s denote the Skorokhod metric on $D[0, 1]$. Then

$$s_A : D[-\infty, \infty] \times D[-\infty, \infty] \ni (f_A, g_A) \longrightarrow s_A(f_A, g_A)$$
$$= s(f_A \circ A^{-1}, g_A \circ A^{-1})$$

defines a metric on $D[-\infty, \infty]$ which makes T to an isometric transformation. Thus, we can identify $D[-\infty, \infty]$ with $D[0, 1]$. Among other things, this isometry states that all theorems for convergence in distribution with respect to $D[0, 1]$ can now be transferred to $D[-\infty, \infty]$ accordingly. So we do not need to consider the limitation by the domain $[0, 1]$ anymore, if the process to be considered is in $D[-\infty, \infty]$.

6.4.1   The Basic MEP

Definition 6.5 Let $(Y_1, X_1), \ldots, (Y_n, X_n)$ be an i.i.d. sequence in $\mathbb{R}^2$ such that $\mathbb{E}(|Y|) < \infty$ and denote the conditional expectation of Y given $X = x$ by $m(x)$, that is,

$$\mathbb{E}(Y \mid X = x) = m(x).$$

Then

$$[-\infty, \infty] \ni x \longrightarrow R_n(x) := n^{-1/2} \sum_{i=1}^{n} \big(Y_i - m(X_i)\big) \, \mathrm{I}_{\{X_i \leq x\}} \in \mathbb{R} \qquad (6.3)$$

defines the *basic marked empirical process* (BMEP).

Note that $R_n(x)$ is defined for $x = \pm\infty$ by

$$R_n(-\infty) = 0 \quad \text{and} \quad R_n(\infty) = n^{-1/2} \sum_{i=1}^{n} \big(Y_i - m(X_i)\big).$$

This extends R_n continuously from $\mathbb{R}$ to $[-\infty, \infty]$ and allows to handle $\sup_{x \in \mathbb{R}} |R_n(x)|$, since $R_n \in D[-\infty, \infty]$.

   Asymptotic analysis of the simple empirical process often uses the transformation of the process to the uniformly empirical process, see Sect. 3.4. A similar procedure is also possible with the BMEP, as described in Stute (1997) and as we will illustrate in detail now.

   Since $F^{-1} \circ F(X) = X$ with probability 1, compare Shorack and Wellner (1986, Chapter 1, Proposition 3, Equation (27)), where F and F^{-1} denote the distribution and quantile function of X, respectively, we get with probability 1

$$R_n(x) = n^{-1/2} \sum_{i=1}^{n} \left(Y_i - m \circ F^{-1} \circ F(X_i) \right) \mathrm{I}_{\{F^{-1} \circ F(X_i) \leq x\}}$$

$$= n^{-1/2} \sum_{i=1}^{n} \left(Y_i - m \circ F^{-1}(F(X_i)) \right) \mathrm{I}_{\{F(X_i) \leq F(x)\}}$$

$$= \hat{R}_n(F(x)),$$

where

$$\hat{R}_n(u) = n^{-1/2} \sum_{i=1}^{n} \left(Y_i - m \circ F^{-1}(F(X_i)) \right) \mathrm{I}_{\{F(X_i) \leq u\}}, \quad \text{for } 0 \leq u \leq 1. \quad (6.4)$$

While $R_n \in D[-\infty, \infty]$, we have $\hat{R}_n \in D[0, 1]$ and we can interpret $\hat{R}_n$ as a BMEP based on the $F(X)$−sample if $m \circ F^{-1}(u) = \mathbb{E}(Y \mid F(X) = u)$, for $\mathbb{P}_{F(X)}$ almost all $0 \leq u \leq 1$.

Lemma 6.6 *Let $Y \in L^2(\Omega, \mathscr{A}, \mathbb{P})$. Denote the distribution and quantile function of X by F and F^{-1}, respectively. With $m(x) = \mathbb{E}(Y \mid X = x)$ and $\sigma^2(x) = VAR(Y \mid X = x)$ we get*

(i) *The conditional expectation of Y given $F(X) = u$, that is $\mathbb{E}(Y \mid F(X) = u)$, is well defined for $\mathbb{P}_{F(X)}$ almost all $0 \leq u \leq 1$ and*

$$\mathbb{E}(Y \mid F(X) = u) = \mathbb{E}(Y \mid X = F^{-1}(u)) = m \circ F^{-1}(u).$$

(ii) *The conditional variance of Y given $F(X) = u$, that is $VAR(Y \mid F(X) = u)$, is well defined for $\mathbb{P}_{F(X)}$ almost all $0 \leq u \leq 1$ and*

$$VAR(Y \mid F(X) = u) = VAR(Y \mid X = F^{-1}(u)) = \sigma^2 \circ F^{-1}(u).$$

(iii) *If F is continuous then $F(X)$ is uniformly distributed on $[0, 1]$ and, with $U = F(X)$, the last equalities read as follows:*

$$\mathbb{E}(Y \mid U = u) = m(F^{-1}(u)), \quad VAR(Y \mid U = u) = \sigma^2(F^{-1}(u)),$$

for $\mathbb{P}_U$ almost all $0 \leq u \leq 1$.

Proof For the first equation, let B be an arbitrarily chosen Borel set of the unit interval. Then

$$\int \mathrm{I}_{\{F(X) \in B\}} \, Y \, d\mathbb{P} = \int \mathrm{I}_{\{F(x) \in B\}} \, \mathbb{E}(Y \mid X = x) \, \mathbb{P}_X(dx)$$

$$= \int \mathrm{I}_{\{F(x) \in B\}} \, \mathbb{E}(Y \mid X = F^{-1} \circ F(x)) \, \mathbb{P}_X(dx)$$

$$= \int \mathrm{I}_{\{u \in B\}} \mathbb{E}(Y \mid X = F^{-1}(u)) \, \mathbb{P}_{F(X)}(du),$$

where the second equality is based on $\mathbb{P}_X(\{x \in \mathbb{R} : F^{-1}(F(x)) = x\}) = 1$, compare Shorack and Wellner (1986, Chapter 1, Proposition 3, Equation (27)). This proves, according to Shorack (2000, Chapter 8, Notation 4.1),

$$m(F^{-1}(u)) = \mathbb{E}(Y \mid F(X) = u), \quad \text{for } \mathbb{P}_{F(X)} \text{ almost all } u.$$

This proves (i). Analogously, part (ii) can be shown, and (iii) is obvious.   □

Remark 6.7 The last lemma tells us that a change of the regressor from X to $F(X)$ causes a change of the regression function from m to $m \circ F^{-1}$, which is now the regression function of Y with respect to $F(X)$. Thus, we can transform the BMEP to $\hat{R}_n(F(x))$, where

$$\hat{R}_n(u) = n^{-1/2} \sum_{i=1}^{n} \left(Y_i - m \circ F^{-1}(F(X_i)) \right) \mathrm{I}_{\{F(X_i) \leq u\}}, \quad \text{for } 0 \leq u \leq 1,$$

which is now the BMEP corresponding to $(Y_1, F(X_1)), \ldots, (Y_n, F(X_n))$. In addition, if F is continuous then $F(X)$ is uniformly distributed on the unit interval and we can set $U_i = F(X_i)$. Now $\hat{R}_n$ is the transformed R_n to the uniform case. It is the counterpart to the uniform empirical process.

As we discussed in Sect. 4.4, the asymptotic behavior of the empirical process is the mathematical backbone in the context of model diagnostics for parametric distribution families of i.i.d. observations in $\mathbb{R}$. The main asymptotic result of the BMEP is given in the next theorem, compare Stute (1997, Theorem 1.1), and it shows that the BMEP has the potential to play the empirical processes counterpart in the regression context. However, in the following theorem, we will not make use of the transformation to the uniform case as it was done in the proof of Stute (1997, Theorem 1.1). The reasons for this are discussed after the proof at the end of this section. Instead, we will refer to Remark 6.4 in the proof.

Theorem 6.8 *Assume that* $\mathbb{E}(Y^2) < \infty$ *and*

$$H : [-\infty, \infty] \ni u \longrightarrow H(u) = \int \mathrm{I}_{\{x \leq u\}} \sigma^2(x) F(\mathrm{d}x) \in \mathbb{R} \tag{6.5}$$

is continuous. Then

$$R_n \longrightarrow R_\infty \quad \text{in distribution in the space } D[-\infty, \infty].$$

R_∞ *is a centered Gaussian process with covariance function*

$$K(s, t) = H(s \wedge t) = \int \mathrm{I}_{\{x \leq s \wedge t\}} \sigma^2(x) F(\mathrm{d}x), \tag{6.6}$$

where F denotes the distribution function of X, $s \wedge t = \min(s, t)$, and $\sigma^2(x) = VAR(Y \mid X = x)$, the conditional variance of Y given $X = x$.

Remark 6.9 The covariance function of the limiting centered Gaussian process R_∞ is identical to the covariance function of the process $B(H)$, where B is a standard Brownian motion on the positive real line with H given under (6.5). Therefore, the paths of R_∞ are continuous.

Corollary 6.10 *If $\mathbb{E}(Y^2) < \infty$ and F is continuous, the continuity assumption (6.5) is fulfilled.*

Proof (of Theorem 6.8) The following proof is based on Stute (1997, Proof of Theorem 1.1) with some adjustments which are discussed in Example 6.12. It is an application of Billingsley (1968, Theorem 15.6).
   Conditioning on $X_1, \ldots, X_n$ guarantees

$$\mathbb{E}(R_n(x)) = n^{-1/2} \sum_{i=1}^{n} \mathbb{E}\big(I_{\{X_i \leq x\}} \mathbb{E}\big((Y_i - m(X_i)) \big| X_i\big)\big) = 0,$$

for every $-\infty \leq x \leq \infty$. Since the terms in the sum of $R_n(x)$ are centered (expectation is 0) and i.i.d., we get in addition that

$$\mathbb{E}(R_n^2(x)) \leq \mathbb{E}\big((Y - m(X))^2\big) \leq \mathbb{E}(Y^2) < \infty.$$

Overall, $R_n(x) \in L_0^2(\Omega, \mathscr{A}, \mathbb{P})$, the space of square-integrable centered functions on $(\Omega, \mathscr{A}, \mathbb{P})$, for $-\infty \leq x \leq \infty$.
   To apply Billingsley (1968, Theorem 15.6), we will show that the finite-dimensional distributions (fidis) of R_n converge to those of R_∞. Take $-\infty \leq x_1, \ldots, x_k \leq \infty$, for $k \in \mathbb{N}$ and apply the multivariate central limit theorem, Billingsley (1995, Theorem 29.5) to get that

$$(R_n(x_1), \ldots, R_n(x_k)) \longrightarrow \mathscr{N}(0, \Sigma), \quad \text{as } n \to \infty,$$

in distribution, where $\Sigma = (\sigma_{i,j})_{1 \leq i, j \leq k}$ is the covariance matrix defined by

$$\sigma_{i,j} = COV(R_n(x_i), R_n(x_j)), \quad \text{for } 1 \leq i, j \leq k.$$

Since

$$COV(R_n(x_i), R_n(x_j)) = \mathbb{E}\big(I_{\{X \leq x_i\}} I_{\{X \leq x_j\}} (Y - m(X))^2\big)$$
$$= \int I_{\{t \leq x_i \wedge x_j\}} \sigma^2(t)\, F(\mathrm{d}t) = K(x_i, x_j),$$

the first part of the proof is done.
   To prove tightness, we adapt Billingsley (1968, (15.21) in Theorem 15.6) according to Remark 6.4 to $D[-\infty, \infty]$.

For $-\infty \le x_1 \le x \le x_2 \le \infty$, set

$$\alpha_i = I_{\{x_1 < X_i \le x\}}\big(Y_i - m(X_i)\big)$$

and

$$\beta_i = I_{\{x < X_i \le x_2\}}\big(Y_i - m(X_i)\big)$$

to obtain

$$\mathbb{E}\Big((R_n(x) - R_n(x_1))^2 (R_n(x_2) - R_n(x))^2\Big) = n^{-2}\mathbb{E}\Big(\Big(\sum_{1 \le i \le n} \alpha_i\Big)^2 \Big(\sum_{1 \le j \le n} \beta_j\Big)^2\Big).$$

Due to the indicator functions involved in the definition of α_i and β_i, $\alpha_i\,\beta_i = 0$. Conditioning on X_i shows that $\mathbb{E}(\alpha_i) = 0 = \mathbb{E}(\beta_i)$, for $1 \le i \le n$. Furthermore, $\alpha_1, \ldots, \alpha_n$ and $\beta_1, \ldots, \beta_n$ are i.i.d. sequences, where, in addition, α_i is independent from β_j, for $1 \le i \ne j \le n$. Overall, this results in

$$n^{-2}\mathbb{E}\Big(\Big(\sum_{1 \le i \le n} \alpha_i\Big)^2 \Big(\sum_{1 \le j \le n} \beta_j\Big)^2\Big) = \frac{n-1}{n}\mathbb{E}(\alpha_1^2)\mathbb{E}(\beta_1^2)$$

$$\le \big(H(x) - H(x_1)\big)\big(H(x_2) - H(x)\big)$$

$$\le \big(H(x_2) - H(x_1)\big)^2.$$

Since H is a nondecreasing, continuous function, the proof is complete.   □

Remark 6.11 The continuity assumption (6.5) in Theorem 6.8 is not dispensable even though it does not appear in Stute (1997, Theorem 1.1). In the proof of Stute (1997, Theorem 1.1), it is noted for the verification of tightness that $\mathbb{E}(Y \mid U = u) = m(F^{-1}(u))$. This then implies the continuity of H, our assumption (6.5). However, the following example shows that $\mathbb{E}(Y \mid U = u) = m(F^{-1}(u))$ does not generally have to be true if F is discontinuous. Nevertheless, in the main application of the theorem continuity of F has to be guaranteed anyway and the missing assumption in Stute (1997, Theorem 1.1) does not affect its importance in statistical application!

Example 6.12 Let U be a uniformly distributed random variable defined on some probability space $(\Omega, \mathscr{A}, \mathbb{P})$. Set $X = I_{\{U \le 0.5\}}$ and $Y = U$. The Bernoulli-distributed random variable X has distribution, respectively, quantile function

$$F(x) = \mathbb{P}(X \le x) = \begin{cases} 0 & : x < 0 \\ 0.5 & : 0 \le x < 1 \\ 1 & : x \ge 1 \end{cases}$$

$$F^{-1}(u) = \begin{cases} 0 & : 0 \le u \le 0.5 \\ 1 & : 0.5 < u \le 1 \end{cases},$$

respectively. Elementary calculation of $\mathbb{E}(Y \mid X = x)$, for $x \in \{0, 1\}$, yields

$$\mathbb{E}(Y \mid X = F^{-1}(u)) = m \circ F^{-1}(u) = 3/4 - F^{-1}(u)/2.$$

Since $\mathbb{E}(Y \mid U = u) = u$, we finally get

$$\mathbb{E}(Y \mid U = u) \neq m \circ F^{-1}(u), \quad \text{for all } 0 \leq u \leq 1.$$

This contradicts

$$\mathbb{E}(Y \mid U = u) = m \circ F^{-1}(u)$$

asserted in Stute (1997, Proof of Theorem 1.1). $\qquad\qquad\qquad\qquad\qquad\square$

6.4.2 The MEP with Estimated Model Parameters Propagating in a Fixed Direction

The result obtained under Theorem 6.8 for the BMEP represents an initial theoretical basis which, however, still has to be extended for statistical applications. If, for example, there is a parameterized regression, then the corresponding parameter must be estimated and instead of the true regression function m we now consider a estimated regression function. If the true m is replaced by the estimated one in the BMEP, then the true errors are replaced by the estimated errors, i.e., by the residuals. This, of course, affects the limit distribution. The extension of the BMEP with estimated parameters goes back to Stute (1997) and we present the result here in our context.

Definition 6.13 Let $(Y_1, X_1), \ldots, (Y_n, X_n)$ be an i.i.d. sequence in $\mathbb{R}^2$ such that $\mathbb{E}(|Y|) < \infty$ and denote the conditional expectation of Y given $X = x$ by $m(x)$. Assume that m belongs to a parametric family

$$\mathcal{M} = \big\{ m(\cdot, \theta) : \theta \in \Theta \big\}$$

such that $m(x) = m(x, \theta_0)$, for some true parameter $\theta_0 \in \Theta \subset \mathbb{R}^p$. Let θ_n be an estimator of θ_0. Then

$$[-\infty, \infty] \ni x \longrightarrow R_n^1(x) := n^{-1/2} \sum_{i=1}^{n} \big(Y_i - m(X_i, \theta_n)\big) \, I_{\{X_i \leq x\}} \in \mathbb{R} \qquad (6.7)$$

defines the *estimated marked empirical process* (EMEP).

The direction of propagation of EMEP, which is determined by the indicator, is given here by $\mathbb{R}$, as with the BMEP itself, since the covariate X is real. Therefore, the process propagates in a fixed direction.

For the analysis of the asymptotic behavior of R_n^1, we now, of course, need further assumptions which we list below:

(i) $n^{1/2}(\theta_n - \theta_0) = n^{-1/2} \sum_{i=1}^n l(X_i, Y_i, \theta_0) + o_{\mathbb{P}}(1)$.

(ii) $\mathbb{E}(l(X_i, Y_i, \theta_0)) = 0$.

(iii) $L(\theta_0) = \mathbb{E}(l(X, Y, \theta_0)l^\top(X, Y, \theta_0))$ exists.

(iv) $w(x, \theta) = \partial m(x, \theta)/\partial \theta = (w_1(x, \theta), \ldots, w_p(x, \theta))^\top$ exists for θ in a neighborhood $V \subset \Theta$ of θ_0 and is continuous with respect to θ.

(v) There exists an F-integrable function $M(x)$ such that $|w_i(x, \theta)| \le M(x)$ for all $\theta \in V \subset \Theta$, $1 \le i \le p$, and V given in 6.4.2(iv).

The first three conditions 6.4.2(i)–(iii) are usually met for least squares or maximum likelihood estimates.

Let $W(t, \theta) = (W_1(t, \theta), \ldots, W_p(t, \theta))^\top$ be defined by

$$W_i(t, \theta) = \mathbb{E}\big(w_i(X, \theta)I_{\{X \le t\}}\big).$$

Lemma 6.14 *Let θ_n converge in probability to θ_0 and assume that $\hat{\theta}_n : \mathbb{R} \to \Theta$ is a measurable function such that $\hat{\theta}_n(x)$ lies for each $x \in \mathbb{R}$ and $n \in \mathbb{N}$ on the line segment that connects θ_n and θ_0. If 6.4.2(iv) and (v) hold, then, for $1 \le i \le p$,*

(i) $\sup_{-\infty \le t \le \infty} \left| \int_{-\infty}^t w_i(x, \hat{\theta}_n(x)) - w_i(x, \theta_0) F_n(dx) \right| = o_{\mathbb{P}}(1)$,

(ii) $\limsup_{n \to \infty} \sup_{-\infty \le t \le \infty} \left| \int_{-\infty}^t w_i(x, \theta_0) (F_n - F)(dx) \right| = 0$ *w.p.1.*

Proof For $\varepsilon, \delta > 0$ we get by the Markov theorem,

$$\mathbb{P}\left(\sup_{-\infty \le t \le \infty} \left| \int_{-\infty}^t w_i(x, \hat{\theta}_n(x)) - w_i(x, \theta_0) F_n(dx) \right| > \varepsilon \right)$$

$$\le \frac{1}{\varepsilon} \mathbb{E}\left(\sup_{|\theta - \theta_0| < \delta} |w_i(X, \theta) - w_i(X, \theta_0)| \right) + \mathbb{P}(|\theta_n - \theta_0| > \delta),$$

for $1 \le i \le p$. Due to 6.4.2(v), the expectation on the right side is finite and the integrand converges to 0 according to 6.4.2(iv) if δ tends to 0. The first assertion now follows from the dominated convergence theorem and the assumed convergence of θ_n to θ_0.

For the second assertion, we fix $K > 0$ and apply 6.4.2(v) to obtain

$$\limsup_{n \to \infty} \sup_{-\infty \le t \le \infty} \left| \int_{-\infty}^t w_i(x, \theta_0) (F_n - F)(dx) \right|$$

$$\le \limsup_{n \to \infty} \sup_{|t| \le K} \left| \int_{-K}^t w_i(x, \theta_0) (F_n - F)(dx) \right|$$

$$+ \limsup_{n \to \infty} \int M(x)I_{\{|x| > K\}} F_n(dx) + \int M(x)I_{\{|x| > K\}} F(dx).$$

According to Theorem 5.66, the first term on the right side is identical to 0 for each fixed K w.p.1. Due to the SLLN, the second term is identical to the third term w.p.1. However, since the third term converges with $K \to \infty$ against 0, the second assertion is proven.   □

The main result of this section is the following theorem, compare Stute (1997, Theorem 1.2).

Theorem 6.15 *Assume* $\mathbb{E}(Y^2) < \infty$, F *is continuous and conditions 6.4.2(i)–6.4.2 (v) are met. Then, under* $m(\cdot) = m(\cdot, \theta_0)$, *we have, uniformly in* x,

$$R_n^1(x) = R_n(x) - n^{1/2} \sum_{i=1}^n W^\top(x, \theta_0) l(X_i, Y_i, \theta_0) + o_\mathbb{P}(1), \quad \text{as } n \to \infty.$$

Furthermore, R_n^1 *converges in* $D[-\infty, \infty]$ *to a centered Gaussian process* R_∞^1 *with covariance function*

$$
\begin{aligned}
K^1(s, t) = {}& K(s, t) + W^\top(s, \theta_0) L(\theta_0) W(t, \theta_0) \\
& - W^\top(s, \theta_0) \mathbb{E}(I_{\{X \le t\}}(Y - m(X, \theta_0)) l(X, Y, \theta_0)) \\
& - W^\top(t, \theta_0) \mathbb{E}(I_{\{X \le s\}}(Y - m(X, \theta_0)) l(X, Y, \theta_0)).
\end{aligned}
$$

Proof By definition,

$$
\begin{aligned}
R_n^1(x) &= n^{-1/2} \sum_{i=1}^n I_{\{X_i \le x\}}[Y_i - m(X_i, \theta_n)] \\
&= R_n(x) - n^{-1/2} \sum_{i=1}^n I_{\{X_i \le x\}}[m(X_i, \theta_n) - m(X_i, \theta_0)].
\end{aligned}
$$

A Taylor expansion of the terms of the sum results in

$$m(X_i, \theta_n) - m(X_i, \theta_0) = (\theta_n - \theta_0)^\top w(X_i, \theta_{ni}),$$

where θ_{ni} is between θ_n and θ_0. Hence,

$$
\begin{aligned}
R_n^1(x) &= R_n(x) - n^{1/2}(\theta_n - \theta_0)^\top n^{-1} \sum_{i=1}^n I_{\{X_i \le x\}} w(X_i, \theta_{ni}) \\
&= R_n(x) - n^{1/2}(\theta_n - \theta_0)^\top n^{-1} \sum_{i=1}^n I_{\{X_i \le x\}}(w(X_i, \theta_{ni}) - w(X_i, \theta_0)) \\
&\quad - n^{1/2}(\theta_n - \theta_0)^\top \left(n^{-1} \sum_{i=1}^n I_{\{X_i \le x\}} w(X_i, \theta_0) - W(x, \theta_0) \right) \\
&\quad - n^{1/2}(\theta_n - \theta_0)^\top W(x, \theta_0) \\
&= R_n(x) - n^{1/2}(\theta_n - \theta_0)^\top W(x, \theta_0) + o_\mathbb{P}(1),
\end{aligned}
$$

uniformly in x, where the last equality follows from Lemma 6.14. Since $W(\cdot, \theta_0)$ is bounded, assumption 6.4.2(i) yields

$$n^{1/2}(\theta_n - \theta_0)^\top W(x, \theta_0) = n^{-1/2} \sum_{i=1}^n l^\top(X_i, Y_i, \theta_0) W(x, \theta_0) + o_\mathbb{P}(1), \qquad (6.8)$$

uniformly in x which shows the first assertion of the theorem.

This representation of R_n^1 shows that the two sequences $(R_n^1)_{n\in\mathbb{N}}$ and $(\hat{R}_n^1)_{n\in\mathbb{N}}$, where

$$\hat{R}_n^1(x) = n^{-1/2} \sum_{i=1}^n \left((Y_i - m(X_i, \theta_0)) \, \mathrm{I}_{\{X_i \leq x\}} - l^\top(Y_i, X_i, \theta_0) W(x, \theta_0) \right),$$

are asymptotically equivalent in the sense of Billingsley (1968, Theorem 4.1). Therefore, we can do the remaining part of the proof with $(\hat{R}_n^1)_{n\in\mathbb{N}}$.

In order to prove tightness of $(\hat{R}_n^1)_{n\in\mathbb{N}}$, it remains to show, by virtue of Theorem 6.8, that the right-hand side of (6.8) is also tight in $D[-\infty, \infty]$. By assumption 6.4.2(ii) and 6.4.2(iii) the sequence $(S_n)_{n\in\mathbb{N}}$, where $S_n = n^{-1/2} \sum_{i=1}^n l(X_i, Y_i, \theta_0)$, tends to a multivariate normal distribution and therefore is tight in $\mathbb{R}^p$. Since $W(\cdot, \theta_0)$ is a bounded deterministic continuous function, the sequence $(S_n^\top W(\cdot, \theta_0))_{n\in\mathbb{N}}$ is tight in $C[-\infty, \infty]$. Since $C-$tightness implies $D-$tightness, we have shown that $(\hat{R}_n^1)_{n\in\mathbb{N}}$ is tight in $D[-\infty, \infty]$.

The convergence of the fidis of $(\hat{R}_n^1)_{n\in\mathbb{N}}$ is a consequence of the multivariate CLT. Hence, it remains to calculate the covariance function $K^1(s, t)$ of R_∞^1 which is identical to the covariance function of the centered process $\hat{R}_n^1$. Recall the definition of $L(\theta_0)$ given under 6.4.2(iii) to get

$$\begin{aligned}
\mathrm{COV}(\hat{R}_n^1(s), \hat{R}_n^1(t)) = {} & \mathbb{E}\left(\mathrm{I}_{\{X \leq s \wedge t\}}(Y - m(X, \theta_0))^2 \right) + W^\top(s, \theta_0) L(\theta_0) W(t, \theta_0) \\
& - W^\top(t) \mathbb{E}\left(\mathrm{I}_{\{X \leq s\}}(Y - m(X, \theta_0)) l(Y, X, \theta_0) \right) \\
& - W^\top(s) \mathbb{E}\left(\mathrm{I}_{\{X \leq t\}}(Y - m(X, \theta_0)) l(Y, X, \theta_0) \right).
\end{aligned}$$

Note that the first term on the right side is the covariance of the BMEP limit process R_∞. $\square$

Remark 6.16 Under the assumptions of Theorem 6.15, Shorack (2000, Chapter 12, Theorem 2.1 (1)) can be directly verified from the covariance function of R_∞^1. This shows that the limiting process R_∞^1 can be realized in $C[-\infty, \infty]$.

6.4.3 The MEP with Estimated Model Parameters Propagating in an Estimated Direction

Previously, all MEPs were based on one-dimensional random variables X, which were used to define the corresponding processes via the indicators $I_{\{X \leq x\}}$. If the input variables X are multidimensional, then the indicator set $(-\infty, x]$ can be replaced by the quadrant with upper right corner x, i.e., by the $\{z \in \mathbb{R}^p : z_i \leq x_i, \text{ for } 1 \leq i \leq p\}$. However, if the model under consideration is a linear or a generalized linear model, then the multidimensional vector X acts on Y by a corresponding linear combination of its components and we can switch to a one-dimensional input, namely, to this linear combination. The corresponding process thus realizes itself again in $D[-\infty, \infty]$. However, we pay a price for this traceability to the one-dimensional case; the direction in which the process evolves is determined by the linear combination. It is thus based on the estimated parameters and therefore propagates in an estimated direction.

Definition 6.17 Let $(Y_1, X_1), \ldots, (Y_n, X_n)$ be an i.i.d. sequence in $\mathbb{R}^{1+p}$ such that $\mathbb{E}(|Y|) < \infty$ and denote the conditional expectation of Y given $X = x$ by $m(x)$. Assume that m belongs to a parametric family

$$\mathcal{M} = \left\{ m(\cdot, \vartheta) : \vartheta = (\beta, \theta) \in \mathbb{R}^p \times \Theta \subset \mathbb{R}^{p+q} \right\}$$

such that $m(x) \equiv m(x, \vartheta_0) = m_0(\beta_0^\top x, \theta_0)$, for some true parameter $(\beta_0, \theta_0) \equiv \vartheta_0 \in \mathbb{R}^p \times \Theta$ and a Borel-measurable function $m_0 : \mathbb{R} \to \mathbb{R}$.

Let $\vartheta_n = (\beta_n, \theta_n)$ be an estimator of ϑ_0. Then

$$[-\infty, \infty] \ni u \longrightarrow \bar{R}_n^1(u) := n^{-1/2} \sum_{i=1}^n \left(Y_i - m_0(\beta_n^\top X_i, \theta_n) \right) I_{\{\beta_n^\top X_i \leq u\}} \in \mathbb{R} \quad (6.9)$$

defines the *estimated marked empirical process in estimated direction* (EMEPE).

Remark 6.18 The specific form $m(x) = m_0(\beta_0^\top x, \theta_0)$ implies that w.p.1

$$\mathbb{E}(Y \mid X) = m(X) = m_0(\beta_0^\top X, \theta_0) = \mathbb{E}(Y \mid \beta_0^\top X), \quad (6.10)$$

i.e., $\mathbb{E}(Y \mid X)$ is measurable with respect to the smaller σ-field $(\beta_0^\top X)^{-1}(\mathscr{B}^*)$, where $\mathscr{B}^*$ denotes the Borel σ-field on $\mathbb{R}$. Be aware that this is a very restrictive condition, because it means that all the information from X concerning $\mathbb{E}(Y \mid X)$ is already stored in the information given by the projection of X onto the line defined by β_0! Note that in the following we will not distinguish between m and m_0, but will always use m, even if m_0 is meant. So instead of writing $m_0(\beta^\top x)$ we will use $m(\beta^\top x)$. Thus, the EMEPE will be

$$[-\infty, \infty] \ni u \longrightarrow \bar{R}_n^1(u) := n^{-1/2} \sum_{i=1}^n \left(Y_i - m(\beta_n^\top X_i, \theta_n) \right) I_{\{\beta_n^\top X_i \leq u\}} \in \mathbb{R}. \quad (6.11)$$

Remark 6.19 If $m(x) = m(\beta_0^\top x, \theta_0)$ applies, then

$$e_i = Y_i - m(\beta_0^\top X_i, \theta_0)$$

denotes the true error. If ϑ_n is an estimator of ϑ_0, then

$$e_i(\vartheta_n) = Y_i - m(\beta_n^\top X_i, \theta_n)$$

defines the estimated error, that is, the residual. Furthermore, according to (6.10),

$$\mathbb{E}(e \mid X) = 0 = \mathbb{E}(e \mid \beta_0^\top X, \theta_0). \tag{6.12}$$

For the conditional variance with respect to $X = x$, we set

$$\sigma^2(x) = \mathbb{E}\big((Y - m(X))^2 \mid X = x\big) = \mathrm{VAR}(Y \mid X = x) \tag{6.13}$$

and define

$$\sigma_{\vartheta_0}^2(t) = \mathbb{E}\big((Y - m(\beta_0^\top X, \theta_0))^2 \mid \beta_0^\top X = t\big) = \mathrm{VAR}_{\vartheta_0}\big(Y \mid \beta_0^\top X = t\big). \tag{6.14}$$

For the functional limit theorem of the EMEPE, we again need some assumptions, which are directly derived from those of Sect. 6.4.2. We also need an additional assumption to control the estimated direction of EMEPE.

(i) $n^{1/2}(\vartheta_n - \vartheta_0) = n^{-1/2} \sum_{i=1}^n l(X_i, Y_i, \vartheta_0) + o_\mathbb{P}(1)$.
(ii) $\mathbb{E}(l(X_i, Y_i, \vartheta_0)) = 0$.
(iii) $L(\vartheta_0) = \mathbb{E}(l(X, Y, \vartheta_0) l^\top(X, Y, \vartheta_0))$ exists and is positive definite.
(iv) $w(x, \vartheta) = \partial m(x, \vartheta)/\partial \vartheta = (w_1(x, \vartheta), \dots, w_{p+q}(x, \vartheta))^\top$ exists for ϑ in a neighborhood $V \subset \mathbb{R}^p \times \Theta$ of ϑ_0 and is continuous with respect to ϑ.
(v) There exists an $\mathbb{P}_X$-integrable function $M(x)$ such that $|w_i(x, \vartheta)| \le M(x)$ for all $\vartheta \in V \subset \mathbb{R}^p \times \Theta$, $1 \le i \le p+q$, and V given in 6.4.3(iv).
(vi) The function

$$H: \quad \mathbb{R}^{p+1} \ni (\beta, u) \longrightarrow H(u, \beta) := \int I_{\{\beta^\top X \le u\}} \sigma^2(X)\, d\mathbb{P} \in \mathbb{R}$$

is uniformly continuous in u at β_0.

Set $W(t) = W(t, \vartheta_0) = (W_1(t, \vartheta_0), \dots, W_{p+q}(t, \vartheta_0))^\top$, where

$$W_i(t) = \mathbb{E}\left(w_i(X, \vartheta_0) I_{\{\beta_0^\top X \le t\}}\right). \tag{6.15}$$

The following technical lemma is of decisive importance for the functional limit theorem of the EMEPE that will follow later.

Lemma 6.20 *Assume that* $\mathbb{E}(Y^2) < \infty$, *6.4.3(vi), and* $m(x) = m(\beta_0^\top x, \theta_0)$ *holds for all* $x \in \mathbb{R}^p$. *Then we get for every* $\varepsilon > 0$:

$$\mathbb{P}\left(\sup_{u \in \mathbb{R}} \sup_{\{\beta : |\beta - \beta_0| \le \delta\}} \left| n^{-1/2} \sum_{i=1}^{n} \left(I_{\{\beta^\top X_i \le u\}} - I_{\{\beta_0^\top X_i \le u\}}\right) e_i \right| \ge \varepsilon \right) \longrightarrow 0,$$

as $\delta \to 0$.

Proof The proof is based on the theory of generalized empirical processes, as presented in the textbooks of van der Vaart and Wellner (1996) and Kosorok (2008), respectively.

For each $\beta \in \mathbb{R}^p$ and $u \in \mathbb{R}$ the set $H = H_{\beta,u} = \{x \in \mathbb{R}^p : \beta^\top x \le u\}$ defines a half-space in $\mathbb{R}^p$. Denote the set of all half-spaces of $\mathbb{R}^p$ by

$$\mathscr{H} = \left\{ H = H_{\beta,u}, \ \beta \in \mathbb{R}^p, u \in \mathbb{R} \right\}.$$

Based on this collection of sets we now define a function class of indicators through

$$\mathscr{F} = \left\{ I_{\{H \times \mathbb{R}\}} : H \in \mathscr{H} \right\}$$

and modify this class by multiplying the individual indicators by the function

$$h : \mathbb{R}^{p+1} \ni (x, y) \longrightarrow h(x, y) = y - m(\beta_0^\top x, \theta_0) \in \mathbb{R}$$

to get

$$\mathscr{F}_h = \left\{ h\, I_{\{H \times \mathbb{R}\}} : H \in \mathscr{H} \right\}.$$

Based on this collection of measurable functions, we consider the generalized empirical process $(\alpha_n(f))_{f \in \mathscr{F}_h}$,

$$\alpha_n(f) = n^{-1/2} \sum_{i=1}^{n} f(X_i, Y_i).$$

Note that according to (6.12) $\mathbb{E}(\alpha_n(f)) = 0$.

The paths of this generalized empirical process are elements of the space $l_\infty(\mathscr{F}_h)$, that is, the space of all function $l : \mathscr{F}_h \ni f \longrightarrow l(f) \in \mathbb{R}$ such that $\sup_{f \in \mathscr{F}_h} |l(f)| \equiv \|l\|_{\mathscr{F}_h} < \infty$. The metric $d_\infty(l_1, l_2) = \|l_1 - l_2\|_{\mathscr{F}_h}$ turns $l_\infty(\mathscr{F}_h)$ into the metric space $(l_\infty(\mathscr{F}_h), d_\infty)$.

First, we note that for every $f \in \mathscr{F}_h$ we have $f(X, Y) \in L^2(\Omega, \mathscr{A}, \mathbb{P})$. Furthermore, for each $f \in \mathscr{F}_h$ and $(x, y) \in \mathbb{R}^{p+1}$, $|f(x, y)| \le |h(x, y)|$, and $h(X, Y) \in L^2(\Omega, \mathscr{A}, \mathbb{P})$. That is, $|h|$ is an envelope of $\mathscr{F}_h$.

In general, there are measurability problems in the study of generalized empirical processes. However, these problems are always negligible if the considered function class is pointwise measurable (PM), see Kosorok (2008, Section 8.2, p. 142). The class $\mathscr{F}_h$ is PM according to Kosorok (2008, Lemma 8.10).

According to van der Vaart and Wellner (1996, Example 3.9.33), the class $\mathscr{H}$ of all half-spaces is a Vapnik-Červonenkis class (VC). The same is obviously true for the class $\mathscr{H}_{\mathbb{R}} = \{H \times \mathbb{R} : H \in \mathscr{H}\}$. Now, apply Kosorok (2008, Lemma 9.8) to get that the subgraphs of the associated indicator functions of $\mathscr{H}_{\mathbb{R}}$ are VC, wherein the subgraph of a real-valued function f defined on some set A is the set $\{(a, t) : t < f(a)\}$. This shows that $\mathscr{F}$ is VC. In addition, $\mathscr{F}_h$ is VC due to Kosorok (2008, Lemma 9.9 (vi)).

Overall, we have now seen that $\mathscr{F}_h$ is a PM VC class with envelope $|h|$ such that $\mathbb{E}(h^2) < \infty$. This shows that $\mathscr{F}_h$ is a $\mathbb{P}_{X,Y}$ Donsker class, see Kosorok (2008, last para., p. 165) and we can apply Kosorok (2008, Lemma 8.17) to get for every $\varepsilon > 0$

$$\mathbb{P}\left(\sup_{f,g \in \mathscr{F}_h : \rho(f,g) \leq \delta} \left|\alpha_n(f) - \alpha_n(g)\right| > \varepsilon\right) \longrightarrow 0, \quad \text{for } \delta \to 0, \tag{6.16}$$

where

$$\rho(f, g) = \left(\mathbb{E}\big((f(X, Y) - g(X, Y))^2\big)\right)^{1/2}.$$

According to (6.16), the proof is complete if we can show that for an arbitrary $\delta > 0$

$$\sup_{u \in \mathbb{R}} \mathbb{E}\left(\big(I_{\{\beta^{\top} X \leq u\}} - I_{\{\beta_0^{\top} X \leq u\}}\big)^2 h^2(X, Y)\right) \leq \delta, \quad \text{for } \beta \to \beta_0. \tag{6.17}$$

Note that

$$\mathbb{E}\left(\big(I_{\{\beta^{\top} X \leq u\}} - I_{\{\beta_0^{\top} X \leq u\}}\big)^2 h^2(X, Y)\right) = \mathbb{E}\left(\big|I_{\{\beta^{\top} X \leq u\}} - I_{\{\beta_0^{\top} X \leq u\}}\big| h^2(X, Y)\right).$$

Denote the integral on the right by $A(\beta, \beta_0, u)$. Then, for $K > 0$, we get by conditioning with respect to X

$$A(\beta, \beta_0, u) \leq \int \big|I_{\{\beta^{\top} x \leq u\}} - I_{\{\beta_0^{\top} x \leq u\}}\big| \sigma^2(x) I_{\{\|x\| \leq K\}} \mathbb{P}_X(dx)$$

$$+ \int \sigma^2(x) I_{\{\|x\| > K\}} \mathbb{P}_X(dx)$$

$$= A_1(\beta, \beta_0, u, K) + A_2(K).$$

Now choose an arbitrary $\gamma > 0$ and note that $|\beta^{\top} x - \beta_0^{\top} x| \leq \|\beta - \beta_0\| \|x\|$, where $\| \cdot \|$ denotes the Euclidean norm on $\mathbb{R}^p$, to get

$$A_1(\beta, \beta_0, u, K) \leq \int \left| I_{\{\beta^\top x \leq u\}} - I_{\{\beta_0^\top x \leq u\}} \right| \sigma^2(x) I_{\{\|x\| \leq K\}} I_{\{|\beta^\top x - \beta_0^\top x| \leq \gamma\}} \mathbb{P}_X(dx)$$

$$+ I_{\{\|\beta - \beta_0\| > \gamma/K\}} \int \sigma^2(x) \mathbb{P}_X(dx)$$

$$\leq \int \left(I_{\{\beta_0^\top x \leq u + \gamma\}} - I_{\{\beta_0^\top x \leq u - \gamma\}} \right) \sigma^2(x) I_{\{\|x\| \leq K\}} I_{\{|\beta^\top x - \beta_0^\top x| \leq \gamma\}} \mathbb{P}_X dx)$$

$$+ I_{\{\|\beta - \beta_0\| > \gamma/K\}} \int \sigma^2(x) \mathbb{P}_X(dx)$$

$$\leq \left(H(u + \gamma, \beta_0) - H(u - \gamma, \beta_0) \right) + I_{\{\|\beta - \beta_0\| > \gamma/K\}} \int \sigma^2(x) \mathbb{P}_X(dx)$$

$$= A_{1,1}(\beta_0, u, \gamma) + A_{1,2}(\beta, \beta_0, \gamma, K).$$

Overall, we have that

$$A(\beta, \beta_0, u) \leq A_{1,1}(\beta_0, u, \gamma) + A_{1,2}(\beta, \beta_0, \gamma, K) + A_2(K).$$

Since $\mathbb{E}(\sigma^2(X)) < \infty$, we can find a $K > 0$ such that $A_2(K) < \delta$. By assumption 6.4.3(vi), H is uniformly continuous in u at β_0 and we therefore can find a $\gamma > 0$ such that for a given $\delta > 0$, $\sup_{|u-v| \leq 2\gamma} |H(u, \beta_0) - H(v, \beta_0)| \leq \delta$. In conclusion, if we take $\|\beta - \beta_0\| < \min(2\gamma, \gamma/K)$ we get

$$\sup_{u \in \mathbb{R}} \mathbb{E} \left(\left(I_{\{\beta^\top X \leq u\}} - I_{\{\beta_0^\top X \leq u\}} \right)^2 h^2(X, Y) \right) \leq 2\delta,$$

which completes the proof of the lemma.   □

Remark 6.21 The proof of the last lemma has shown that $\mathscr{H}$ is a PM VC class. Thus, it is also a Glivenko-Cantelli (GC) class, that is, w.p.1

$$\sup_{H \in \mathscr{H}} \left| 1/n \sum_{i=1}^n I_{\{X_i \in H\}} - \int I_{\{X \in H\}} d\mathbb{P} \right| \longrightarrow 0, \text{ as } n \to \infty.$$

Interpret $\mathscr{H}$ as the class of indicator functions based on the half-spaces and multiply each indicator by a function w, such that $\mathbb{E}(|w(X)|) < \infty$, then Kosorok (2008, Corollary 9.27) guarantees that

$$\sup_{H \in \mathscr{H}} \left| 1/n \sum_{i=1}^n w(X_i) I_{\{X_i \in H\}} - \int w(X) I_{\{X \in H\}} d\mathbb{P} \right| \longrightarrow 0, \text{ as } n \to \infty,$$

w.p.1.

The main result of this section is the following theorem, compare Stute and Zhu (2002, Theorem 1).

Theorem 6.22 *Assume $\mathbb{E}(Y^2) < \infty$, F_{β_0}, the distribution function of $\beta_0^\top X$, is continuous, conditions 6.4.3(i) – 6.4.3(vi) are met, and $m(x) = m(\beta_0^\top x, \theta_0)$ holds for* *all $x \in \mathbb{R}^p$. Then, $\bar{R}_n^1$ converges in $D[-\infty, \infty]$ to a centered Gaussian process $\bar{R}_\infty^1 = R_\infty - W^\top V$, where V is a centered $(p+q)$−dimensional normal vector with covariance $L(\vartheta_0)$, W is defined in (6.15), and R_∞ is a centered Gaussian process with covariance function*

$$K(s, t) = \mathbb{E}(R_\infty(s) R_\infty(t)) = \int I_{\{u \le s \wedge t\}} \sigma_{\vartheta_0}^2(u) F_{\beta_0}(du).$$

The covariance between R_∞ and $W^\top V$ is given by

$$COV(R_\infty(s), W^\top(t)V) = W^\top(t) \mathbb{E}\left((Y - m(\beta_0^\top X, \theta_0))l(X, Y, \vartheta_0)I_{\{\beta_0^\top X \le s\}}\right),$$
$$(6.18)$$

and the covariance function of $\bar{R}_\infty^1$ by

$$\begin{aligned}
\bar{K}^1(s, t) = K(s, t) &+ W^\top(s)L(\vartheta_0)W(t) \\
&- W^\top(s)\mathbb{E}(I_{\{\beta_0^\top X \le t\}}(Y - m(\beta_0^\top X, \theta_0))l(X, Y, \vartheta_0)) \quad (6.19) \\
&- W^\top(t)\mathbb{E}(I_{\{\beta_0^\top X \le s\}}(Y - m(\beta_0^\top X, \theta_0))l(X, Y, \vartheta_0)).
\end{aligned}$$

Proof As the proof will show, the EMEPE is stochastically equivalent to an EMEP in which the estimated direction of evolution, β_n, is replaced by the true direction β_0. To do this, we first define the associated EMEP R_n^1

$$R_n^1(u) = n^{-1/2} \sum_{i=1}^n (Y_i - m(X_i, \vartheta_n))I_{\{\beta_0^\top X_i \le u\}}, \quad \text{for } u \in [-\infty, \infty].$$

Note that we change the notation $m(\beta^\top X, \theta)$ back to $m(X, \vartheta)$, since the subsequent proof is closely based on Theorem 6.15 and this theorem uses the notation $m(X, \vartheta)$. Related to R_n^1 is the BMEP R_n, which is defined by

$$R_n(u) = n^{-1/2} \sum_{i=1}^n (Y_i - m(X_i, \vartheta_0))I_{\{\beta_0^\top X_i \le u\}}, \quad \text{for } u \in [-\infty, \infty].$$

Due to (6.10), R_n is a BMEP with respect to the input $\beta_0^\top X_1, \ldots, \beta_0^\top X_n$. Since F_{β_0} is continuous and $\mathbb{E}(Y^2) < \infty$, we can apply Corollary 6.10 and Theorem 6.8 to get that R_n tends in distribution to the centered Gaussian process R_∞ in $D[-\infty, \infty]$ with covariance function

$$K(s, t) = \int I_{\{u \le s \wedge t\}} \sigma_{\vartheta_0}^2(u) F_{\beta_0}(du).$$

The asymptotics of EMEP R_n^1 can be obtained as in the proof from Theorem 6.15 and we derive that R_n^1 tends in distribution in $D[-\infty, \infty]$ to a centered Gaussian process R_∞^1 with covariance function

$$K^1(s,t) = K(s,t) + W^\top(s,\vartheta_0)L(\vartheta_0)W(t,\vartheta_0)$$
$$- W^\top(s,\vartheta_0)\mathbb{E}(I_{\{\beta_0^\top X \leq t\}}(Y - m(X,\vartheta_0))l(X,Y,\vartheta_0))$$
$$- W^\top(t,\vartheta_0)\mathbb{E}(I_{\{\beta_0^\top X \leq s\}}(Y - m(X,\vartheta_0))l(X,Y,\vartheta_0)).$$

Now take the true error $e_i = Y_i - m(\beta_0^\top X_i, \theta_0)$ and split $R_n^1(u) - \bar{R}_n^1(u)$ as follows:

$$R_n^1(u) - \bar{R}_n^1(u) = n^{-1/2}\sum_{i=1}^n e_i\left(I_{\{\beta_0^\top X_i \leq u\}} - I_{\{\beta_n^\top X_i \leq u\}}\right)$$
$$+ n^{-1/2}\sum_{i=1}^n \left(m(\beta_n^\top X_i,\theta_n) - m(\beta_0^\top X_i,\theta_0)\right)\left(I_{\{\beta_n^\top X_i \leq u\}} - I_{\{\beta_0^\top X_i \leq u\}}\right)$$
$$= A_1(\beta_n,\vartheta_0,u) + A_2(\vartheta_n,\vartheta_0,u).$$

According to Lemma 6.20, since $\vartheta_n \to \vartheta_0$ in probability,

$$\sup_{u\in\mathbb{R}}|A_1(\beta_n,\vartheta_0,u)| \longrightarrow 0, \quad \text{as } n\to\infty,$$

in probability. For $A_2(\vartheta_n,\vartheta_0,u)$, we use a Taylor expansion and derive by Lemma 6.14, similar as in the proof of Theorem 6.15, that

$$A_2(\vartheta_n,\vartheta_0,u) = n^{1/2}(\vartheta_n - \vartheta_0)^\top n^{-1}\sum_{i=1}^n w(X_i,\vartheta_0)\left(I_{\{\beta_n^\top X_i \leq u\}} - I_{\{\beta_0^\top X_i \leq u\}}\right) + o_\mathbb{P}(1),$$

uniformly in u, as $n\to\infty$. Since $n^{1/2}(\vartheta_n - \vartheta_0)$ tends to a normal distribution, it remains to show that

$$\sup_{u\in\mathbb{R}}\left|n^{-1}\sum_{i=1}^n w_k(X_i,\vartheta_0)\left(I_{\{\beta_n^\top X_i \leq u\}} - I_{\{\beta_0^\top X_i \leq u\}}\right)\right| \longrightarrow 0, \quad \text{as } n\to\infty,$$

in probability, for $1 \leq k \leq p+q$. For this, assume that $|\beta_n - \beta_0| < \gamma$ for $\gamma > 0$. Then, for $1 \leq k \leq p+q$ the supremum is bounded from above by

$$\sup_{u\in\mathbb{R},|\beta-\beta_0|<\gamma}\left|n^{-1}\sum_{i=1}^n w_k(X_i,\vartheta_0)I_{\{\beta^\top X_i \leq u\}} - \mathbb{E}\left(w_k(X,\vartheta_0)I_{\{\beta^\top X \leq u\}}\right)\right|$$
$$+ \left|n^{-1}\sum_{i=1}^n w_k(X_i,\vartheta_0)I_{\{\beta_0^\top X_i \leq u\}} - \mathbb{E}\left(w_k(X,\vartheta_0)I_{\{\beta_0^\top X \leq u\}}\right)\right|$$
$$+ \sup_{u\in\mathbb{R},|\beta-\beta_0|<\gamma}\mathbb{E}\left(M(X)|I_{\{\beta^\top X \leq u\}} - I_{\{\beta_0^\top X \leq u\}}|\right).$$

According to Remark 6.21, the first two terms in the above bound tend to 0. Since $\beta_n \to \beta_0$ in probability, as $n\to\infty$, the third term tends to 0 with the same argumentation that was used to prove (6.17). This finally completes the proof of the theorem.   □

6.5   Mathematical Framework: Bootstrap of Marked Empirical Processes

This section examines the asymptotics of bootstrap variants of the BMEP and EMEP processes in the GLM context. At first, this is done, in general, without using a special resampling method and without distinguishing between parametric and semi-parametric models. Specifications of the theoretical results obtained with respect to these two concrete models are given at the end of this section.

Let us recall Definition 6.17 of the EMEPE $\bar{R}_n^1$ and the proof of Theorem 6.22. There it was shown that $\bar{R}_n^1$ is asymptotically equivalent to the particular EMEP

$$R_n^1(u) = n^{-1/2} \sum_{i=1}^n \left(Y_i - m(\beta_n^\top X_i, \theta_n)\right) I_{\{\beta_0^\top X_i \leq u\}}.$$

The corresponding bootstrap analog to this EMEP is given in the following definition.

Definition 6.23   Assume the setup of Definition 6.17, let $(Y_{1,n}^*, X_1), \ldots, (Y_{n,n}^*, X_n)$ be the bootstrap data according to some resampling scheme such that $\mathbb{E}_n^*(Y_{i,n}^*) = m(X_i, \vartheta_n)$, where $\vartheta_n = (\beta_n, \theta_n)$ is the estimate of ϑ_0 based on the original data. Denote with $\vartheta_n^* = (\beta_n^*, \theta_n^*)$ the estimated parameter based on the bootstrap data. Then

$$[-\infty, \infty] \ni u \longrightarrow R_n^{1*}(u) = n^{-1/2} \sum_{i=1}^n \left(Y_{i,n}^* - m(\beta_n^{*\top} X_i, \theta_n^*)\right) I_{\{\beta_n^\top X_i \leq u\}} \quad (6.20)$$

defines the *bootstrapped estimated marked empirical process*.

Remark 6.24   For a direct transfer of EMEPE into the bootstrap world, instead of the indicator $I_{\{\beta_n^\top X_i \leq u\}}$, one would have to actually use the indicator $I_{\{\beta_n^{*\top} X_i \leq u\}}$ in Definition 6.23. But, as already noted, EMEPE and EMEP are stochastically equivalent for the original data. Furthermore, the bootstrap version of EMEP has the big advantage that in Monte Carlo simulations to determine corresponding statistics, the values of $\beta_n^\top X_1, \ldots, \beta_n^\top X_n$ only have to be sorted once and not separately for each individual bootstrap dataset, which would be necessary in the case of the indicator $I_{\{\beta_n^{*\top} X_i \leq u\}}$. Due to this performance advantage, we have only considered the EMEP variant for the bootstrap procedure here.

Note that

$$
\begin{aligned}
R_n^{1*}(u) &= n^{-1/2} \sum_{i=1}^{n} \left(Y_{i,n}^* - m(\beta_n^{*\top} X_i, \theta_n^*) \right) \mathrm{I}_{\{\beta_n^{*\top} X_i \leq u\}} \\
&= n^{-1/2} \sum_{i=1}^{n} \left(Y_{i,n}^* - m(\beta_n^\top X_i, \theta_n) \right) \mathrm{I}_{\{\beta_n^{*\top} X_i \leq u\}} \\
&\quad - n^{-1/2} \sum_{i=1}^{n} \left(m(\beta_n^{*\top} X_i, \theta_n^*) - m(\beta_n^\top X_i, \theta_n) \right) \mathrm{I}_{\{\beta_n^{*\top} X_i \leq u\}} \\
&= R_n^*(u) - S_n^*(u).
\end{aligned}
$$

Within the bootstrap world, the first process on the right side, that is,

$$
R_n^*(u) = n^{-1/2} \sum_{i=1}^{n} \left(Y_{i,n}^* - m(\beta_n^\top X_i, \theta_n) \right) \mathrm{I}_{\{\beta_n^{*\top} X_i \leq u\}}, \tag{6.21}
$$

can be interpreted as a bootstrap version of a BMEP, since $\mathbb{E}_n^*(Y_{i,n}^*) = m(\beta_n^\top X_i, \theta_n)$. The second process

$$
S_n^*(u) = n^{-1/2} \sum_{i=1}^{n} \left(m(\beta_n^{*\top} X_i, \theta_n^*) - m(\beta_n^\top X_i, \theta_n) \right) \mathrm{I}_{\{\beta_n^{*\top} X_i \leq u\}} \tag{6.22}
$$

deals with the influence of parameter estimation in m.

The two bootstrap methods considered so far have two things in common. First, the X_i from the underlying dataset is taken directly into the bootstrap dataset, i.e., $X_{i,n}^* = X_i$. So $X_{i,n}^*$ in the bootstrap dataset is deterministic and not random like in the original dataset! Second, the corresponding $Y_{i,n}^*$ has the property $\mathbb{E}_n^*(Y_{i,n}^*) = m(\beta_n^\top X_i, \theta_n)$.

The goal in this chapter is to prove that w.p.1, R_n^{1*} converges toward the same limit process $\bar{R}_\infty^1$ as $\bar{R}_n^1$ does.

To get a more compact notation, we will write $m(x, \vartheta)$ for $m(\beta^\top x, \theta)$ in different places, where $\vartheta = (\beta, \theta)$.

In the forthcoming proofs, we will base ourselves on arguments which require a special condition and which we now summarize in advance in the following definition.

Definition 6.25 Let V be a compact neighborhood of ϑ_0 and

$$
h: \quad \mathbb{R}^{p+1} \times V \ni (x, y, \vartheta) \longrightarrow h(x, y, \vartheta) \in \mathbb{R}
$$

a measurable function such that $h(x, y, \vartheta)$ is continuous in $\vartheta = (\beta, \theta)$ for all $\vartheta \in V$ and $(x, y) \in \mathbb{R}^{p+1}$. We call such a function h *uniformly dominated by M over V at*

ϑ_0 if there exists a $\mathbb{P}_{X,Y}-$ integrable function M such that $|h(x, y, \vartheta)| \leq M(x, y)$ for all $\vartheta \in V$ and $(x, y) \in \mathbb{R}^{p+1}$.

In the following two sections, we will sometimes use a technical argument in the proofs, which we next formulate here as a lemma. The proof of this lemma is based in its technique on the proof of Lemma 6.20.

Lemma 6.26 *Let h be uniformly dominated by M over V at ϑ_0 and assume that*

$$H : \mathbb{R} \ni u \longrightarrow H(u) = \mathbb{E}\big(|h(X, Y, \vartheta_0)|I_{\{\beta_0^\top X \leq u\}}\big) \in \mathbb{R}$$

is uniformly continuous in u. Then we get

(i) As $n \to \infty$,

$$\sup_{\vartheta \in V, u \in \mathbb{R}} \left| \frac{1}{n} \sum_{i=1}^n h(X_i, Y_i, \vartheta) I_{\{\beta^\top X_i \leq u\}} - \mathbb{E}\big(h(X, Y, \vartheta)I_{\{\beta^\top X \leq u\}}\big) \right| \longrightarrow 0, \quad w.p.1.$$

(ii) As $\varepsilon \to 0$,

$$\sup_{\|\vartheta - \vartheta_0\| \leq \varepsilon, u \in \mathbb{R}} \left| \mathbb{E}\big(h(X, Y, \vartheta)I_{\{\beta^\top X \leq u\}}\big) - \mathbb{E}\big(h(X, Y, \vartheta_0)I_{\{\beta_0^\top X \leq u\}}\big) \right| \longrightarrow 0.$$

(iii) If $\vartheta_n \to \vartheta_0$ w.p.1, then, as $n \to \infty$,

$$\sup_{u \in \mathbb{R}} \left| \frac{1}{n} \sum_{i=1}^n h(X_i, Y_i, \vartheta_n) I_{\{\beta_n^\top X_i \leq u\}} - \mathbb{E}\big(h(X, Y, \vartheta_0)I_{\{\beta_0^\top X \leq u\}}\big) \right| \longrightarrow 0,$$

w.p.1.

Proof Theorem 5.66 guarantees that

$$\mathscr{G} = \big\{ h(\cdot, \cdot, \vartheta) \, : \, \vartheta \in V \big\}$$

is a PM-GC class (pointwise measurable Glivenko-Cantelli class) with integrable envelope M. As already pointed out in the proof of Lemma 6.20, the collection

$$\mathscr{F} = \big\{ I_{\{H \times \mathbb{R}\}} \, : \, H \text{ is half-space in } \mathbb{R}^p \big\}$$

is a PM-VC class and therefore a PM-GC class. In summary, we then get from Kosorok (2008, Corollary 9.27) that

$$\mathscr{F} = \big\{ h(\cdot, \cdot, \vartheta) I_{\{\beta^\top \cdot \leq u\}} \, : \, (\beta, \theta) = \vartheta \in V \text{ and } u \in \mathbb{R} \big\}$$

is a PM-GC class which completes the proof of part (i) of the lemma.

For (ii), first observe that

$$\sup_{\|\vartheta-\vartheta_0\|\le\varepsilon,\,u\in\mathbb{R}}\left|\mathbb{E}\big(h(X,Y,\vartheta)\mathrm{I}_{\{\beta^\top X\le u\}}\big)-\mathbb{E}\big(h(X,Y,\vartheta_0)\mathrm{I}_{\{\beta_0^\top X\le u\}}\big)\right|$$

$$\le\mathbb{E}\Big(\sup_{\|\vartheta-\vartheta_0\|\le\varepsilon}\big|h(X,Y,\vartheta)-h(X,Y,\vartheta_0)\big|\Big)$$

$$+\sup_{\|\beta-\beta_0\|<\varepsilon,\,u\in\mathbb{R}}\mathbb{E}\big(\big|h(X,Y,\vartheta_0)\big|\,\big|\mathrm{I}_{\{\beta^\top X\le u\}}-\mathrm{I}_{\{\beta_0^\top X\le u\}}\big|\big).$$

The assumptions, according to the dominated convergence theorem, guarantee that the first term on the right side converges to 0 as $\varepsilon \to 0$. Denote the expectation appearing in the second term on the right side by $A(\beta, u, \varepsilon)$ and choose $K > 0$ to get

$$A(\beta,u,\varepsilon)\le\mathbb{E}\big(\big|h(X,Y,\vartheta_0)\big|\,\big|\mathrm{I}_{\{\beta^\top X\le u\}}-\mathrm{I}_{\{\beta_0^\top X\le u\}}\big|\mathrm{I}_{\{\|X\|\le K\}}\big)$$

$$+\mathbb{E}\big(\big|h(X,Y,\vartheta_0)\big|\mathrm{I}_{\{\|X\|>K\}}\big)$$

$$=A_1(\beta,u,\varepsilon,K)+A_2(K).$$

Next select $\gamma > 0$ to get

$$A_1(\beta,u,\varepsilon,K)\le\mathbb{E}\big(\big|h(X,Y,\vartheta_0)\big|\,\big|\mathrm{I}_{\{\beta^\top X\le u\}}-\mathrm{I}_{\{\beta_0^\top X\le u\}}\big|\mathrm{I}_{\{\|X\|\le K\}}\mathrm{I}_{\{|\beta^\top X-\beta_0^\top X|\le\gamma\}}\big)$$

$$+\mathrm{I}_{\{\|\beta-\beta_0\|>\gamma/K\}}\mathbb{E}\big(\big|h(X,Y,\vartheta_0)\big|\big)$$

$$\le\mathbb{E}\big(\big|h(X,Y,\vartheta_0)\big|\,\big|\mathrm{I}_{\{\beta_0^\top X\le u+\gamma\}}-\mathrm{I}_{\{\beta_0^\top X\le u-\gamma\}}\big|\big)$$

$$+\mathrm{I}_{\{\|\beta-\beta_0\|>\gamma/K\}}\mathbb{E}\big(\big|h(X,Y,\vartheta_0)\big|\big)$$

$$=\big(H(u+\gamma)-H(u-\gamma)\big)+\mathrm{I}_{\{\|\beta-\beta_0\|>\gamma/K\}}\mathbb{E}\big(\big|h(X,Y,\vartheta_0)\big|\big)$$

$$=A_{1,1}(u,\gamma)+A_{1,2}(\beta,\gamma,K).$$

All in all, this means that we have

$$A(\beta,u,\varepsilon)\le A_{1,1}(u,\gamma)+A_{1,2}(\beta,\gamma,K)+A_2(K).$$

Now fix $\delta > 0$. Since $\mathbb{E}(|h(X,Y,\vartheta_0)|) < \infty$, we can find a $K > 0$ such that $A_2(K) < \delta$. H is uniformly continuous and we can therefore find a $\gamma > 0$ such that, uniformly in u, $A_{1,1} < \delta$. If we take $\varepsilon < \min(\gamma, \gamma/K)$, then $A_{1,2}(\beta,\gamma,K) = 0$, and we get for such an ε that $A(\beta, u, \varepsilon) < 2\delta$. This shows that

$$\sup_{\|\beta-\beta_0\|<\varepsilon,\,u\in\mathbb{R}}A(\beta,u,\varepsilon)\longrightarrow 0,$$

as $\beta \to \beta_0$. Overall, this proves part (ii) of the lemma.

Since $\vartheta_n \longrightarrow \vartheta_0$ w.p.1, part (iii) now follows directly from (i) and (ii). This completes the proof of the lemma.   □

6.5.1 Bootstrap of the BMEP

To prove a corresponding functional limit theorem for the bootstrap version of the BMEP we will make use of the following assumptions.

(i) $\mathbb{E}_n^*(Y_{i,n}^*) = m(\beta_n^\top X_i, \theta_n) \equiv m(X_i, \vartheta_n)$, where we set as before $\vartheta_n = (\beta_n, \theta_n)$. There exists a $\delta > 0$ and a non-negative function

$$h_e : \mathbb{R}^p \times \mathbb{R} \times \mathbb{R}^p \times \Theta \ni (x, y, \beta, \theta) \equiv (x, y, \vartheta) \longrightarrow h_e(x, y, \vartheta) \in \mathbb{R}$$

such that $\mathbb{E}_n^*(|Y_{i,n}^* - m(X_i, \vartheta_n)|^{2+\delta}) = h_e(X_i, Y_i, \vartheta_n)$ and h_e is uniformly dominated by M_e over V at ϑ_0 for some function M_e and a compact neighborhood V of ϑ_0.

(ii) There exists a non-negative function

$$h_v : \mathbb{R}^p \times \mathbb{R} \times \mathbb{R}^p \times \Theta \ni (x, y, \beta, \theta) \equiv (x, y, \vartheta) \longrightarrow h_v(x, y, \vartheta) \in \mathbb{R}$$

such that $\mathrm{VAR}_n^*(Y_{i,n}^*) = h_v(X_i, Y_i, \vartheta_n)$ and for all $u \in \mathbb{R}$

$$\mathbb{E}\big(h_v(X, Y, \vartheta_0)\mathrm{I}_{\{\beta_0^\top X \le u\}}\big) = \int \mathrm{I}_{\{t \le u\}}\sigma_{\vartheta_0}^2(t)\, F_{\beta_0}(dt),$$

where F_{β_0} is the distribution function of $\beta_0^\top X$ and $\sigma_{\vartheta_0}^2$ is defined under (6.14). Furthermore, h_v is uniformly dominated by M_v over V at ϑ_0 for some function M_v and a compact neighborhood V of ϑ_0 and the function

$$H_v : \mathbb{R} \times V \ni (u, \beta, \theta) \equiv (u, \vartheta) \longrightarrow H_v(u, \vartheta) := \mathbb{E}\big(\mathrm{I}_{\{\beta^\top X \le u\}}h_v(X, Y, \vartheta)\big)$$

is uniformly continuous in u at ϑ_0.

(iii) $\vartheta_n \longrightarrow \vartheta_0$, as $n \to \infty$, w.p.1.

The first two conditions seem somewhat unusual at first glance. They specify conditions for the bootstrap moments, which depend on the respective resampling procedure. Thus, we can treat the two resampling methods with only one theorem.

Theorem 6.27 *Assume that conditions 6.5.1(i), 6.5.1(ii), and 6.5.1(iii) are met. Then, w.p.1, the process R_n^* converges in $D[-\infty, \infty]$ to a centered Gaussian process R_∞ with covariance function*

$$K(s, t) = \mathbb{E}\big(R_\infty(s)\, R_\infty(t)\big) = \int \mathrm{I}_{\{u \le s \wedge t\}}\sigma_{\vartheta_0}^2(u)\, F_{\beta_0}(du).$$

Proof To prove the assertion we use again Billingsley (1968, Theorem 15.6).

For this, we first show that the fidis of R_n^* converge in distribution to those of R_∞. Let $k \in \mathbb{N}$ and take $-\infty \leq t_1 < \ldots < t_k \leq \infty$. According to Cramér-Wold, see Billingsley (1968, Theorem 7.7), we have to show that, w.p.1, for every $0 \neq a \in \mathbb{R}^k$

$$\sum_{j=1}^k a_j R_n^*(t_j) \longrightarrow \mathcal{N}(0, a^\top \Sigma a), \quad \text{as } n \to \infty,$$

in distribution, where $\Sigma = (\sigma_{j,\ell})_{1 \leq j,\ell \leq k}$ and $\sigma_{j,\ell} = \mathrm{COV}(R_\infty(t_j), R_\infty(t_\ell)) = K(t_j, t_\ell)$.

Set

$$Z_n^* = \sum_{j=1}^k a_j R_n^*(t_j) = n^{-1/2} \sum_{i=1}^n \left((Y_{i,n}^* - m(X_i, \vartheta_n)) \Big(\sum_{j=1}^k a_j \mathrm{I}_{\{\beta_n^\top X_i \leq t_j\}} \Big) \right)$$

$$\equiv \sum_{i=1}^n \xi_{i,n}^* A_{i,n},$$

where $\xi_{i,n}^* = n^{-1/2}(Y_{i,n}^* - m(X_i, \vartheta_n))$. Note that $\xi_{1,n}^*, \ldots, \xi_{n,n}^*$ are independent and centered, because of 6.5.1(i). Furthermore, $A_{1,n}, \ldots, A_{n,n}$ are deterministic with respect to $\mathbb{P}_n^*$.

We first consider the variance of Z_n^* and get

$$\mathrm{VAR}_n^*(Z_n^*) = \sum_{1 \leq j,\ell \leq k} a_j \Big(1/n \sum_{i=1}^n \mathrm{I}_{\{\beta_n^\top X_i \leq t_j \wedge t_\ell\}} \mathrm{VAR}_n^*(Y_{i,n}^*) \Big) a_\ell$$

$$= \sum_{1 \leq j,\ell \leq k} a_j \Big(\frac{1}{n} \sum_{i=1}^n \mathrm{I}_{\{\beta_n^\top X_i \leq t_j \wedge t_\ell\}} h_v(X_i, Y_i, \vartheta_n) \Big) a_\ell,$$

where the last equality follows from 6.5.1(ii). Now apply Lemma 6.26 to get that w.p.1

$$\frac{1}{n} \sum_{i=1}^n \mathrm{I}_{\{\beta_n^\top X_i \leq t_j \wedge t_\ell\}} h_v(X_i, Y_i, \vartheta_n) \longrightarrow \int \mathrm{I}_{\{u \leq t_j \wedge t_\ell\}} \sigma_{\vartheta_0}^2(u) \, F_{\beta_0}(du) = K(t_j, t_\ell),$$

as $n \to \infty$, that is,

$$\mathrm{VAR}_n^*(Z_n^*) \longrightarrow a^\top \Sigma a, \quad \text{as } n \to \infty, \text{ w.p.1.} \tag{6.23}$$

Since Σ is positive semi-definite, $a^\top \Sigma a \geq 0$. If $a^\top \Sigma a = 0$, Chebyshev's inequality guarantees that $Z_n^* = o_{\mathbb{P}_n^*}(1)$ and we have that w.p.1,

$$Z_n^* \longrightarrow \mathcal{N}(0, a^\top \Sigma a), \quad \text{as } n \to \infty.$$

In this case, $\mathcal{N}(0, a^\top \Sigma a) = \mathcal{N}(0, 0)$ is a degenerated normal distribution. Now assume that $a^\top \Sigma a > 0$. To prove the asymptotic normality of Z_n^*, Serfling (1980, Corollary to Theorem 1.9.3) can be applied and we have to show that the Lyapunov condition

$$\frac{1}{\mathrm{VAR}_n^*(Z_n^*)^{(2+\nu)/2}} \sum_{i=1}^n \mathbb{E}_n^*\left(\left|\xi_{i,n}^* A_{i,n}\right|^{2+\nu}\right) \longrightarrow 0, \quad \text{as } n \to \infty \tag{6.24}$$

is fulfilled w.p.1, for some $\nu > 1$, where the null set does not depend on a.

Since $a^\top \Sigma a > 0$, (6.23), and $|A_{i,n}| \le \|a\|\, k$, the Lyapunov condition (6.24) is, therefore, fulfilled if we can prove that

$$\sum_{i=1}^n \mathbb{E}_n^*\left(\left|\xi_{i,n}^*\right|^{2+\delta}\right) = \frac{1}{n^{1+\delta/2}} \sum_{i=1}^n \mathbb{E}_n^*\left((Y_{i,n}^* - m(X_i, \vartheta_n))^{2+\delta}\right)$$

$$= \frac{1}{n^{\delta/2}} \frac{1}{n} \sum_{i=1}^n h_e(X_i, Y_i, \vartheta_n)$$

$$\longrightarrow 0, \quad \text{as } n \to \infty, \text{ w.p.1,}$$

where $\delta > 0$ and h_e are chosen according to assumption 6.5.1(i). The assumed properties of h_e together with the w.p.1 convergence $\vartheta_n \to \vartheta_0$ now yield according to Theorem 5.66

$$\sup_{\vartheta \in V} \left|\frac{1}{n} \sum_{i=1}^n h_e(X_i, Y_i, \vartheta) - \mathbb{E}(h_e(X, Y, \vartheta_0))\right| \longrightarrow 0, \quad \text{as } n \to \infty, \text{ w.p.1,}$$

where V is chosen according to 6.5.1(i). This proves the convergence of the finite-dimensional distributions against $\mathcal{N}(0, \Sigma)$.

It remains to show that $(R_n^*)_{n \in \mathbb{N}}$ is tight. Since $D[-\infty, \infty]$ can be identified with $D[0, 1]$, compare Remark 6.4, we can adjust Billingsley (1968, Theorem 15.6) accordingly to prove tightness. For this let $-\infty \le u_1 \le u \le u_2 \le \infty$. As in the proof of Theorem 6.8, we get from Lemma 6.26 that w.p.1

$$\limsup_{n \to \infty} \mathbb{E}_n^*\left((R_n^*(u) - R_n^*(u_1))^2 (R_n^*(u_2) - R_n^*(u))^2\right)$$

$$\le \limsup_{n \to \infty} \left(\frac{1}{n} \sum_{i=1}^n \mathbb{E}_n^*\left((Y_{i,n}^* - m(X_i, \vartheta_n))^2 \mathbb{I}_{\{u_1 < \beta_n^\top X_i \le u_2\}}\right)\right)^2$$

$$= \limsup_{n \to \infty} \left(\frac{1}{n} \sum_{i=1}^n \mathbb{E}_n^*\left(h_v(X_i, Y_i, \vartheta_n)\mathbb{I}_{\{u_1 < \beta_n^\top X_i \le u_2\}}\right)\right)^2$$

$$= \left(H_v(u_2, \vartheta_0) - H_v(u_1, \vartheta_0)\right)^2.$$

Note that $H_v(\cdot, \vartheta_0)$ is uniformly continuous.

With a small adaptation in the proof of Billingsley (1968, Theorem 15.6), more precisely under Billingsley (1968, (15.30) in the proof of Theorem 15.6), this last result now yields that, with w.p.1, $(R_n^*)_{n \in \mathbb{N}}$ is tight.   □

6.5.2 Bootstrap of the EMEP

Additionally to the assumptions 6.5.1(i), 6.5.1(ii), and 6.5.1(iii) of Section 6.5.1, we need further conditions to handle the process S_n^*.

(iv) $n^{1/2}(\vartheta_n^* - \vartheta_n) \longrightarrow Z$ in distribution, as $n \to \infty$, w.p.1, where Z is a zero mean multivariate distribution with covariance matrix $L(\vartheta_0)$.

(v) $L(\vartheta_0) = \mathbb{E}(l(X, Y, \vartheta_0)l^\top(X, Y, \vartheta_0))$ exists and is positive definite.

(vi) $n^{1/2}(\vartheta_n^* - \vartheta_n) = n^{-1/2} \sum_{i=1}^n l(X_i, Y_{i,n}^*, \vartheta_n) + o_{\mathbb{P}_n^*}(1)$, as $n \to \infty$, w.p.1.

(vii) $\mathbb{E}_n^*(l(X_i, Y_{i,n}^*, \vartheta_n)) = 0$ and there exists a $\delta > 0$ and a non-negative function

$$h_{l,e} : \mathbb{R}^p \times \mathbb{R} \times \mathbb{R}^p \times \Theta \ni (x, y, \beta, \theta) \equiv (x, y, \vartheta) \longrightarrow h_{l,e}(x, y, \vartheta) \in \mathbb{R}$$

such that $\mathbb{E}_n^*(\|l(X_i, Y_{i,n}^*, \vartheta_n)\|^{2+\delta}) = h_{l,e}(X_i, Y_i, \vartheta_n)$. Furthermore, $h_{l,e}$ is uniformly dominated over V at ϑ_0 for some function $M_{l,e}$ and a compact neighborhood V at ϑ_0.

(viii) The covariance matrix

$$L_n^*(\vartheta_n) = \frac{1}{n} \sum_{i=1}^n \mathbb{E}_n^*\big(l(X_i, Y_{i,n}^*, \vartheta_n)l^\top(X_i, Y_{i,n}^*, \vartheta_n)\big) \longrightarrow L(\vartheta_0), \quad \text{as } n \to \infty, \text{w.p.1.}$$

(ix) For every $x \in \mathbb{R}^p$, $w(x, \vartheta) = \partial m(x, \vartheta)/\partial \vartheta = (w_1(x, \vartheta), \dots, w_{p+q}(x, \vartheta))^\top$ exists and is continuous with respect to ϑ for every ϑ in a neighborhood of ϑ_0 (not depending on x).

(x) For $1 \leq i \leq p + q$, $w_i(x, \vartheta)$ is uniformly dominated by some M_w over V at ϑ_0.

(xi) The function

$$W : \quad \mathbb{R} \times V_\beta \ni (u, \beta) \longrightarrow W(u, \beta) = \mathbb{E}\big(w(X, \vartheta_0)\mathrm{I}_{\{\beta^\top X \leq u\}}\big) \in \mathbb{R}^{p+q}$$

is uniformly continuous in u at β_0, where $V_\beta = \{\beta : (\beta, \theta_0) \in V\}$ and V is given under 6.5.2(ix).

(xii) There exists a function

$$h_{cov} : \mathbb{R}^p \times \mathbb{R} \times \mathbb{R}^p \times \Theta \ni (x, y, \beta, \theta) \equiv (x, y, \vartheta) \longrightarrow h_{cov}(x, y, \vartheta) \in \mathbb{R}^{p+q}$$

such that $\mathbb{E}_n^*\big((Y_{i,n}^* - m(X_i, \vartheta_n))\, l(X_i, Y_{i,n}^*, \vartheta_n)\big) = h_{cov}(X_i, Y_i, \vartheta_n)$ and for all $u \in \mathbb{R}$

$$\mathbb{E}\big(h_{cov}(X, Y, \vartheta_0) \mathrm{I}_{\{\beta_0^\top X \leq u\}}\big) = \mathbb{E}\big((Y - m(\beta_0^\top X, \theta_0))\, l(X, Y, \vartheta_0)\, \mathrm{I}_{\{\beta_0^\top X \leq u\}}\big).$$

Furthermore, each component $h_{cov,r}$, where $1 \leq r \leq p+q$, is uniformly dominated by $M_{cov,r}$ over V at ϑ_0 for some function $M_{cov,r}$ and a compact neighborhood V of ϑ_0, and the function

$$H_{cov} : \mathbb{R} \times V \ni (u, \beta, \theta) \equiv (u, \vartheta) \longrightarrow H_{cov}(u, \vartheta)$$
$$= \mathbb{E}\big(\mathrm{I}_{\{\beta^\top X \leq u\}} h_{cov}(X, Y, \vartheta)\big) \in \mathbb{R}^{p+q}$$

is uniformly continuous in u at ϑ_0.

In the following two remarks, we examine the validity of the moment conditions stated above for the resampling procedures used in the parametric and semiparametric bootstraps, respectively.

Remark 6.28 According to the Resampling Scheme 5.42 for the parametric case, $Y_{i,n}^*$ has density

$$f(y|\theta_{X_i}(\beta_n), \phi_n) = \exp\left(\frac{\theta_{X_i}(\beta_n)y - \zeta(\theta_{X_i}(\beta_n))}{\phi_n}\right) h(y, \phi_n),$$

where β_n and ϕ_n are the MLE corresponding to the original dataset and $\theta_x(\beta) = (g \circ \zeta')^{-1}(\beta^\top x)$. Now apply (5.19) to get

$$\mathrm{VAR}_n^*(Y_{i,n}^*) = h_v(X_i, Y_i, \vartheta_n) = \phi_n \zeta''(\theta_{X_i}(\beta_n)).$$

This representation of h_v can be used to find conditions that guarantee the validity of assumption 6.5.1(ii). The situation is similar with assumption 6.5.1(i).

Various assumptions state that for some function u

$$\mathbb{E}_n^*\big(u(X_i, Y_{i,n}^*, \vartheta_n)\big) = h(X_i, Y_i, \vartheta_n)$$

is uniformly dominated by a function M over a compact neighborhood V of ϑ_0. In case of the parametric bootstrap, we have

$$\mathbb{E}_n^*\big(u(X_i, Y_{i,n}^*, \vartheta_n)\big) = \int u(X_i, y, \vartheta_n) f(y|\theta_{X_i}(\beta_n), \phi_n) v(dy),$$

which is only a function of X_i and ϑ_n. Looking at the density of $Y_{i,n}^*$ reveals that one could also write it as

$$\exp\Big(K_1(X_i, \vartheta_n)y + c(y, \phi_n)\Big) K_2(X_i, \vartheta_n)$$

which even simplifies further, for instance, for the normal, Poisson, Bernoulli, gamma, and inverse Gaussian distribution to

$$\exp\Big(K_1(X_i, \vartheta_n)y + K_3(\phi_n)c(y)\Big) K_2(X_i, \vartheta_n).$$

Therefore, if $\|X_i\|$ is bounded by some K, one can try to shrink the neighborhood V and obtain the bound

$$\mathbb{E}_n^*\big(u(X_i, Y_{i,n}^*, \vartheta_n)\big) \le \int I_{\{\|X_i\|<K\}} u(X_i, y, \vartheta_n) \exp\Big(C_1 y + C_3 c(y)\Big) C_2 \nu(\mathrm{d}y).$$

On the basis of such a representation, conditions can then be formulated that ultimately guarantee the required integrability conditions.

Finally, note that Corollary 5.62 already provides a linear expansion and assumption 6.5.2(vi) and 6.5.2(viii) as well as $\mathbb{E}_n^*(l(X_i, Y_{i,n}^*, \vartheta_n)) = 0$ from assumption 6.5.2(vii).

Remark 6.29 According to the Resampling scheme 5.64 a wild bootstrap is used and

$$Y_{i,n}^* = m(X_i, \vartheta_n) + \tau_i \big(Y_i - m(X_i, \vartheta_n)\big),$$

where τ_i is a Rademacher variable, that is, $\mathbb{P}(\tau = 1) = 1/2 = \mathbb{P}(\tau = -1)$, also independent of X_i and Y_i.

Various assumptions state that for some function u

$$\mathbb{E}_n^*\big(u(X_i, Y_{i,n}^*, \vartheta_n)\big) = h(X_i, Y_i, \vartheta_n)$$

is uniformly dominated by a function M over a compact neighborhood V of ϑ_0. Obviously,

$$\mathbb{E}_n^*\big(u(X_i, Y_{i,n}^*, \vartheta_n)\big) = u(X_i, Y_i, \vartheta_n) I_{\{\tau_i = -1\}} + u(X_i, 2m(X_i, \vartheta_n) - Y_i, \vartheta_n) I_{\{\tau_i = 1\}}$$

.

On the basis of such a representation, conditions can then be formulated that ultimately guarantee the required integrability conditions.

Finally, note that Corollary 5.81 already provides a linear expansion and assumption 6.5.2(vi) and 6.5.2(viii) as well as $\mathbb{E}_n^*(l(X_i, Y_{i,n}^*, \vartheta_n)) = 0$ from assumption 6.5.2(vii).

The following lemma shows that condition 6.5.2(iv) is a consequence of conditions 6.5.1(iii), 6.5.2(v), 6.5.2(vi), 6.5.2(vii), and 6.5.2(viii). In order to obtain a more compact notation, we have retained it in the list of conditions.

Lemma 6.30 *Assume that conditions 6.5.1(iii), 6.5.2(v), 6.5.2(vi), 6.5.2(vii), and 6.5.2(viii) hold. Then, w.p.1,*

$$n^{-1/2}(\vartheta_n^* - \vartheta_n) \longrightarrow Z, \quad as \; n \to \infty,$$

where Z is multivariate normally distributed with zero mean and covariance matrix $L(\vartheta_0)$.

Proof Due to 6.5.2(vi) and Cramér-Wold, see Billingsley (1968, Theorem 7.7), we have to show that, w.p.1, for every $0 \ne a \in \mathbb{R}^{p+q}$

$$Z_n^* = n^{-1/2} \sum_{i=1}^n a^\top l(X_i, Y_{i,n}^*, \vartheta_n) \longrightarrow \mathcal{N}(0, a^\top L(\vartheta_0)a), \quad \text{as } n \to \infty,$$

in distribution. According to Serfling (1980, Corollary to Theorem 1.9.3), this follows if we can show that for some $\nu > 0$ the Lyapunov condition

$$\frac{1}{\mathrm{VAR}_n^*(Z_n^*)^{(2+\nu)/2}} \sum_{i=1}^n \mathbb{E}_n^* \left(\left| n^{-1/2} a^\top l(X_i, Y_{i,n}^*, \vartheta_n) \right|^{2+\nu} \right) \longrightarrow 0, \quad \text{as } n \to \infty, \text{w.p.1}$$

holds, where the null set does not depend on a.

For the variance, we get from 6.5.2(viii)

$$\mathrm{VAR}_n^*(Z_n^*) = \frac{1}{n} \sum_{i=1}^n a^\top \mathbb{E}_n^* \left(l(X_i, Y_{i,n}^*, \vartheta_n) l^\top(X_i, Y_{i,n}^*, \vartheta_n) \right) a = a^\top L_n^*(\vartheta_n) a$$
$$\longrightarrow a^\top L(\vartheta_0)a,$$

as $n \to \infty$, w.p.1, where the null set does not depend on a. Since $L(\vartheta_0)$ is positive definite and $a \neq 0$, $a^\top L(\vartheta_0)a > 0$. Thus, the Lyapunov condition is fulfilled if we can show that w.p.1

$$\frac{1}{n^{1+\nu/2}} \sum_{i=1}^n \mathbb{E}_n^* \left(\left| a^\top l(X_i, Y_{i,n}^*, \vartheta_n) \right|^{2+\nu} \right) \longrightarrow 0, \quad \text{as } n \to \infty.$$

Apply 6.5.2(vii) and choose $\nu = \delta$ to get

$$\frac{1}{n^{\delta/2}} \frac{1}{n} \sum_{i=1}^n \mathbb{E}_n^* \left(\left| a^\top l(X_i, Y_{i,n}^*, \vartheta_n) \right|^{2+\delta} \right) \leq \frac{\|a\|^{2+\delta}}{n^{\delta/2}} \frac{1}{n} \sum_{i=1}^n h_{l,e}(X_i, Y_i, \vartheta_n).$$

Corollary 5.67 together with assumption 6.5.1(iii) completes the proof.   □

As we have outlined in the introduction to this chapter,

$$R_n^{1*}(u) = R_n^*(u) + S_n^*(u),$$

where $S_n^*(u)$ is defined in (6.22). The main part now is to handle the process S_n^*.

Note that assumptions 6.5.2(iv) and 6.5.1(iii) imply

$$\mathbb{P}_n^*(\|\vartheta_n^* - \vartheta_0\| > \varepsilon) \longrightarrow 0, \quad \text{as } n \to \infty, \text{w.p.1}, \tag{6.25}$$

for $\varepsilon > 0$. Except for an $o_{\mathbb{P}_n^*}(1)$ term we can therefore assume that ϑ_n^* and ϑ_n are in the neighborhood V from assumption 6.5.2(ix) and we can apply Taylor's expansion to get

$$m(x, \vartheta_n^*) = m(x, \vartheta_n) + (\vartheta_n^* - \vartheta_n)^\top w(x, \hat{\vartheta}_n^*(x)),$$

where $\hat{\vartheta}_n^*(x)$ is in the line segment connecting ϑ_n^* and ϑ_n. Now, as under (6.15), we set $W(t) = W(t, \vartheta_0) = (W_1(t, \vartheta_0), \ldots, W_{p+q}(t, \vartheta_0))^\top$, where

$$W_i(t) = W_i(t, \vartheta_0) = \mathbb{E}\left(w_i(X, \vartheta_0)\mathrm{I}_{\{\beta_0^\top X \leq t\}}\right).$$

If we insert this in S_n^*, then the following decomposition is obtained.

$$
\begin{aligned}
S_n^*(u) &= n^{1/2}\big(\vartheta_n^* - \vartheta_n\big)^\top n^{-1} \sum_{i=1}^n w(X_i, \hat{\vartheta}_n^*(x))\mathrm{I}_{\{\beta_n^\top X_i \leq u\}} + o_{\mathbb{P}_n^*}(1) \\
&= n^{1/2}\big(\vartheta_n^* - \vartheta_n\big)^\top W(u, \vartheta_0) \qquad\qquad\qquad\qquad (6.26) \\
&\quad + n^{1/2}\big(\vartheta_n^* - \vartheta_n\big)^\top n^{-1} \sum_{i=1}^n \big(w(X_i, \hat{\vartheta}_n^*(X_i)) - w(X_i, \vartheta_0)\big)\mathrm{I}_{\{\beta_n^\top X_i \leq u\}} \\
&\quad + n^{1/2}\big(\vartheta_n^* - \vartheta_n\big)^\top \Big(n^{-1} \sum_{i=1}^n w(X_i, \vartheta_0)\mathrm{I}_{\{\beta_n^\top X_i \leq u\}} - W(u, \vartheta_0)\Big) \\
&\quad + o_{\mathbb{P}_n^*}(1).
\end{aligned}
$$

Lemma 6.31 *Let $\hat{\vartheta}_n^* : \mathbb{R}^p \to V$ be a measurable function such that $\hat{\vartheta}_n^*(x)$ lies for each $x \in \mathbb{R}^p$ in the line segment that connects ϑ_0^* and ϑ_0 and assume that 6.5.1(iii), 6.5.2(iv), 6.5.2(ix), 6.5.2(x), and 6.5.2(xi) hold. Then, w.p.1, for $1 \leq j \leq p+q$, as $n \to \infty$,*

(i) $\sup_{u\in\mathbb{R}} \left|n^{-1} \sum_{i=1}^n w_j(X_i, \vartheta_0)\mathrm{I}_{\{\beta_n^\top X_i \leq u\}} - W_j(u, \vartheta_0)\right| \longrightarrow 0,$

(ii) $\sup_{u\in\mathbb{R}} \left|n^{-1} \sum_{i=1}^n \big(w_j(X_i, \hat{\vartheta}_n^*(X_i)) - w_j(X_i, \vartheta_0)\big)\mathrm{I}_{\{\beta_n^\top X_i \leq u\}}\right| = o_{\mathbb{P}_n^*}(1).$

Proof Since $w_j(X, \vartheta_0)$ is integrable and the collection of half-spaces in $\mathbb{R}^p$ forms a GC class, we get from Kosorok (2008, Corollary 9.27) that w.p.1

$$\sup_{\beta\in\mathbb{R}^p, u\in\mathbb{R}} \left|n^{-1} \sum_{i=1}^n w_j(X_i, \vartheta_0)\mathrm{I}_{\{\beta^\top X_i \leq u\}} - \mathbb{E}\big(w_j(X, \vartheta_0)\mathrm{I}_{\{\beta^\top X \leq u\}}\big)\right| \longrightarrow 0, \quad \text{as } n \to \infty.$$

Therefore, we obtain from 6.5.1(iii) that for every $\varepsilon > 0$

$$
\begin{aligned}
&\limsup_{n\to\infty} \sup_{u\in\mathbb{R}} \left|n^{-1} \sum_{i=1}^n w_j(X_i, \vartheta_0)\mathrm{I}_{\{\beta_n^\top X_i \leq u\}} - W_j(u, \vartheta_0)\right| \\
&\leq \limsup_{n\to\infty} \sup_{\beta\in\mathbb{R}^p, u\in\mathbb{R}} \left|n^{-1} \sum_{i=1}^n w_j(X_i, \vartheta_0)\mathrm{I}_{\{\beta^\top X_i \leq u\}} - \mathbb{E}\big(w_j(X, \vartheta_0)\mathrm{I}_{\{\beta^\top X \leq u\}}\big)\right| \\
&\quad + \sup_{\|\beta-\beta_0\|<\varepsilon, u\in\mathbb{R}} \left|\mathbb{E}\big(w_j(X, \vartheta_0)\mathrm{I}_{\{\beta^\top X \leq u\}}\big) - W_j(u, \vartheta_0)\right| \\
&= \sup_{\|\beta-\beta_0\|<\varepsilon, u\in\mathbb{R}} \left|\mathbb{E}_n\big(w_j(X, \vartheta_0)\mathrm{I}_{\{\beta^\top X \leq u\}}\big) - W_j(u, \vartheta_0)\right|,
\end{aligned}
$$

w.p.1. But the last term on the right side tends to 0, as $\varepsilon \to 0$, under the stated assumptions, with similar arguments as we used in the proof of Lemma 6.26. For the second part, we get from (6.25) that

$$\sup_{u \in \mathbb{R}} \left| n^{-1} \sum_{i=1}^{n} \left(w_j(X_i, \hat{\vartheta}_n^*(X_i)) - w_j(X_i, \vartheta_0) \right) \mathrm{I}_{\{\beta_n^\top X_i \leq u\}} \right|$$

$$\leq n^{-1} \sum_{i=1}^{n} \sup_{\|\vartheta - \vartheta_0\| < \varepsilon} \left| w_j(X_i, \vartheta) - w_j(X_i, \vartheta_0) \right| + o_{\mathbb{P}_n^*}(1).$$

Now, by condition 6.5.2(x),

$$n^{-1} \sum_{i=1}^{n} \sup_{\|\vartheta - \vartheta_0\| < \varepsilon} \left| w_j(X_i, \vartheta) - w_j(X_i, \vartheta_0) \right|$$

$$\longrightarrow \mathbb{E} \left(\sup_{\|\vartheta - \vartheta_0\| < \varepsilon} \left| w_j(X_i, \vartheta) - w_j(X_i, \vartheta_0) \right| \right),$$

as $n \to \infty$, w.p.1. Due to the assumptions 6.5.2(ix) and 6.5.2(x), the last expectation tends to 0, as $\varepsilon \to 0$, by an application of the dominated convergence theorem. This proves the lemma.   □

Under the assumptions of Lemma 6.31 we get from (6.26) that uniformly in u

$$S_n^*(u) = n^{1/2} \left(\vartheta_n^* - \vartheta_n \right)^\top W(u, \vartheta_0) + o_{\mathbb{P}_n^*}(1), \quad \text{w.p.1}.$$

Now, use the asymptotic linear representation of ϑ_n^* of condition 6.5.2(vi) for further modification of S_n^* to get

$$S_n^*(u) = n^{-1/2} \sum_{i=1}^{n} l^\top(X_i, Y_{i,n}^*, \vartheta_n) W(u) + o_{\mathbb{P}_n^*}(1), \quad \text{w.p.1}, \qquad (6.27)$$

uniformly in u. Here and in the rest of this section we use $W(u)$ for $W(u, \vartheta_0)$.

Theorem 6.32 *Assume that conditions 6.5.1(i)–6.5.1(iii) and 6.5.2(v)–6.5.2(xii) hold. Then, w.p.1, R_n^{1*} converges in $D[-\infty, \infty]$ to a centered Gaussian process $\bar{R}_\infty^1$ with covariance function*

$$\bar{K}^1(s, t) = K(s, t) + W^\top(s) L(\vartheta_0) W(t)$$
$$- W^\top(s) \mathbb{E}(I_{\{\beta_0^\top X \leq t\}} (Y - m(\beta_0^\top X, \theta_0)) l(X, Y, \vartheta_0))$$
$$- W^\top(t) \mathbb{E}(I_{\{\beta_0^\top X \leq s\}} (Y - m(\beta_0^\top X, \theta_0)) l(X, Y, \vartheta_0)),$$

where $K(s, t)$ is the covariance function of the BMEP given in Theorem 6.27.

Proof Due to the assumed conditions, we can use the representation of S_n^* obtained under (6.27) to get that the two sequences $(R_n^{1*})_{n \in \mathbb{N}}$ and $(\hat{R}_n^{1*})_{n \in \mathbb{N}}$, where

$$\hat{R}_n^{1*}(u) = n^{-1/2} \sum_{i=1}^{n} \left(\left(Y_{i,n}^* - m(\beta_n^\top X_i, \theta_n) \right) \mathrm{I}_{\{\beta_n^\top X_i \leq u\}} - l^\top(X_i, Y_{i,n}^*, \vartheta_n) W(u) \right),$$

are asymptotically equivalent in the sense of Billingsley (1968, Theorem 4.1). To prove the assertion, we apply Billingsley (1968, Theorem 15.6) to $(\hat{R}_n^{1*})_{n \in \mathbb{N}}$. Note that

$$\hat{R}_n^{1*}(u) = R_n^*(u) - n^{-1/2} \sum_{i=1}^{n} l^\top(X_i, Y_{i,n}^*, \vartheta_n) W(u)$$

and $(R_n^*)_{n \in \mathbb{N}}$ is tight in $D[-\infty, \infty]$ according to Theorem 6.27. Furthermore, the proof of Lemma 6.30 shows that $n^{-1/2} \sum_{i=1}^{n} l^\top(X_i, Y_{i,n}^*, \vartheta_n)$ converges to a zero mean multivariate normal distribution with covariance matrix $L(\vartheta_0)$, w.p.1. By assumption 6.5.2(xi), $W(\cdot)$ is continuous. Thus, $n^{-1/2} \sum_{i=1}^{n} l^\top(X_i, Y_{i,n}^*, \vartheta_n) W(u)$ is tight in $C[-\infty, \infty]$ and therefore also tight in $D[-\infty, \infty]$. All in all, the tightness of $(\hat{R}_n^{1*})_{n \in \mathbb{N}}$ results, w.p.1.

It remains to show that the fidis of $\hat{R}_n^{1*}$ converge in distribution to those of $\bar{R}_\infty^1$. For this, let $k \in \mathbb{N}$, take $-\infty \leq u_1 < \ldots < u_k \leq \infty$, and $0 \neq a \in \mathbb{R}^k$. To apply Cramér-Wold, we have to show that w.p.1

$$Z_n^* = \sum_{j=1}^{k} a_j \hat{R}_n^{1*}(u_j) \longrightarrow \mathcal{N}(0, a^\top \Sigma a), \quad \text{for } n \to \infty,$$

in distribution, where $\Sigma = (\sigma_{r,s})_{1 \leq r,s \leq k}$ and $\sigma_{r,s} = \mathrm{COV}(\bar{R}_\infty^1(u_r), \bar{R}_\infty^1(u_s)) = \bar{K}^1(u_r, u_s)$. A simple rearrangement of the terms in Z_n^* results in

$$Z_n^* = \sum_{i=1}^{n} \frac{Y_{i,n}^* - m(X_i, \vartheta_n)}{\sqrt{n}} \sum_{j=1}^{k} a_j \mathrm{I}_{\{\beta_n^\top X_i \leq u_j\}} - \frac{l^\top(X_i, Y_{i,n}^*, \vartheta_n)}{\sqrt{n}} \sum_{j=1}^{k} a_j W(u_j)$$

$$= \sum_{i=1}^{n} \xi_{i,n}^* A_{i,n} - \eta_{i,n}^{*\top} B,$$

where $\xi_{i,n}^* = n^{-1/2}(Y_{i,n}^* - m(X_i, \vartheta_n))$ and $\eta_{i,n}^* = n^{-1/2} l(X_i, Y_{i,n}^*, \vartheta_n)$. These variables are centered and $(\xi_{1,n}^*, \eta_{1,n}^*), \ldots, (\xi_{n,n}^*, \eta_{n,n}^*)$ are independent. Furthermore, $A_{i,n}$ and B are deterministic with respect to $\mathbb{P}_n^*$. For the variance of Z_n^*, this results in

$$\text{VAR}_n^*(Z_n^*) = \sum_{i=1}^n A_{i,n}^2 \text{VAR}_n^*(\xi_{i,n}^*) + \sum_{i=1}^n B^\top \mathbb{E}_n^*\big(\eta_{i,n}^* \eta_{i,n}^{*\top}\big) B$$

$$- 2B^\top \sum_{i=1}^n \mathbb{E}_n^*(\xi_{i,n}^* \eta_{i,n}^*) A_{i,n}.$$

As we have seen in the proof of Theorem 6.27,

$$\sum_{i=1}^n A_{i,n}^2 \text{VAR}_n^*(\xi_{i,n}^*) \longrightarrow \sum_{1\le r,s\le k} a_r K(u_s, u_r) a_s, \quad \text{as } n \to \infty, \text{ w.p.1.}$$

Assumption 6.5.2(viii) guarantees that w.p.1, as $n \to \infty$,

$$\sum_{i=1}^n B^\top \mathbb{E}_n^*\big(\eta_{i,n}^* \eta_{i,n}^{*\top}\big) B \longrightarrow B^\top L(\vartheta_0) B = \sum_{1\le r,s\le k} a_s W^\top(u_s) L(\theta_0) W(u_r) a_r.$$

For the last term, conditions 6.5.1(iii), 6.5.2(xii) together with Lemma 6.26 imply that, w.p.1, as $n \to \infty$,

$$B^\top \sum_{i=1}^n \mathbb{E}_n^*(\xi_{i,n}^* \eta_{i,n}^*) A_{i,n}$$

$$= \sum_{1\le r,s\le k} a_r W^\top(u_r) \frac{1}{n} \sum_{i=1}^n h_{cov}(X_i, Y_i, \vartheta_n) \mathrm{I}_{\{\beta_n^\top X_i \le u_s\}} a_s$$

$$\longrightarrow \sum_{1\le r,s\le k} a_r W^\top(u_r) \mathbb{E}\big((Y - m(\beta_0^\top X, \theta_0)) l(X, Y, \vartheta_0) \mathrm{I}_{\{\beta_0^\top X \le u_s\}}\big) a_s.$$

All in all this shows that w.p.1, as $n \to \infty$

$$\text{VAR}_n^*(Z_n^*) \longrightarrow \sum_{1\le r,s\le k} a_r \bar{K}^1(u_r, u_s) a_s = a^\top \Sigma a.$$

If $a^\top \Sigma a = 0$, Chebyshev's inequality implies that $Z_n^* = o_{\mathbb{P}_n^*}(1)$ and we have that

$$Z_n^* \longrightarrow \mathcal{N}(0, a^\top \Sigma a), \quad \text{as } n \to \infty.$$

Now assume that $a^\top \Sigma a > 0$. According to Serfling (1980, Corollary to Theorem 1.9.3), the validity of the Lyapunov condition

$$\frac{1}{\text{VAR}_n^*(Z_n^*)^{(2+v)/2}} \sum_{i=1}^n \mathbb{E}_n^*\big(|\xi_{i,n}^* A_{i,n} - B^\top \eta_{i,n}^*|^{2+v}\big) \longrightarrow 0, \quad \text{as } n \to \infty, \text{ w.p.1,}$$

for some $\nu > 0$, implies the asymptotic normality of Z_n^*. Note that

$$
\mathbb{E}_n^* \big(|\xi_{i,n}^* A_{i,n} - B^\top \eta_{i,n}^*|^{2+\nu} \big)
$$

$$
= \sum_{i=1}^{n} \Big(\mathbb{E}_n^* \big(|\xi_{i,n}^* A_{i,n} - B^\top \eta_{i,n}^*|^{2+\nu} \big)^{1/(2+\nu)} \Big)^{2+\nu}
$$

$$
\leq \sum_{i=1}^{n} \Big(\mathbb{E}_n^* \big(|\xi_{i,n}^* A_{i,n}|^{2+\nu} \big)^{1/(2+\nu)} + \mathbb{E}_n^* \big(|B^\top \eta_{i,n}^*|^{2+\nu} \big)^{1/(2+\nu)} \Big)^{2+\nu}
$$

$$
\leq 2^{2+\nu} \sum_{i=1}^{n} \max \Big(\mathbb{E}_n^* \big(|\xi_{i,n}^* A_{i,n}|^{2+\nu} \big), \mathbb{E}_n^* \big(|B^\top \eta_{i,n}^*|^{2+\nu} \big) \Big)
$$

$$
\leq 2^{2+\nu} \Big(\sum_{i=1}^{n} \mathbb{E}_n^* \big(|\xi_{i,n}^* A_{i,n}|^{2+\nu} \big) + \sum_{i=1}^{n} \mathbb{E}_n^* \big(|B^\top \eta_{i,n}^*|^{2+\nu} \big) \Big).
$$

Conditions 6.5.1(i) and 6.5.2(vii) allow us to apply the same arguments used to verify the Lyapunov condition in the proof of Theorem 6.27. This completes the proof. □

Remark 6.33 Note that $\bar{K}^1$ matches the covariance given under (6.19). Thus, the bootstrap version of the EMEP converges to the same process as the EMEPE does.

6.6   Exercises

Exercise 6.1   The Kolmogorov-Smirnov (D_n) and Cramér-von Mises (W_n^2) statistics are used in the GOF test. If you want to use another statistics, which property is necessary so that all GOF-related theorems hold true.

Exercise 6.2   At which point in the mathematical framework of the marked empirical process is the fact necessary that at least one of the covariates is a continuous random variable.

Exercise 6.3   Compare the performance of the GOF test using the Kolmogorov-Smirnov and Cramér-von Mises statistics. For instance, extend the plots shown in Fig. 6.18.

Exercise 6.4   Plot the $p-$values of the GOF test based on the Kolmogorov-Smirnov (KS) statistics against the $p-$values of the GOF test based on the Cramér-von Mises (CvM) statistics. Make sure that each $p-$value pair was generated on the same original and bootstrap datasets.

Investigate a situation where the p-value based on the KS is small and the p-value based on CvM is large and vice versa. Can you modify one of the datasets in order to make the difference between the p-values even larger?

References

Billingsley P (1968) Convergence of probability measures. Wiley, New York

Billingsley P (1995) Probability and measure, 3rd edn. Wiley Series in Probability and Mathematical Statistics. Wiley, New York

Dikta G, Kvesic M, Schmidt C (2006) Bootstrap approximations in model checks for binary data. J Am Stat Assoc 101(474):521–530

Khmaladze EV (1982) Martingale approach in the theory of goodness-of-fit tests. Theory of Probability & Its Applications 26(2):240–257

Kosorok M (2008) Introduction to empirical processes and semiparametric inference. Springer series in statistics. Springer, New York

Nikabadze A, Stute W (1997) Model checks under random censorship. Stat Probab Lett 32(3):249–259

Serfling RJ (1980) Approximation theorems of mathematical statistics. Wiley Series in Probability and Mathematical Statistics. Wiley, New York

Shorack GR (2000) Probability for statisticians. Springer Texts in Statistics. Springer, New York

Shorack GR, Wellner JA (1986) Empirical processes with applications to statistics. Wiley Series in Probability and Mathematical Statistics. Wiley, New York

Stute W (1997) Nonparametric model checks for regression. Ann Stat 25(2):613–641

Stute W, Zhu LX (2002) Model checks for generalized linear models. Scandinavian Journal of Statistics Theory and Applications 29(3):535–545

Stute W, González Manteiga W, Presedo Quindimil M (1998) Bootstrap approximations in model checks for regression. J Am Stat Assoc 93(441):141–149

van der Vaart AW, Wellner JA (1996) Weak Convergence and Empirical Processes: With Applications to Statistics. Springer Series in Statistics, Springer, New York

van Heel M, Dikta G, Braekers R (2019) Bootstrap based goodness-of-fit tests for binary multivariate regression models. Technical report, Fachhochschule Aachen

Appendix A
boot Package

A helpful tool for bootstrapping is the boot package which comes preinstalled with R.

```
rownames(installed.packages(priority= "recommended"))
```

```
##   [1] "boot"        "class"        "cluster"     "codetools"
##   [5] "foreign"     "KernSmooth"   "lattice"     "MASS"
##   [9] "Matrix"      "mgcv"         "nlme"        "nnet"
##  [13] "rpart"       "spatial"      "survival"
```

The functions from the boot package can be used after loading the library

```
library(boot)
```

In this section, we do not describe the whole package, but only what is important for this book. Note, that one can find many different packages for bootstrapping on CRAN. These packages must be installed by the user manually through the command

```
install.packages("packagename")
```

A.1 Ordinary Bootstrap

Suppose we have a sample $X_1, \ldots, X_n \sim F$ of independent random variables and a test statistic $T_0 = T(X_1, \ldots, X_n)$. Denote by F_n the edf of $X_1, \ldots, X_n$. A common task is to generate independent random variables $X_{i1}^*, \ldots, X_{in}^* \sim F_n, 1 \leq i \leq m$ and calculate $T_i^* = T(X_{i1}^*, \ldots, X_{in}^*)$. This can easily be accomplished by the function "boot". The test statistic must be implemented as an R-function that has the two arguments one for the original sample and one for an index vector. This index vector

© Springer Nature Switzerland AG 2021
G. Dikta and M. Scheer, *Bootstrap Methods*,
https://doi.org/10.1007/978-3-030-73480-0

is generated by "boot" and passed to our R-function. Denote by $j_1, \ldots, j_n$ the index vector, then $X_{j_1}, \ldots, X_{j_n}$ are independent with distribution function F_n. Lets look at an example.

R-Example A.1 We generate 20 normal distributed random variables with mean 5 and standard deviation 2 and use the arithmetic mean as the test statistic T. Then we let the function "boot" calculate $m = 100$ bootstrap replicates of T.

```
arithMean <- function(originalSample, indexVector){
  mean(originalSample[indexVector])
}
```

```
set.seed(1234) # setting the seed for reproducability
x <- rnorm(20, mean=5, sd=2) # the original sample
print(b <- boot::boot(data=x, statistic=arithMean, R=100))
```

```
##
## ORDINARY NONPARAMETRIC BOOTSTRAP
##
##
## Call:
## boot::boot(data = x, statistic = arithMean, R = 100)
##
##
## Bootstrap Statistics :
##      original       bias    std. error
## t1* 4.529284 0.01409941    0.3707043
```

The object b returned by "boot" contains the arithmetic mean of the original sample and the arithmetic means of the 100 bootstrap samples.

```
b$t0
```

```
## [1] 4.529284
```

```
head(as.vector(b$t))
```

```
## [1] 4.553685 4.871633 4.937805 4.458266 4.707033 3.966022
```

Plotting b results in two plots. The first shows a histogram for the 100 calculated test statistics with the test statistic of the original sample as a dashed vertical line. The second plot is a Q–Q plot of the 100 ordered test statistics against normal quantiles, cf. Fig. A.1.

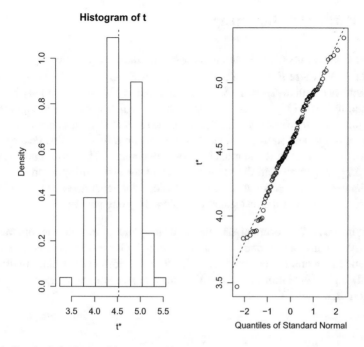

Fig. A.1 Standard plot for an object returned by boot()

```
plot(b)
```

In order to see what the function "boot" does, we reproduce the 100 bootstrap replicates of *T* manually.

```
set.seed(1234) # setting the seed for reproducability
x <- rnorm(20, mean=5, sd=2) # the original sample
n <- length(x)
m <- 100
indices <- sample.int(n=n, size=n*m, replace=TRUE)
dim(indices) <- c(m, n)
repsOfT <- sapply(1:100, function(i){
  arithMean(x, indices[i,])
})
print(all(repsOfT == b$t))
```

```
## [1] TRUE
```

As can be seen from the last R-code the function "boot" generates, by default, all *m* × *n* indices at once. One can force "boot" to generate random indices separately for every single bootstrap replication by passing simple = TRUE to "boot".

A.2   Parametric Bootstrap

Another common task is to generate independent random variables $X^*_{i1}, \ldots, X^*_{in} \sim \hat{F}$, $1 \leq i \leq m$, where $\hat{F}$ is a parametric estimate of F. Afterward, like in the ordinary bootstrap, we calculate $T^*_i = T(X^*_{i1}, \ldots, X^*_{in})$. In the case of the ordinary bootstrap, the function boot() generated random indices, which were passed together with the original sample to our implementation of the test statistic. Now, beside the implementation of our test statistic, we have to implement a function that generates data according to $\hat{F}$. This function must have two parameters. The first argument should be the original sample and the second argument for other information needed like the estimated parameter for $\hat{F}$. Since "boot" does not generate any random indices, our implementation of the test statistic requires only one parameter.

R-Example A.2 The original sample is 10 independent normal random variables $X_1, \ldots, X_{10}$ with mean 3 and standard deviation 2. Our test statistic is the trimmed arithmetic mean and the bootstrap samples follow a normal distribution with mean $\bar{X}_{10}$ and standard deviation s^2_{10}, where $\bar{X}_{10}$ and s^2_{10} are the empirical mean and standard deviation of $X_1, \ldots, X_{10}$.

```
set.seed(1234)
x <- rnorm(10, mean = 3, sd = 2)

generateData <- function(originalSample, paraEstimates){
  rnorm(length(originalSample), paraEstimates[1],
    paraEstimates[2])
}

trimmedMean <- function(x){
  mean(x, trim = 0.1)
}

# pass the estimated model parameter to the argument mle
boot::boot(data = x, statistic = trimmedMean, R = 100,
  sim = "parametric", ran.gen=generateData,
  mle = c(mean(x), sd(x)))


  ##
  ## PARAMETRIC BOOTSTRAP
  ##
  ##
  ## Call:
  ## boot::boot(data = x, statistic = trimmedMean, R = 100,
  ## sim = "parametric",
  ##       ran.gen = generateData, mle = c(mean(x), sd(x)))
  ##
  ##
```

```
## Bootstrap Statistics :
##      original        bias    std. error
## t1* 3.325981  -0.0157458     0.318165
```

A.3   Confidence Intervals

The function "boot.ci" takes an object returned by "boot" and calculates various confidence intervals.

```
arithMean <- function(originalSample, indexVector){
  mean(originalSample[indexVector])
}
```

```
set.seed(1234) # setting the seed for reproducability
x <- rnorm(20, mean=5, sd=2) # the original sample
b <- boot::boot(data=x, statistic=arithMean, R=999)
boot::boot.ci(b, conf=0.9, type=c("norm","basic", "perc", "bca"))
```

```
## BOOTSTRAP CONFIDENCE INTERVAL CALCULATIONS
## Based on 999 bootstrap replicates
##
## CALL :
## boot::boot.ci(boot.out = b, conf = 0.9, type = c("norm",
## "basic",
##      "perc", "bca"))
##
## Intervals :
## Level          Normal                   Basic
## 90%     ( 3.926,  5.119 )      ( 3.969,  5.160 )
##
## Level        Percentile                 BCa
## 90%     ( 3.899,  5.089 )      ( 3.780,  5.041 )
## Calculations and Intervals on Original Scale
```

There is also another type of confidence intervals that can be calculated with "boot.ci". In order to obtain these so-called studentized confidence interval, we have to calculate the variance of every bootstrap sample $X_{i1}^*, \ldots, X_{in}^*$ and for the original sample and pass them to "boot.ci". We illustrate this in the following example.

R-Example A.3 Again, we generate 20 normal distributed random variables with mean 5 and standard deviation 2 and use the arithmetic mean as the test statistic T. Then we let the function "boot" calculate $m = 999$ bootstrap replicates of T and the variance of the bootstrap sample $X_{i1}^*, \ldots, X_{in}^*, 1 \leq i \leq m$.

```
arithMean <- function(originalSample, indexVector){
  bootstrapSample = originalSample[indexVector]
  c(mean(bootstrapSample), var(bootstrapSample))
}


set.seed(1234) # setting the seed for reproducability
x <- rnorm(20, mean=5, sd=2) # the original sample
b <- boot::boot(data=x, statistic=arithMean, R=999)
# note b$t[,2] contains the variance estimate var(bootstrapSample)
# from the function arithMean()
boot::boot.ci(b, conf=0.9, type="stud",
              var.t0=var(x), var.t=b$t[,2])



  ## BOOTSTRAP CONFIDENCE INTERVAL CALCULATIONS
  ## Based on 999 bootstrap replicates
  ##
  ## CALL :
  ## boot::boot.ci(boot.out = b, conf = 0.9, type = "stud",
  ## var.t0 = var(x),
  ##     var.t = b$t[, 2])
  ##
  ## Intervals :
  ## Level     Studentized
  ## 90%    ( 3.849,  5.171 )
  ## Calculations and Intervals on Original Scale
```

Appendix B
`simTool` Package

An R-Package that facilitates simulation studies. It disengages the researcher from administrative source code.

The `simTool` package is designed for statistical simulations that have two components. One component generates the data and the other one analyzes the data. The main aims of the `simTool` package are the reduction of the administrative source code (mainly loops and management code for the results) and a simple applicability of the package that allows the user to quickly learn how to work with the `simTool` package. Parallel computing is also supported. Finally, convenient functions are provided to summarize the simulation results.

The workflow is quite easy and natural. One defines two data.frames (or tibbles), the first one represents the functions that generate the datasets and the second one represents the functions that analyze the data. They should follow three rules:

- the first column (a character vector) defines the functions to be called.
- the other columns are the parameters that are passed to function specified in the first column.
- the entry NA will not be passed to the function specified in the first column.

These two data.frames are passed to "eval_tibbles" which conducts the simulation. Afterward, the results can nicely be displayed as a data.frame. We now define the data generation functions for our first simulation.

```
print(dg <- dplyr::bind_rows(
  expand_tibble(fun = "rexp", n = c(10L, 20L), rate = 1:2),
  expand_tibble(fun = "rnorm", n = c(10L, 20L), mean = 1:2)
))


## # A tibble: 8 x 4
##    fun       n  rate  mean
##    <chr> <int> <int> <int>
## 1 rexp     10     1    NA
## 2 rexp     20     1    NA
```

© Springer Nature Switzerland AG 2021
G. Dikta and M. Scheer, *Bootstrap Methods*,
https://doi.org/10.1007/978-3-030-73480-0

```
## 3 rexp        10      2      NA
## 4 rexp        20      2      NA
## 5 rnorm       10      NA      1
## 6 rnorm       20      NA      1
## 7 rnorm       10      NA      2
## 8 rnorm       20      NA      2
```

This data.frame represents 8 R-functions. For instance, the second row represents a function that generates 20 exponential distributed random variables with rate 1. Since mean=NA in the second row, this parameter is not passed to "rexp". Similar, we define the data.frame for data analyzing functions.

```
print(pg <- dplyr::bind_rows(
  expand_tibble(proc = "min"),
  expand_tibble(proc = "mean", trim = c(0.1, 0.2))
))
```

```
## # A tibble: 3 x 2
##    proc   trim
##    <chr> <dbl>
## 1 min     NA
## 2 mean    0.1
## 3 mean    0.2
```

The following pseudo-code shows what the package in principle does

```
1.   convert dg to R-functions   {g_1, ..., g_k}
2.   convert pg to R-functions   {f_1, ..., f_L}
3.   initialize result object
4.   append dg and pg to the result object
5.   t1 = current.time()
6.   for g in   {g_1, ..., g_k}
7.     for r in 1:replications (optionally in a
                               parallel manner)
8.       data = g()
9.       for f in  {f_1, \ldots, f_L}
10.        append f(data) to the result object (opt.
                  apply a post-analyze-function)
11.      optionally append data to the result object
12.   optionally summarize the result object over all
         replications but separately for
         f_1, ..., f_L (and optional group variables)
13. t2 = current.time()
14. Estimate the number of replications per hour from
      t1 and t2
```

The object returned by "eval_tibbles" is a list of class eval_tibbles.

```
dg <- expand_tibble(fun = "rnorm", n = 10, mean = 1:2)
pg <- expand_tibble(proc = "min")
eg <- eval_tibbles(data_grid = dg, proc_grid = pg,
                   replications = 2)
eg
```

```
## # A tibble: 4 x 6
##   fun       n mean replications proc  results
##   <chr> <dbl> <int>        <int> <chr>   <dbl>
## 1 rnorm    10    1            1 min    -0.189
## 2 rnorm    10    1            2 min    -0.440
## 3 rnorm    10    2            1 min    -0.546
## 4 rnorm    10    2            2 min     0.927
## Number of data generating functions: 2
## Number of analyzing procedures: 1
## Number of replications: 2
## Estimated replications per hour: 87028786
## Start of the simulation: 2021-01-23 14:05:42
## End of the simulation: 2021-01-23 14:05:42
```

As stated in command line 12 we can summarize the result objects over all replications but separately for all data analyzing functions.

```
dg <- expand_tibble(fun = "runif", n = c(10, 20, 30))
pg <- expand_tibble(proc = c("min", "max"))
eval_tibbles(
  data_grid = dg, proc_grid = pg, replications = 1000,
  summary_fun = list(mean = mean)
)
```

```
## # A tibble: 6 x 6
##   fun       n replications summary_fun proc   value
##   <chr> <dbl>        <int> <chr>       <chr>  <dbl>
## 1 runif    10            1 mean        min   0.0885
## 2 runif    10            1 mean        max   0.910
## 3 runif    20            1 mean        min   0.0488
## 4 runif    20            1 mean        max   0.953
## 5 runif    30            1 mean        min   0.0317
## 6 runif    30            1 mean        max   0.970
## Number of data generating functions: 3
## Number of analyzing procedures: 2
## Number of replications: 1000
## Estimated replications per hour: 49413706
## Start of the simulation: 2021-01-23 14:05:42
```

```
## End of the simulation: 2021-01-23 14:05:42
```

```
eval_tibbles(
  data_grid = dg, proc_grid = pg, replications = 1000,
  summary_fun = list(mean = mean, sd = sd)
)
```

```
## # A tibble: 12 x 6
##    fun       n replications summary_fun proc    value
##    <chr> <dbl>        <int> <chr>       <chr>   <dbl>
## 1  runif    10            1 mean        min    0.0925
## 2  runif    10            1 mean        max     0.909
## 3  runif    10            1 sd          min    0.0814
## 4  runif    10            1 sd          max    0.0855
## 5  runif    20            1 mean        min    0.0465
## 6  runif    20            1 mean        max     0.951
## 7  runif    20            1 sd          min    0.0427
## 8  runif    20            1 sd          max    0.0450
## 9  runif    30            1 mean        min    0.0313
## 10 runif    30            1 mean        max     0.969
## 11 runif    30            1 sd          min    0.0304
## 12 runif    30            1 sd          max    0.0299
## Number of data generating functions: 3
## Number of analyzing procedures: 2
## Number of replications: 1000
## Estimated replications per hour: 48842125
## Start of the simulation: 2021-01-23 14:05:42
## End of the simulation: 2021-01-23 14:05:42
```

Sometimes the analyzing functions return quite complicated objects like a model fit.

```
regData <- function(n, SD) {
  x <- seq(0, 1, length = n)
  y <- 10 + 2 * x + rnorm(n, sd = SD)
  tibble(x = x, y = y)
}
eval_tibbles(
  expand_tibble(fun = "regData", n = 5L, SD = 1:2),
  expand_tibble(proc = "lm", formula = c("y~x", "y~I(x^2)")),
  replications = 2
)
```

```
## # A tibble: 8 x 7
##    fun       n   SD replications proc  formula  results
```

```
##    <chr>   <int> <int>      <int> <chr> <chr>      <list>
## 1 regData    5     1           1  lm    y~x        <lm>
## 2 regData    5     1           1  lm    y~I(x^2)   <lm>
## 3 regData    5     1           2  lm    y~x        <lm>
## 4 regData    5     1           2  lm    y~I(x^2)   <lm>
## 5 regData    5     2           1  lm    y~x        <lm>
## 6 regData    5     2           1  lm    y~I(x^2)   <lm>
## 7 regData    5     2           2  lm    y~x        <lm>
## 8 regData    5     2           2  lm    y~I(x^2)   <lm>
## Number of data generating functions: 2
## Number of analyzing procedures: 2
## Number of replications: 2
## Estimated replications per hour: 656228
## Start of the simulation: 2021-01-23 14:05:42
## End of the simulation: 2021-01-23 14:05:42
```

The parameter post_analyze (if specified) is applied directly after the result was generated (see command line 10). Note, "purrr::compose" can be very handy if your post-analyzing-function can be defined by a few single functions:

```
eval_tibbles(
  expand_tibble(fun = "regData", n = 5L, SD = 1:2),
  expand_tibble(proc = "lm", formula = c("y~x", "y~I(x^2)")),
  post_analyze = purrr::compose(function(mat)
    mat["(Intercept)", "Estimate"], coef, summary.lm),
  replications = 2
)
```

```
## # A tibble: 8 x 7
##    fun      n     SD replications proc  formula    results
##    <chr>  <int> <int>      <int> <chr> <chr>        <dbl>
## 1 regData    5     1           1  lm    y~x          10.3
## 2 regData    5     1           1  lm    y~I(x^2)     10.5
## 3 regData    5     1           2  lm    y~x          10.6
## 4 regData    5     1           2  lm    y~I(x^2)     10.6
## 5 regData    5     2           1  lm    y~x          10.7
## 6 regData    5     2           1  lm    y~I(x^2)     10.7
## 7 regData    5     2           2  lm    y~x          10.4
## 8 regData    5     2           2  lm    y~I(x^2)     10.5
## Number of data generating functions: 2
## Number of analyzing procedures: 2
## Number of replications: 2
## Estimated replications per hour: 483826
## Start of the simulation: 2021-01-23 14:05:42
## End of the simulation: 2021-01-23 14:05:42
```

Sometimes the result object is a data.frame itself:

```
presever_rownames <- function(mat) {
  rn <- rownames(mat)
  ret <- tibble::as_tibble(mat)
  ret$term <- rn
  ret
}


eval_tibbles(
  expand_tibble(fun = "regData", n = 5L, SD = 1:2),
  expand_tibble(proc = "lm", formula = c("y~x", "y~I(x^2)")),
  post_analyze = purrr::compose(
    presever_rownames, coef, summary, identity),
  replications = 3
)
```

```
## # A tibble: 24 x 11
##     fun      n      SD replications proc  formula Estimate
##     <chr> <int> <int>        <int> <chr> <chr>      <dbl>
## 1 regD...     5     1            1 lm    y~x         9.97
## 2 regD...     5     1            1 lm    y~x         1.90
## 3 regD...     5     1            1 lm    y~I(x^...   10.3
## 4 regD...     5     1            1 lm    y~I(x^...    1.66
## 5 regD...     5     1            2 lm    y~x         10.1
## 6 regD...     5     1            2 lm    y~x          1.40
## 7 regD...     5     1            2 lm    y~I(x^...   10.2
## 8 regD...     5     1            2 lm    y~I(x^...    1.53
## 9 regD...     5     1            3 lm    y~x         9.61
## 10 regD...    5     1            3 lm    y~x          1.81
## # ... with 14 more rows, and 4 more variables: `Std.
## #   Error` <dbl>, `t value` <dbl>, `Pr(>|t|)` <dbl>,
## #   term <chr>
## Number of data generating functions: 2
## Number of analyzing procedures: 2
## Number of replications: 3
## Estimated replications per hour: 465502
## Start of the simulation: 2021-01-23 14:05:42
## End of the simulation: 2021-01-23 14:05:42
```

To summarize the replications, it is necessary to additional group the calculations with respect to another variable. This variable can be passed to group_for_summary.

```
eval_tibbles(
  expand_tibble(fun = "regData", n = 5L, SD = 1:2),
  expand_tibble(proc = "lm",
                formula = c("y~x", "y~I(x^2)")),
  post_analyze = purrr::compose(
```

```
    presever_rownames, coef, summary, identity),
  summary_fun = list(mean = mean, sd = sd),
  group_for_summary = "term",
  replications = 3
)
```

```
## # A tibble: 16 x 12
##      fun       n    SD replications summary_fun proc  formula
##      <chr> <int> <int>        <int> <chr>       <chr> <chr>
##  1 regD...     5     1            1 mean        lm    y~x
##  2 regD...     5     1            1 mean        lm    y~x
##  3 regD...     5     1            1 mean        lm    y~I(x^...
##  4 regD...     5     1            1 mean        lm    y~I(x^...
##  5 regD...     5     1            1 sd          lm    y~x
##  6 regD...     5     1            1 sd          lm    y~x
##  7 regD...     5     1            1 sd          lm    y~I(x^...
##  8 regD...     5     1            1 sd          lm    y~I(x^...
##  9 regD...     5     2            1 mean        lm    y~x
## 10 regD...     5     2            1 mean        lm    y~x
## 11 regD...     5     2            1 mean        lm    y~I(x^...
## 12 regD...     5     2            1 mean        lm    y~I(x^...
## 13 regD...     5     2            1 sd          lm    y~x
## 14 regD...     5     2            1 sd          lm    y~x
## 15 regD...     5     2            1 sd          lm    y~I(x^...
## 16 regD...     5     2            1 sd          lm    y~I(x^...
## # ... with 5 more variables: term <chr>, Estimate <dbl>,
## #   'Std. Error' <dbl>, 't value' <dbl>, 'Pr(>|t|)' <dbl>
## Number of data generating functions: 2
## Number of analyzing procedures: 2
## Number of replications: 3
## Estimated replications per hour: 327024
## Start of the simulation: 2021-01-23 14:05:42
## End of the simulation: 2021-01-23 14:05:42
```

Sometimes it is handy to access the parameter constellation that was used during the data generation in the (post) data analyzing phase. Of course, one could write wrapper functions for every data generating function and append the parameter constellation from the data generation as attributes to the dataset, but the purpose of this package is to reduce such administrative source code. Hence, if the (post) data analyzing function has an argument .truth, then "eval_tibbles" will manage that handover. A brief example should explain this. Suppose we want to estimate the bias of the empirical quantile estimator if the data is normally distributed.

```
dg <- expand_tibble(fun = c("rnorm"), mean = c(1,1000),
                    sd = c(1,10), n = c(10L, 100L))
pg <- expand_tibble(proc = "quantile", probs = 0.975)
post_ana <- function(q_est, .truth){
  tibble::tibble(bias = q_est - stats::qnorm(
    0.975, mean = .truth$mean, sd = .truth$sd))
}
eval_tibbles(dg, pg, replications = 10^3,
             discard_generated_data = TRUE,
```

```
                     ncpus = 2,
                     post_analyze = post_ana,
                     summary_fun = list(mean = mean))
```

```
## # A tibble: 8 x 9
##   fun    mean    sd     n replications summary_fun proc
##   <chr> <dbl> <dbl> <int>        <int> <chr>       <chr>
## 1 rnorm     1     1    10            1 mean        quan...
## 2 rnorm  1000     1    10            1 mean        quan...
## 3 rnorm     1    10    10            1 mean        quan...
## 4 rnorm  1000    10    10            1 mean        quan...
## 5 rnorm     1     1   100            1 mean        quan...
## 6 rnorm  1000     1   100            1 mean        quan...
## 7 rnorm     1    10   100            1 mean        quan...
## 8 rnorm  1000    10   100            1 mean        quan...
## # ... with 2 more variables: probs <dbl>, bias <dbl>
## Number of data generating functions: 8
## Number of analyzing procedures: 1
## Number of replications: 1000
## Estimated replications per hour: 1807516
## Start of the simulation: 2021-01-23 14:05:43
## End of the simulation: 2021-01-23 14:05:45
```

If we want to do the analysis for different distributions, we could modify our post data analyzing function, but we can also simply add a .truth-column to the data generating grid. In this case, the information from the .truth-column is directly passed to the .truth-parameter:

```
dg <- dplyr::bind_rows(
  expand_tibble(fun = c("rnorm"), mean = 0, n = c(10L, 100L),
                .truth = qnorm(0.975)),
  expand_tibble(fun = c("rexp"), rate = 1, n = c(10L, 100L),
                .truth = qexp(0.975, rate = 1)),
  expand_tibble(fun = c("runif"), max = 2, n = c(10L, 100L),
                .truth = qunif(0.975, max = 2))
)
pg <- expand_tibble(proc = "quantile", probs = 0.975)
post_ana <- function(q_est, .truth){
  ret <- q_est - .truth
  names(ret) <- "bias"
  ret
}
eval_tibbles(dg, pg, replications = 10^3,
             discard_generated_data = TRUE,
             ncpus = 2,
             post_analyze = post_ana,
             summary_fun = list(mean = mean))
```

```
## # A tibble: 6 x 11
##    fun    mean     n .truth rate   max replications
##    <chr> <dbl> <int>  <dbl> <dbl> <dbl>       <int>
## 1 rnorm     0    10   1.96    NA    NA           1
## 2 rnorm     0   100   1.96    NA    NA           1
## 3 rexp     NA    10   3.69     1    NA           1
## 4 rexp     NA   100   3.69     1    NA           1
## 5 runif    NA    10   1.95    NA     2           1
## 6 runif    NA   100   1.95    NA     2           1
## # ... with 4 more variables: summary_fun <chr>, proc <chr>,
## #    probs <dbl>, bias <dbl>
## Number of data generating functions: 6
## Number of analyzing procedures: 1
## Number of replications: 1000
## Estimated replications per hour: 3886143
## Start of the simulation: 2021-01-23 14:05:46
## End of the simulation: 2021-01-23 14:05:46
```

In the same fashion one could write a data analyzing function with a parameter .truth. To go even a step further, we store the analytic quantile function in the .truth-column:

```
dg <- dplyr::bind_rows(
  expand_tibble(
    fun = c("rnorm"), mean = 0, n = c(10L, 1000L),
    .truth = list(function(prob) qnorm(prob, mean = 0))),
  expand_tibble(
    fun = c("rexp"), rate = 1, n = c(10L, 1000L),
    .truth = list(function(prob) qexp(prob, rate = 1))),
  expand_tibble(
    fun = c("runif"), max = 2, n = c(10L, 1000L),
    .truth = list(function(prob) qunif(prob, max = 2)))
)
bias_quantile <- function(x, prob, .truth) {
  est <- quantile(x, probs = prob)
  ret <- est - .truth[[1]](prob)
  names(ret) <- "bias"
  ret
}
pg <- expand_tibble(proc = "bias_quantile", prob = c(0.9, 0.975))
eval_tibbles(dg, pg, replications = 10^3,
             discard_generated_data = TRUE,
             ncpus = 1,
             summary_fun = list(mean = mean))


## # A tibble: 12 x 11
##     fun    mean     n .truth rate   max replications
##     <chr> <dbl> <int> <list> <dbl> <dbl>       <int>
```

```
## 1  rnorm     0    10 <fn>      NA    NA           1
## 2  rnorm     0    10 <fn>      NA    NA           1
## 3  rnorm     0  1000 <fn>      NA    NA           1
## 4  rnorm     0  1000 <fn>      NA    NA           1
## 5  rexp     NA    10 <fn>       1    NA           1
## 6  rexp     NA    10 <fn>       1    NA           1
## 7  rexp     NA  1000 <fn>       1    NA           1
## 8  rexp     NA  1000 <fn>       1    NA           1
## 9  runif    NA    10 <fn>      NA     2           1
## 10 runif    NA    10 <fn>      NA     2           1
## 11 runif    NA  1000 <fn>      NA     2           1
## 12 runif    NA  1000 <fn>      NA     2           1
## # ... with 4 more variables: summary_fun <chr>, proc <chr>,
## #   prob <dbl>, bias <dbl>
## Number of data generating functions: 6
## Number of analyzing procedures: 2
## Number of replications: 1000
## Estimated replications per hour: 2150355
## Start of the simulation: 2021-01-23 14:05:47
## End of the simulation: 2021-01-23 14:05:48
```

But one should keep in mind that if one calculates the quantile during the (post) analyzing phase that this happens on replication level. To be more precise lets look at an excerpt of the pseudo-code from the beginning of the vignette:

```
6.  for g in  {g_1, ..., g_k}
7.    for r in 1:replications (optionally
                              in a parallel manner)
8.      data = g()
9.      for f in  {f_1, \ldots, f_L}
10.       append f(data) to the result object (opt.
                apply a post-analyze-function)
```

No matter if one extends the data analyzing function $f\_1, \ldots, f\_L$ or the post-analyze-function with an argument .truth the calculation are made for every single replication during Step 10. Hence, the operations are not vectorized!

Finally, by specifying ncpus larger than 1 a cluster objected is created for the user.

```
eval_tibbles(
  data_grid = dg, proc_grid = pg, replications = 10,
  ncpus = 2, summary_fun = list(mean = mean)
)
```

```
## # A tibble: 12 x 11
##     fun    mean     n .truth  rate   max replications
```

```
##     <chr> <dbl> <int> <list> <dbl> <dbl>          <int>
##  1 rnorm     0    10 <fn>     NA    NA              1
##  2 rnorm     0    10 <fn>     NA    NA              1
##  3 rnorm     0  1000 <fn>     NA    NA              1
##  4 rnorm     0  1000 <fn>     NA    NA              1
##  5 rexp     NA    10 <fn>      1    NA              1
##  6 rexp     NA    10 <fn>      1    NA              1
##  7 rexp     NA  1000 <fn>      1    NA              1
##  8 rexp     NA  1000 <fn>      1    NA              1
##  9 runif    NA    10 <fn>     NA     2              1
## 10 runif    NA    10 <fn>     NA     2              1
## 11 runif    NA  1000 <fn>     NA     2              1
## 12 runif    NA  1000 <fn>     NA     2              1
## # ... with 4 more variables: summary_fun <chr>, proc <chr>,
## #   prob <dbl>, bias <dbl>
## Number of data generating functions: 6
## Number of analyzing procedures: 2
## Number of replications: 10
## Estimated replications per hour: 63536
## Start of the simulation: 2021-01-23 14:05:49
## End of the simulation: 2021-01-23 14:05:49
```

As it is stated in command line 7, the replications are parallelized. In our case, this means that roughly every CPU conducts 5 replications.

The parameter cluster_seed must be an integer vector of length 6 and serves the same purpose as the function set.seed. By default, cluster_seed equals rep(12345, 6). Note, in order to reproduce the simulation study it is also necessary that ncpus does not change.

Further information about the `simTool`-package is on the package-web-site. [1]

---

[1] http://marselscheer.github.io/simTool/index.html

Appendix C
bootGOF Package

Our package helps to perform goodness-of-fit tests according to Chap. 6. In order to illustrate how the package can be applied we will reproduce some of the results from that chapter. More detailed information about the package can be found on https://github.com/MarselScheer/bootGOF. The package supports the classes `lm` and `glm`. Hence, the normal model with log-transformed ridership fitted in Sect. 6.1.2, compare R-object `fit_lognormal`, can easily be tested by calling

```
library(bootGOF)
set.seed(123, kind ="Mersenne-Twister", normal.kind ="Inversion")
gof_test <- bootGOF::GOF_model(
  model = fit_lognorm,
  data = ridership,
  nmb_boot_samples = 100,
  simulator_type = "parametric",
  y_name = "y",
  Rn1_statistic = bootGOF::Rn1_CvM$new())
gof_test$get_pvalue()
```

```
## [1] 0.05
```

This is the same p-value as we obtained in Sect. 6.1.2. All models of class `lm` and `glm` are covered by this function. However, semi-parametric models can also be treated by the package but additional information must be passed. The reason why semi-parametric models have to be handled differently is that the linear component that is necessary for the test is not always a natural component of such models. Consider again the simple model from Sect. 6.2

$$Y = \sin(aX) + \varepsilon,$$

where X is uniformly distributed and ε is normally distributed. After fitting a model with a least square estimator the linear component aX cannot be extracted in general from the model fit directly because the fitting algorithm is not really aware of that

© Springer Nature Switzerland AG 2021
G. Dikta and M. Scheer, *Bootstrap Methods*,
https://doi.org/10.1007/978-3-030-73480-0

linear component. Usually, such fitting algorithms treat the equation in a more general way like $Y = m(a, X) + \varepsilon$. However, the goodness-of-fit test explicitly uses such a linear component. Therefore, the package has to know how to extract it from the model object. We generate a dataset to illustrate how the package can be applied in such a situation.

```
set.seed(123,kind ="Mersenne-Twister",normal.kind ="Inversion")
gen_data <- function(N = 200, sd = 0.2)   {
  dplyr::mutate(
    data.frame(X = runif(N, min = 6, max = 14)),
    mu = sin(0.5 * X),
    epsilon = rnorm(N, sd = sd),
    Y = mu + epsilon)
}
nonlinear <- gen_data()
```

As in Sect. 6.2 we use the following least square estimator

```
set.seed(123,kind ="Mersenne-Twister",normal.kind ="Inversion")
library(minpack.lm)
fit <- minpack.lm::nlsLM(Y ~ sin(a * X),
  data = nonlinear,
  start = c(a = 0.5),
  control = nls.control(maxiter = 500))
fit
```

```
## Nonlinear regression model
##   model: Y ~ sin(a * X)
##    data: nonlinear
##        a
## 0.4988
##   residual sum-of-squares: 7.362
##
## Number of iterations to convergence: 2
## Achieved convergence tolerance: 1.49e-08
```

In order to create a goodnes-of-fit-test, we have to use "GOF_model_test", which expect three interfaces. The first interface requires that we implement three functions "yhat", "y_minus_yhat" and "beta_x_covariates", which are the predictions for the dependent variable (also called target-variable), the residuals on the scale of the dependent variable and the inner product of the estimated parameters and the independent variables (also called covariates or features). The only thing that does not work out of the box and requires a dedicated implementation is "beta_x_covariates" because that is the linear component aX. Furthermore, the object returned by "minpack.lm::nlsLM" does not contain the original dataset but that dataset is necessary to calculate the inner product. Hence, we make a list that contains the model fit and the data that was used to fit the model.

```
fit_and_data <- list(fit = fit, data = nonlinear)
```

Now we can implement the interface

```r
library(R6)
my_nls_info_extractor <- R6::R6Class(
  classname = "my_nls_info_extractor",
  inherit = GOF_model_info_extractor,
  public = list(
    yhat = function(model) {
      predict(object = model$fit)
    },
    y_minus_yhat = function(model) {
      residuals(object = model$fit)
    },
    beta_x_covariates = function(model) {
      a_hat <- coef(object = model$fit)
      X <- model$data$X
      ret <- a_hat * X
      return(ret)
    }
  ))
my_info_extractor <- my_nls_info_extractor$new()
```

Clearly, only "beta_x_covariates" requires really some implementation efforts. Since we did not make an assumption about the distribution of ε, we cannot use a parametric resampling scheme. However, we can apply the wild bootstrap that uses only the predictions and the residuals. The class "GOF_sim_wild_rademacher" implements this wild bootstrap but needs an info extractor to obtain the preditions and residuals. Since we already implemented that interface we can reuse it:

```r
my_simulator <- GOF_sim_wild_rademacher$new(
  gof_model_info_extractor = my_info_extractor
)
```

Finally, we need to implement the interface "GOF_model_trainer" which requires a function "refit" that is able to update the model object by refitting it to a new dataset. R already provides the necessary function, i.e., "stats::update". However, we combined the fitted model with the dataset in a list. Since the package will bootstrap multiple datasets and refit the model to the new data sets, we need to take this list into account:

```r
my_nls_trainer <- R6::R6Class(
  classname = "GOF_nls_trainer",
  inherit = GOF_model_trainer,
  public = list(
    refit = function(model, data) {
      fit <- update(object = model$fit, data = data)
      ret <- list(fit = fit, data = data)
      return(ret)
    }))
```

```
my_trainer <- my_nls_trainer$new()
```

Now we can invoke the goodness-of-fit test by providing all three implemented interfaces to "GOF_model_test":

```
set.seed(123,kind ="Mersenne-Twister",normal.kind ="Inversion")
gof_test <- GOF_model_test$new(
  model = fit_and_data,
  data = nonlinear,
  nmb_boot_samples = 500,
  y_name = "Y",
  Rn1_statistic = Rn1_CvM$new(),
  gof_model_info_extractor = my_info_extractor,
  gof_model_resample = GOF_model_resample$new(
    gof_model_simulator = my_simulator,
    gof_model_trainer = my_trainer
  )
)
gof_test$get_pvalue()
```

```
## [1] 0.852
```

As expected, we obtain a rather large *p*-value because we used the correct model for fitting the data. Again, objects of class lm or glm can be easily tested without knowledge about the three interfaces. But they allow the user to also apply the goodness-of-fit test to models that are not directly supported by the package. See the vignettes of the package for more details about the architecture and the three interfaces.

Appendix D
Session Info

```
sessionInfo()
```

```
## R version 3.6.2 (2019-12-12)
## Platform: x86_64-pc-linux-gnu (64-bit)
## Running under: Debian GNU/Linux 10 (buster)
##
## Matrix products: default
## BLAS/LAPACK: /usr/lib/x86_64-linux-gnu/libopenblasp-r0.3.5.so
##
## locale:
##  [1] LC_CTYPE=en_US.UTF-8       LC_NUMERIC=C
##  [3] LC_TIME=en_US.UTF-8        LC_COLLATE=en_US.UTF-8
##  [5] LC_MONETARY=en_US.UTF-8    LC_MESSAGES=C
##  [7] LC_PAPER=en_US.UTF-8       LC_NAME=C
##  [9] LC_ADDRESS=C               LC_TELEPHONE=C
## [11] LC_MEASUREMENT=en_US.UTF-8 LC_IDENTIFICATION=C
##
## attached base packages:
## [1] stats4    stats     graphics  grDevices datasets
## [6] utils     methods   base
##
## other attached packages:
##  [1] R6_2.4.1         minpack.lm_1.2-1 bootGOF_0.1.0
##  [4] GGally_1.4.0     webshot_0.5.2    profvis_0.3.6
##  [7] dplyr_0.8.3      xtable_1.8-4     simTool_1.1.4
## [10] codetools_0.2-16 tidyr_1.0.0      lubridate_1.7.4
## [13] readr_1.3.1      cowplot_1.0.0    ggplot2_3.2.1
## [16] boot_1.3-23      knitr_1.26
##
## loaded via a namespace (and not attached):
##  [1] tidyselect_0.2.5 xfun_0.11
##  [3] purrr_0.3.3      reshape2_1.4.3
##  [5] colorspace_1.4-1 vctrs_0.2.1
##  [7] htmltools_0.4.0  utf8_1.1.4
##  [9] rlang_0.4.2      pillar_1.4.3
## [11] glue_1.3.1       withr_2.1.2
```

© Springer Nature Switzerland AG 2021
G. Dikta and M. Scheer, *Bootstrap Methods*,
https://doi.org/10.1007/978-3-030-73480-0

```
## [13] RColorBrewer_1.1-2 lifecycle_0.1.0
## [15] plyr_1.8.5          stringr_1.4.0
## [17] munsell_0.5.0       gtable_0.3.0
## [19] htmlwidgets_1.5.1   evaluate_0.14
## [21] labeling_0.3        parallel_3.6.2
## [23] fansi_0.4.0         highr_0.8
## [25] Rcpp_1.0.3          checkmate_2.0.0
## [27] renv_0.9.3          backports_1.1.5
## [29] scales_1.1.0        farver_2.0.1
## [31] hms_0.5.2           digest_0.6.23
## [33] stringi_1.4.3       grid_3.6.2
## [35] cli_2.0.0           tools_3.6.2
## [37] magrittr_1.5        lazyeval_0.2.2
## [39] tibble_2.1.3        crayon_1.3.4
## [41] pkgconfig_2.0.3     zeallot_0.1.0
## [43] MASS_7.3-51.4       ellipsis_0.3.0
## [45] assertthat_0.2.1    reshape_0.8.8
## [47] compiler_3.6.2
```

Index

A
Algorithm
    Box-Muller, 16
    rejection, 16
Alternative, 48

B
Bike sharing data, 108
Bootstrap
    approximation, 3
    classical, 4, 21
    empirical process, 35
    model based, 78
    sample, 22
Bootstrap of the estimated marked empirical
    process, 214

C
Classical bootstrap, 4
    central limit theorem, 31
    weak law of large numbers, 29
Cramér-von Mises statistic, 60
    MEP, 167
Critical value, 48

D
Distance
    Cramér-von Mises, 60
    Kolmogorov-Smirnov, 60
Distribution function
    empirical, 4

E
Empirical distribution function, 4

Empirical process, 34
    bootstrap, 35
    estimated, 60
    uniform, 34
Error
    type 1, 48
Estimated empirical process, 60
Exponential family with dispersion parameter, 121

G
Generalized linear model
    parametric, 123
    semi-parametric, 142

H
Hypothesis, 48
    alternative, 48
    null, 48

K
Kolmogorov-Smirnov statistic, 60
    MEP, 167
Kullback-Leibler information, 123
    modified, 124

L
Least Square Estimator (LSE), 77

M
Mallow's p−metric, 39

© Springer Nature Switzerland AG 2021
G. Dikta and M. Scheer, *Bootstrap Methods*,
https://doi.org/10.1007/978-3-030-73480-0

Marked empirical process, 198, 203, 207
    basic, 198
    BMEP, 198
    EMEP, 203
    EMEPE, 207
    estimated parameters, 203
        bootstrap, 214
        estimated direction, 207
Monte Carlo, 23

N
Null hypothesis, 48

P
Parametric generalized linear model, 123
p-value, 48

Q
Quantile function, 11

R
Rademacher random variables, 96
Regression model
    estimated residuals, 77
    fixed design, 75
    homoscedastic, 75
    model based bootstrap, 78

residuals, 75
Rejection region, 48
Residuals, 75
    centered estimated residuals, 78
    estimated residuals, 77
Rosenblatt Transformation, 19

S
Semi-parametric generalized linear model, 142

T
Test
    one-sample, 49
    two-sample
        location model, 53
Type 1 error, 48

U
Uniform distribution, 11
    on an interval, 11
    standard, 11
Uniformly dominated, 216

W
Wild bootstrap, 96

Printed in the United States
by Baker & Taylor Publisher Services